TRENDS IN NURSING RESEARCH

TRENDS IN NURSING RESEARCH

ADAM J. RYAN
AND
JACK DOYLE
EDITORS

Nova Science Publishers, Inc.
New York

NOTICE TO THE READER

The Publisher has taken reasonable care in the preparation of this book, but makes no expressed or implied warranty of any kind and assumes no responsibility for any errors or omissions. No liability is assumed for incidental or consequential damages in connection with or arising out of information contained in this book. The Publisher shall not be liable for any special, consequential, or exemplary damages resulting, in whole or in part, from the readers' use of, or reliance upon, this material. Any parts of this book based on government reports are so indicated and copyright is claimed for those parts to the extent applicable to compilations of such works.

Independent verification should be sought for any data, advice or recommendations contained in this book. In addition, no responsibility is assumed by the publisher for any injury and/or damage to persons or property arising from any methods, products, instructions, ideas or otherwise contained in this publication.

This publication is designed to provide accurate and authoritative information with regard to the subject matter covered herein. It is sold with the clear understanding that the Publisher is not engaged in rendering legal or any other professional services. If legal or any other expert assistance is required, the services of a competent person should be sought. FROM A DECLARATION OF PARTICIPANTS JOINTLY ADOPTED BY A COMMITTEE OF THE AMERICAN BAR ASSOCIATION AND A COMMITTEE OF PUBLISHERS.

Library of Congress Cataloging-in-Publication Data

Trends in nursing research / [edited by] Adam J. Ryan and Jack Doyle.
     p. ; cm.
  Includes bibliographical references and index.
  ISBN 978-1-60456-642-0 (hardcover)
  1. Nursing. I. Ryan, Adam J. II. Doyle, Jack, 1957-
  [DNLM: 1. Nursing. 2. Nurse-Patient Relations. 3. Nursing Care. 4. Nursing Process. WY 100 T794 2008]
  RT42.T74 2008
  610.73--dc22
                              2008014844

Published by Nova Science Publishers, Inc. ✦ New York

Contents

Preface

This book focuses on the latest research in the field of nursing. Nursing is the protection, promotion, and optimization of health and abilities, prevention of illness and injury, alleviation of suffering through the diagnosis and treatment of human response, and advocacy in the care of individuals, families, communities, and populations. Definitions of nursing have evolved to acknowledge six essential features of professional nursing: Provision of a caring relationship that facilitates health and healing, Attention to the range of human experiences and responses to health and illness within the physical and social environments, Integration of objective data with knowledge gained from an appreciation of the patient or group's subjective experience, Application of scientific knowledge to the processes of diagnosis and treatment through the use of judgement and critical thinking, Advancement of professional nursing knowledge through scholarly inquiry, and Influence on social and public policy to promote social justice.

Chapter 1 - This chapter presents the methodological journey and findings of a study exploring the meaning of nurse-patient intimacy in oncology care settings. The 'data' for this study is provided by the dialogue that took place through feminist conversational interviewing with thirty oncology patients, interviewed once, and twenty-three oncology nurses, interviewed twice, over a ten month period.

The study findings reveal nurse-patient intimacy as a process, which begins when the nurse and patient first meet, and nurse empathy for the patient follows identification. This identification is influenced by the patient's characteristics and response to their cancer and its treatment. Reciprocal self-disclosure characterises the intimacy that develops in the context of the nurse assuming a 'professional friend' role in a homely atmosphere where care is delivered. The outcome of intimacy is satisfaction for the nurse, but also emotional effects. Peer support among nurses in sustaining intimacy with patients is also revealed.

At first glance, it would appear that utilising phenomenological and feminist approaches simultaneously is philosophically and methodologically unsound. After all, many feminists consider phenomenology an essentialist doctrine, and essentialism is a central target of feminist criticism. However, such arguments fail to acknowledge the various phenomenological approaches available to researchers.

The phenomenological approach adopted for this study was guided by the work of phenomenologist Gadamer, whose work is also referred to as philosophical hermeneutics or interpretive phenomenology. Gadamer views the research interview as a dialogue between researcher and participant, and like feminist research, the dialogue becomes a shared project. Moreover, intimacy between study participants and researcher is espoused in feminist research, and with interpretive phenomenology, the researcher is the instrument, which suggests intimacy in the interview process.

Therefore, in the context of this study, 'feminist' is viewed as a qualitative approach, in which the subjectivity of both the researcher and participants, is central, and a close and mutual relationship between researcher and participant is seen as important. Furthermore, a diffusion of power between study participants and researcher is paramount in feminist research. Similarly, with hermeneutic understanding, the researcher and participants work together to reach a shared understand of the phenomenon being explored.

The methodological approach presented is this chapter is representative of the inter-disciplinary nature of qualitative inquiry. Moreover, in the context of the literature surrounding nurse-patient intimacy, the views of nurse theorists, such as Travelbee and Peplau are not sufficient alone. Therefore, the views of philosophers such as Scheler and Stein and moral theologian Campbell, are also provided to support the interpretations revealed in the study findings.

The hybrid nature of the methodological influences adopted in this study therefore reflects the qualitative researcher adopting the role of bricoleur, and mirrors the characteristics of the qualitative researcher who has to be flexible, responsive and reflexive. This hybrid approach is not surprising since nursing gains its theoretical underpinnings from diverse philosophical and theoretical standpoints.

Chapter 2 - Nurses are aware that the profession of nursing is holistic, that every action taken in the care of a patient has consequences, and they like to believe that those consequences have a positive impact on the patient and their family's ultimate health. For nurses, gaining an understanding of patients' expectations regarding spiritual care is essential to entering into a truly holistic, caring relationship with patients. The purpose of this phenomenolo-gical study was to explore the expectations patients have of nurses and how patients describe good nursing care. Specifically, questions were posed to reveal participants' perceptions of spiritual care provided by their nurses. Using Paterson's and Zderad's framework of humanistic nursing, 11 participants were interviewed. Data were analyzed using the Giorgi method of repetitive reflection. Findings suggested that participants appreciated nursing presence, being there, as having a positive influence on their health and well being, and elements of nursing presence were used to describe good nursing care. In fact, the spiritual element of nursing presence, being with, comprised the most defining characteristics of good nursing care, but, paradoxically, was not expected. Sharing of self by nurses was appreciated from the participants' perspective. All participants were able to define spirituality, most frequently in terms of religiosity; and religious elements of spirituality were not expected, nor welcomed, by most participants. Participants revealed that they perceived nurses to be busy, and this perceived lack of time was offered as a rationale for not expecting spiritual care.

Chapter 3 - Background: Evidence of disparities in child and adolescent immunization rates are abundant in the literature (Niederhauser and Stark, 2005). These disparities occur in different ethnic groups, races, and socioeconomic classes. However, there is a lack of studies that examine factors associated with under-immunization rates in Asian and Pacific Islander (API) children and adolescents.

Community Health Centers (CHCs), who serve predominantly poor and minority populations, are in an ideal position to minimize gaps in child and adolescent immunization rates. The purpose of this study was to identify factors associated with under-immunization in racially and ethnically diverse children who seek health care services at a CHC in Hawaii. The setting for this study was at an urban CHC in downtown Honolulu that provides health care to a multi-ethnic population including many API immigrant families.

Methods: This was a cross-sectional descriptive design study. A sample of 400 children and adolescents, ages birth to 21 years, who received care at the CHC during a 12 month period of time, were randomly selected for participation in the study. Of the 400 who were selected, 369 medical records were available to review during the 1 month data collection period. The data collected from the medical records included age of child or adolescent (in months), gender, ethnicity, total household income, insurance status and type and date of childhood immunizations. For this study, a child was considered not up-to-date on their immunizations if they did not have the recommended immunization within one month of the due date. This study was approved by the Committee on Human Subjects, University of Hawaii at Manoa.

Results: The overall immunization rates for this sample was 41% up-to-date, 30% not up-to-date and 29% had no record of immunizations in their medical record. For the final analysis, the not-up-to-date and no record were merged into one category and considered not-up-to-date. There were 38% male and 62% female medical records reviewed. The total household income mean was $887 (range $0-$5153, SD $871). Sixty-three percent had insurance coverage, 35% had no insurance and 2% had no insurance information in the medical record. In the bi-variate analysis ethnicity (x^2 12.274, p= .015), insurance status (x^2 18.994, p= .000) and total household income (x^2 9.167, p= .010) were significantly associated with up-to-date status. In the logistic regression analysis, total family income and insurance status was associated with up-to-date status; when conducting the analysis with all three variables ethnicity was not significantly associated with immunization status.

Discussion: Overall the majority of children and adolescents in this study had sub-optimal immunization rates. The findings in this study are similar to findings in other studies of poor and ethnically diverse children and adolescents; immunization rates are significantly associated with having insurance, having a higher total family income and among the different ethnic groups. Interventions targeting increasing immunization rates in poor and ethnically diverse children are necessary to decrease disparities in this important public health intervention.

Chapter 4 - *Introduction*: Cardiovascular disease (CVD) remains a significant worldwide health problem leading to premature death and chronic illness with Coronary heart disease (CHD) accounts for 52% of CVD cases with 16 million cases of CHD in the US. One of the treatment options for those with CHD is Coronary Artery Bypass Surgery (CABG). The aim of the surgery is to alleviate symptoms such as angina and breathlessness, prevent further Myocardial Infarctions (MIs) and reduce the progression of CHD.

METHOD and AIM OF STUDY: A study was undertaken in the United Kingdom five years after CABG. Patients from a previous study agreed to participate in a follow-up study five years after cardiac surgery. Participants were asked to complete a quality of life questionnaire, the Short-Form 36 (SF-36) and questionnaires on their psychological well-being (anxiety and depression symptoms). Neuropsychological assessment was also performed at the follow-up. The assessments of psychological well-being and neuropsychological tests were previously completed prior to surgery.

Results: One hundred and nine patients were interviewed face-to-face. The SF-36 component summaries of the patients indicated that their physical (PCS) and mental (MCS) health was relatively good (45.8 and 53.6, respectively, with 0 = worst health and 100 = best health and 50 being the mean score). Lower PCS scores were associated with comorbid illness. Psychological well-being (anxiety and depression) was found to correlate with the SF-36 physical and mental component summaries ($p < .001$) at the time of follow-up.

Deficits in neuropsychological scores five years post CABG were found in 28% of the patients with no correlation between the SF-36 component summaries and the neuropsychological assessment five years after CABG suggesting that these deficits do not interfere with patient perceived HRQoL.

Discussion: The significance of psychological well-being were highlighted in the hierarchical regression analysis with pre-operative angina scores and the following data five years post CABG; comorbid illness, anxiety and depressive symptoms and physical activity, accounting for 37% of the variance in PCS. Pre-operative anxiety, interim myocardial infarction and the following data five years post CABG: age, diet scores, anxiety, and depression symptoms, accounted for 60% of the variance in MCS.

Conclusion: The findings demonstrate that patient perceived HRQoL five years after CABG is generally good. However, it is negatively affected the presence of anxiety or depression symptoms at follow-up. The findings have implications for healthcare professionals and highlight the importance of anxiety and depression after surgical revascularisation.

Chapter 5 - This chapter describes a research model developed and used by the author, the 3-D Health Services Research Model (3-D HSR Model). The model provides a framework for the design and interpretation of research data to support evidence-based practice in community health settings. The model incorporates the following three research approaches: population-based data analysis, process evaluations, and outcome evaluations. The model consists of the following three aspects: 1) the interpretation of population-based data to identify major health issues affecting a defined community, 2) the selection of effective interventions to enhance the health of the community, and 3) the integration of evaluative research, specifically a process evaluation to ascertain the extent the intervention was delivered as intended and an outcome evaluation to determine the measurable impact the intervention had on the community's health issues. The 3-D HSR model includes key approaches from both epidemiology and health services research. For example, epidemiologic research approaches provide the foundation in the identification of major health issues in a community through the analysis of selected population-based datasets, data from state vital statistics, and mortality and morbidity data on communicable and other diseases collected and reported by county, state, national, and international public health agencies. The model is consistent with the concepts from health services research and Nursing-Health Services Research as described by Jones and Mark in 2005. In addition, the model supports the scope of nursing research as outlined in the 2006 American Association of Colleges of Nursing (AACN) Position Statement on Nursing Research.

A case example is included to illustrate the application of the model to a current national health issue: assuring that children have access to continuous, quality, primary health care. The case example, original research by the author as principle investigator, is an analysis of a population-based dataset, the National Survey of Children's Health, to identify factors through regression analysis of U.S. children at risk for not having access to continuous, quality primary health care.

Chapter 6 - Nurses value providing high quality care, and adoption of evidence-based practices offer opportunities to make measurable improvements in healthcare outcomes. For this reason, providing evidence-based care has become the standard for quality in our healthcare system, yet research shows that patients only receive evidence-based care about half the time (Asch et al., 2006; Clark, 2005; Mangione-Smith et al., 2007; McGlynn et al., 2003; McInerny, Cull, and Yudkowsky, 2005; Peterson et al., 2006; Shrank et al., 2006; Zuckerman, Stevens, Inkelas, and Halfon, 2004). While the body of research in this area is growing, a great deal of work is still needed to better understand how to improve use of evidence-based healthcare at the practitioner and organizational levels.

Chapter 7 - Age frequently carries the burden of diseases, many of which in turn are associated with discomfort and various complaints. Chronic pain is such a common complaint and is an important issue in the care of older people, and perhaps the most important problem in their daily lives. It is known to, alone or together with other factors, negatively affect an older person's quality of life. Examples of covariates to chronic pain are functional limitations, fatigue, sleeping problems, and depressed mood/depression. All these factors have been found to be more prevalent among people with chronic pain, but studies about these topics (in relation to pain) in older people are sparce, especially those focusing on fatigue and sleeping problems. Also the need for care and treatment is found to increase with increased degree of pain, especially among those with musculoskeletal pain. Despite this, studies focusing on chronic pain, pain management, and quality of life among older people (especially the oldest and frailest) are limited, and a pharmacological approach to diminishing pain dominates in the literature. A broad view is needed when studying pain as well as when caring for people in pain. This is especially important when the pain cannot be fully removed, and relief from suffering through other factors leading to increased quality of life is a more realistic option.

Chapter 8 - Nursing education in Spain is developing rapidly in accordance with the European Union growth and within an international globalization movement. The purpose of this chapter is to provide an overview of nursing education in Spain. A brief history of modern nursing education is presented together with its recent reform and a view of recent developments.

Since nursing education was integrated at the university level in 1977, the only academic recognition for this education in Spain was the three year diploma degree. Nurses had to move to other disciplines in order to achieve academic growth or forward their nursing studies abroad. Over these years, there have been numerous attempts to achieve the Bachelor in Nursing Science.

In 1998 eight Nursing Universities of Spain began to offer graduated –level advanced programs of 2 academic years , 120 European Credit transfer System (ECTS) . The degree upon completion of this advanced program is the master of nursing science. This program includes nursing research, teaching, management, and advanced care.

Recently in January 2005, the Spanish Government published the guidelines for undergraduate, master's and doctoral levels (BOE, 55/2005). Finally, as a result of the Bologna Process, nursing is being fully recognized as a higher education discipline, and its curriculum is being organized within the framework of undergraduate and graduate education.

At the same time, in May 2005, the Ministries of Health and Education approved the proposal of the specialities in Nursing (BOE,450/2005). These specialities determined the areas of Nursing care; family and community health nursing, nursing midwifery, mental health nursing, elderly nursing, health work nursing, medical care nursing and paediatric nursing. These specialities will improve patient care as well as the continuing education already available.

Chapter 9 - Disruptive behaviors can have a profound effect on staff perceptions, attitudes and reactions that affect decision making and communication flow. Feelings of anger, hostility and frustration lead to impaired relationships, confused expectations, and unclear roles and responsibilities which can impede the transfer of vital information that can adversely affect patient outcomes of care. Health care organizations need to be aware of the significance of disruptive behaviors and develop appropriate policies, standards and procedures to effectively deal with this serious issue.

Chapter 10 - Diets rich in fresh fruits and vegetables protect against chronic, degenerative disease. This is suggested to be related to their high antioxidant content. Up to 40% of all cancers may be preventable by diet, and risk of other age-related diseases, such as heart disease, dementia, diabetes, has a strong dietary link also. Incidence of age-related disease is increasing, for most there is no cure, and treatment is difficult, expensive and often ineffective. Therefore disease prevention is a global issue of increasing importance.

Today's student nurses are tomorrow's primary healthcare professionals and role models for health promotion and good dietary habits. However, in a cross-sectional non-experimental dietary study of 274 nursing students (228 females, 46 males), results showed low daily intake of fluid, dairy products and fruits and vegetables (<2 portions) in the majority, and 40% never took breakfast. Interestingly, study of dietary habits of registered nurses yielded similar findings. Of 251 nurses (208 female, 43 male), >50% reported dining out and eating fast food regularly. Skipping meals, fewer family meals, and high intake of fast foods are habits that are likely to result in lower intake of 'healthy' food including fruits, vegetables and dairy products. Sixty-five percent of nurses studied ate <2 portions of fruits and vegetables per day, a worryingly low intake when the recommended intake for optimal health is 5 or more/day, and 63% took no milk or other dairy products. Dairy products are a major source of dietary calcium, and low consumption of calcium is associated with higher risk of osteoporosis and bone fracture in later life. Interestingly, the self-perceived nutritional status was deemed satisfactory by most nursing students and nurses, even though study findings indicate dietary practices are far from optimal.

Thirty-six older persons in the local Chinese community were surveyed on dietary-related behaviour and lifestyle. Results showed that 40% lived alone and ate alone on a regular basis. They took few fruits and vegetable per day, no dairy or bean curd products, and inadequate fluid. Half were overweight or obese.

Results indicate low intake of antioxidant-rich food among nursing students, nurses and older persons in Hong Kong. Nurses must be trained to be knowledgeable about the relationship between diet and health and be ready and willing to lead by example, and therefore diet and health inter-relationships should be made explicit components of the nursing curriculum. Also, it is important to communicate to members of the public the importance of diet in prevention of age-related disease and promotion of healthy ageing.

In: Trends in Nursing Research
Editors: Adam J. Ryan and Jack Doyle

ISBN 978-1-60456-642-0
© 2009 Nova Science Publishers, Inc.

Chapter 1

Exploring the Meaning of Nurse-Patient Intimacy in Oncology Care Settings: Utilisation of Phenomenology and Feminism

Mura Dowling
National University of Irealnd, Galway

Abstract

This chapter presents the methodological journey and findings of a study exploring the meaning of nurse-patient intimacy in oncology care settings. The 'data' for this study is provided by the dialogue that took place through feminist conversational interviewing with thirty oncology patients, interviewed once, and twenty-three oncology nurses, interviewed twice, over a ten month period.

The study findings reveal nurse-patient intimacy as a process, which begins when the nurse and patient first meet, and nurse empathy for the patient follows identification. This identification is influenced by the patient's characteristics and response to their cancer and its treatment. Reciprocal self-disclosure characterises the intimacy that develops in the context of the nurse assuming a 'professional friend' role in a homely atmosphere where care is delivered. The outcome of intimacy is satisfaction for the nurse, but also emotional effects. Peer support among nurses in sustaining intimacy with patients is also revealed.

At first glance, it would appear that utilising phenomenological and feminist approaches simultaneously is philosophically and methodologically unsound. After all, many feminists consider phenomenology an essentialist doctrine, and essentialism is a central target of feminist criticism. However, such arguments fail to acknowledge the various phenomenological approaches available to researchers.

The phenomenological approach adopted for this study was guided by the work of phenomenologist Gadamer, whose work is also referred to as philosophical hermeneutics or interpretive phenomenology. Gadamer views the research interview as a dialogue between researcher and participant, and like feminist research, the dialogue becomes a shared project. Moreover, intimacy between study participants and researcher is espoused in feminist research, and with interpretive phenomenology, the researcher is the instrument, which suggests intimacy in the interview process.

Therefore, in the context of this study, 'feminist' is viewed as a qualitative approach, in which the subjectivity of both the researcher and participants, is central, and a close and mutual relationship between researcher and participant is seen as important. Furthermore, a diffusion of power between study participants and researcher is paramount in feminist research. Similarly, with hermeneutic understanding, the researcher and participants work together to reach a shared understand of the phenomenon being explored.

The methodological approach presented is this chapter is representative of the interdisciplinary nature of qualitative inquiry. Moreover, in the context of the literature surrounding nurse-patient intimacy, the views of nurse theorists, such as Travelbee and Peplau are not sufficient alone. Therefore, the views of philosophers such as Scheler and Stein and moral theologian Campbell, are also provided to support the interpretations revealed in the study findings.

The hybrid nature of the methodological influences adopted in this study therefore reflects the qualitative researcher adopting the role of *bricoleur,* and mirrors the characteristics of the qualitative researcher who has to be flexible, responsive and reflexive. This hybrid approach is not surprising since nursing gains its theoretical underpinnings from diverse philosophical and theoretical standpoints.

Introduction

The birth of this study arose from a need to address questions regarding caring in the nurse-patient relationship. The methodological journey taken in the creation of this study began and ended with a decision to utilise insights from philosophical hermeneutics (also known as interpretive phenomenology) after the work of Gadamer (1989). However, along that journey a feminist perspective was also adopted. In the context of this study, 'feminist' means that a qualitative approach, in which the subjectivity of both the researcher and participants, is central, and a close and mutual relationship between researcher and participant is seen as important, in the context of a pronounced interest in ethics (Alvesson and Skoldberg 2000). One might rightly ask how philosophical hermeneutics espoused by Gadamer (1989), and a feminist approach to knowledge development, is connected. However, as clearly outlined below, "feminist work has an interpretive dimension" (Nielsen 1990, p. 8). It is important to point out at this juncture that this work is not a piece of feminist research, but a study that has borrowed from feminist research methodologies in data gathering, specifically interviewing. This distinction is important, since a feminist project would be a political and politicised one, with its aim being to say something (political) about gender (in the case of Women's Studies, more often, specifically about women) in order to challenge or change existing assumptions or epistemologies. A piece of feminist research on this topic would, for example, have argued that there is something integrally different about the way men and women experience intimacy in the nurse-patient relationship, and this study does not and cannot do this.

It is important also to highlight the research presented in this chapter is representative of the inter-disciplinary nature of qualitative inquiry. This is evident in the inclusion of, for instance, the views of Habermas, who also influences current debates on subjects far removed from nursing, such as literature and cultural studies. Moreover, the views of nurse theorists, such as Travelbee and Peplau are not sufficient alone, to support the study discussion. This necessitated the inclusion of the views of philosophers such as Scheler and Stein and moral theologian Campbell, to provide support for the interpreted findings, suggesting that the study insights gleaned, have relevance not only to other intimate consumer-health care provider relationships, but to intimate relationships generally.

Exploration of Pre-Judgements

The following section represents a flavour of the reading and writing that was undertaken in the early stages of the study in order to identify pre-understandings surrounding the concept of intimacy. Gadamer asserts that pre-judgements or prejudices have a special importance in interpretation, and are not something that should be or can be disposed of (Pascoe 1996), and that the past has a profoundly pervasive power in the phenomenon of understanding (Linge 1976). Therefore, identification of my own personal pre-understandings on the topic of nurse-patient intimacy was considered central to the study.

There is a silence that shrouds the use of the term intimacy in nursing and this silence had implications for the method of data collection and approach utilised in this study. There is also a lack of conceptual clarity of intimacy from a nursing perspective (Williams 2001a), therefore, conducting a concept analysis was the most appropriate way to start the study. Rodgers' cyclical model of concept analysis (Rodgers 1989,1993) was employed in conducting the analysis of intimacy in nursing, because the principal aim of the analysis was to clarify the concept for this research study.

The sample of literature identified from the literature search undertaken for the concept analysis (25 qualitative studies, 3 quantitative studies, 6 theoretical papers, 2 literature reviews, 4 commentaries/anecdotal and 1 concept analysis), was reviewed to identify data relevant to the attributes, antecedents, consequences, surrogate terms, and related concepts, along with the references of intimacy.

The purpose of identifying the references of a concept is to clarify the range of events and circumstances over which the application of the concept is considered fitting (Rodgers 1989). Humanistic philosophy of the 1960's penetrated nursing theory and promoted the concept of a relationship between the nurse and the patient as achievable (Aranda 2001). This 'new' nursing ideology argues that a one-to-one relationship between the nurse and patient is the foundation of nursing practice (Salvage 1990).

Antecedents to intimacy identified were "space, privacy and time" (Allan 2001, p. 56) and the requirement of "nurse readiness" (nurse communication caring) and "client comfort" (client negotiating for comfort) (Schubert 1989, p.126). The attributes of intimacy were revealed to be reciprocal self-disclosure in the presence of passivity, which is a positive motivation to surrender control (Dignam 1998). Consequences (outcomes) of intimacy is a "high degree of knowing self and other", and the outcome of knowing one another (nurse and client) provides "the condition for mutual connectedness" (Schubert 1989, p.141). Intimacy is also revealed as "professionally rewarding" for nurses (Ramos 1992, 503), but "can result in increased vulnerability to suffer both emotional and physical pain" (Loftus and McDowell 2000, p. 517). Related terms identified were 'involvement', 'closeness 'and 'engagement' with surrogate terms revealed as 'sexuality' and 'sex' (Dowling 2003).

Others have also found reciprocity (Timmerman 1991) and self-disclosure (Timmerman 1991, Kadner 1994) to be important in intimacy in nursing. However, this concept analysis also reveals that self-awareness is necessary for self-disclosure. Timmerman (1991) also provided a definition of intimacy following her concept analysis. However, this concept analysis, utilising Rodgers' evolutionary model (1989), did not achieve in providing a definition, suggesting that intimacy in nursing is an evolving concept. This fits with the philosophical foundations of the evolutionary approach, which places prominence on concept analysis as a basis for further inquiry and concept development, "rather than an end point itself" (Rodgers 1993, p. 88).

This analysis resulted in an understanding of the concept of intimacy as it applies to the nurse-patient relationship, and a clear association between intimacy and caring became evident, which directed subsequent reading on love, caring and intimacy.

Caring, love and intimacy are at the heart of the therapeutic relationships nurses engage in with patients and represents everyday nursing practice, which is complex and often taken-for-granted (McLeod 1994). 'New' nursing ideology is one that recognises the one-to-one relationship between the nurse and patient as being the foundation of nursing practice. Bradshaw (1995), however, argues that the empowerment of 'New Nursing' is dependent on what she calls a destruction of 'Old Nursing', and she questions whether nursing has really advanced if the psychodynamic approach to nursing care has marginalised the practical tasks and techniques of physical care.

Morse et al., (1990) exposed five viewpoints on caring, namely: caring as a therapeutic intervention; caring as an affect; caring as a moral imperative; caring as an interpersonal relationship, and caring as a human trait. The view of caring in nursing as an interpersonal interaction probably has the greatest relationship with intimacy (Dowling 2004a). This viewpoint revolves around it being a mutual attempt of caring between the nurse and the patient. Gadow (1980) argues that the interpersonal context for care evolves as a creation of both the patient and the nurse, in other words, whole person with whole person. For caring to occur, both the nurse and patient must communicate openly with trust and respect for each other (Morse et al., 1990), and the nurse must engage with the patient in order to respond meaningfully (Morse et al., 1992). Caring, therefore, equates with involvement (Forrest 1989). Reciprocity is also a central attribute of intimacy in nursing (Dowling 2003). However, Reiman (1976) argues that the mutual revealing of personal information is not what controls intimacy; it merely deepens and nurtures the caring that powers the intimacy.

The viewpoint of caring as a human trait also relates closely to intimacy as caring as part of being human (Morse et al. 1990). Moreover, Griffin (1983) argues that the nurse develops an increased awareness of personal worth by caring for patients. This perspective on caring has its origins in existential philosophy (McCance et al., 1997), and suggests a distinct type of subjective relationship between the nurse and patient, related to what the German religious philosopher Buber (1878-1965) termed an I-Thou relationship (Buber 1955/2002). However, this type of relationship is the antithesis to the expected 'professional' relationship between nurses and patients.

Of the five perspectives on caring proposed by Morse et al. (1990), the view of caring as a moral imperative holds the greatest relevance for nurses (Dowling 2004a). This is because the foundation of a caring relationship is essentially a moral one, upon which the other four perspectives rest. Moreover, patients are vulnerable and depend on a relationship of trust (Bradshaw 1995). Nevertheless, it is important to note at this point that being a patient brings with it the burden of an intensified sensitivity (van Kaam 1959), and perhaps nurses are drawn more to care for individuals who are needy of such care.

Returning to the discussion of 'new' nursing, evidence of the influence of sociology on this topic is apparent as 'new' nursing aimed to 'humanise' nursing care by its attention to a 'bio-psycho-social' model in which a humanistic concern with communication prevails (Mulholland 1997). However, expression of the nurse–patient relationship as central to nursing practice pre-dates 'new' nursing ideology, in the work of, for instance, Peplau (1952). More recently, Barker has proposed the Tidal Model, based on a series of studies exploring various views of nursing (Barker 2001). His model incorporates tenets of Peplau's work, as well as the therapeutic use of self (that is, how the nurse uses his/her personal qualities in her/his relationships with patients they are caring for) as proposed by Nurse Theorist Joyce Travelbee (1971).

Involvement is a related concept of intimacy (Dowling 2003). However, Williams (2001b), questions whether theoretical writings regarding intimacy in practice actually represent over-involvement. Morse (1991) describes the over-involved relationship as one where the patient and nurse mutually respect, trust and care for each other. The use of the term 'care' in this context suggests an emotional investment by the patient in his/her relationship with the nurse. This description of over-involvement is interesting in light of the theoretical views proposed by 'new' nursing. Perhaps the issue is not with mutual trust and respect between the nurse and patient, but with the inclusion of caring for each other. Such mutual caring may be perceived as the antithesis to the expected professional relationship between nurses and patients. Moreover, the use of the term 'over-involvement' suggests a nurse who is not in control (Dowling 2006a).

Parsons (1951) presents a multidimensional scheme for classifying relationships containing five dichotomous pattern variables, which, he argues, structures all social action (Lidz 2000). These patterns reflect the reality of intimacy in nursing practice (Dowling 2006a). Dowling (2006a) argues that nurses are encouraged to find what could be termed as a safe equilibrium and are expected to care with empathy and kindness but, at the same time, maintain a degree of emotional detachment. In this context a balanced relationship suggests the presence of reciprocity, where the nurse would self-disclose some personal details that s/he considered appropriate, such as if they had experienced the death of a parent, when asked for such information by a bereaved patient. Dowling (2006a) also argues that it is perhaps only nurses who are truly self-aware that can really engage in intimate relationships with their patients. Self-disclosure requires an acute degree of self-awareness when a distressed patient probes the nurse with questions in order to ascertain the nurse's personal experience of coping with stressful events. In such a case, the nurse must measure his/her self-disclosure carefully, since the outcome of his/her sharing may have either a positive or negative effect on the patient. However, self-awareness and knowledge of the self develops over time with experience. Moreover, the risks of self-disclosure appear greater if the nurse has not developed self-awareness. This issue is also closely related to how the nurse communicates with patients, which in turn affects the development of intimacy.

Context: Nurse-Patient Communication in Cancer Care Settings

The importance of effective communication between health care professionals and patients is a key aspect of a good cancer service (DoH 1995 [Calman-Hine Report]). However, communication between nurses and their patients is complex, particularly when the patient is experiencing a diagnosis of cancer, which evokes fear and anxiety in most people (Maguire 1995, Sawyer 2000).

When nurse-patient patient communication in cancer is effective, it can result not only in psychological benefits for patients, but also physical benefits, with improved pain control and adherence to often difficult treatment regimens (Wilkinson, Gambles and Roberts 2002). However, May (1990), in a review of the literature, reports that nurses spend minimal time engaging in verbal communication, employ strategies to avoid communication and control their interactions with patients. Moreover, it is reported that nurses focus on the physical tasks of care and give little attention to patients' emotional and psychological issues (Macleod Clark 1982, Bond 1983, Booth et al., 1996). More specifically to cancer, it has been demonstrated that nurses' communication skills have revealed little improvement over a twenty year span (Bailey and Wilkinson 1998, Wilkinson, et al., 1999), and that nurses control their communication with cancer patients to keep the level of disclosure at a superficial level (Wilkinson 1991). It is also reported that nurses' use of blocking behaviours increases, the more patients' disclose feelings (Booth et al., 1996). When nurses fail to meet patients' emotional needs, dissatisfaction in communication results (Suominen, Leini-Kilpi and Laippala 1995, Krishnasamy 1996).

Communication in oncology care settings is influenced by many factors. One such influence is how communication is established at the time of diagnosis, where developing the nurse-patient relationship is paramount in order for nurses to effectively support patients throughout their cancer journey (Furlong and O'Toole 2006). At diagnosis, a variety of responses is set in motion, with initial shock, disbelief and denial, feelings of anxiety and depression, anger and guilt, and finally a sense of adaptation to the demands of treatment (Massie and Holland 1989). However, if the patient is not equipped with sufficient emotional reserves, the result may be psychological distress (Kruijver et al., 2000). It is imperative therefore, that oncology nurses maintain openness in their approach to communicating with patients.

Emotions Surrounding Communication in Cancer

Emotions feature strongly in nurse-patient communication in cancer care (Northouse and Northouse 1987, Maguire and Faulkner 1988). Communicating with patients with life-threatening illness, such as cancer is "not easy, and the demands on health care professionals are immense" (Wilkinson et al., 1999, p.342). Nurses report an awareness of using blocking and distancing tactics with cancer patients, arising from anxiety over their communication with patients (Webster 1981). Health care professionals may develop feelings of helplessness and anxiety when they feel inadequately prepared to communicate effectively with patients (Wong, Lee and Mok 2001). Nurses may fear that probing patients for information on how they are feeling may cause the patient to experience emotional distress (Bailey and Wilkinson 1998). Doctors too, are reported to avoid truth-telling practice with oncology patients, especially when faced with families request to 'do not tell' (Ozdogan et al., 2006). However, ineffective communication results in the patient experiencing elevated anxiety, a sense of uncertainty and diminished satisfaction with their care (Wilkinson et al., 2002).

Communicative Behaviours

There has been much research conducted on communication in oncology care settings, with two types of communicative actions revealed as important for cancer patients, these being instrumental (such as informing patients about their illness and treatment), and affective (such as giving comfort and building trust). Affective communicative behaviours reflect the psychosocial aspects of nursing care that feature prominently in oncology nursing (Wettergren 1996). However, research evidence points to nurses' attention on instrumental communicative actions in favour of affective communicative behaviours.

Krishanamy (1996) suggests that cancer patients perceive nurses' communicative behaviours conveying the provision of companionship and intimacy as supportive. Nevertheless, it is also important to note that cancer patients report the importance of emotionally supportive behaviours, such as listening, only when their need for instrumental support is met, through nurses' clinical know-how (Larson 1984). Similar preferences of patients for instrumental behaviours over affective communicative behaviours is also reported elsewhere (von Essen and Sjoden 1991, Larsson et al., 1998). However, recent findings reported by Liu, Mok and Wong (2006) suggest that oncology patients value nurses' affective communicative actions when they are experienced in tandem with nurses' instrumental caring behaviours.

Of relevance also is a nurse's attitude to cancer. Cancer can represent immense fear and emotion for some nurses (Morton 1996), and doctors and nurses may fear that talking openly about the patient's cancer may result in issues raised that are too difficult to face (Maguire 1985). This is not surprising as the time around diagnosis is often a devastating for cancer patients (Denny and McGuigan 1999). Moreover, it is argued that what is labelled as 'blocking' in cancer care communication is actually an attempt to maintain optimism (Jarrett and Payne 2000), and an attempt to survive confronting emotionally charged situations with cancer patients (Kruijver et al., 2000).

Jarrett and Payne (1995) suggested that the contribution of patients to nurse-patient communication is a neglected aspect that requires further attention. They subsequently undertook to investigate cancer patients' influence on nurse-patient communication using an ethnomethodological approach (Jarrett and Payne 2000). Their study revealed that thoughts considered negative were viewed as harmful to the ward atmosphere and the patient's coping responses, and suggested that patients and relatives are also active participants in creating a "cheerful, positive and constructive atmosphere" (Jarrett and Payne 2000, p. 89). They also reported that both nurses and patients undertook self comparison during communication as a means to achieve optimism (Jarrett and Payne 2000).

Communication in cancer is therefore influenced by many factors. These factors range from patients' response to their diagnosis, to the care setting where they receive treatment. The view of Slevin (1987) is interesting in that he argues that "communication is inherently neither good nor bad. In order to be effective and helpful it needs to be appropriate to the patient and his [sic] circumstances" (p. 59). Slevin's focus on the need for "effective" communication is noteworthy. This means that nurses must use communication skills that suit the patient's particular needs at that time. This requires a need for oncology nurses to develop a heightened sense of self-awareness of, not only their communication behaviours, but also, their emotional response and attitude to cancer.

Research Framework

This study adopted a phenomenological approach. Phenomenology has become a dominant factor in the pursuit of knowledge development in nursing, and presents "credible displays of living knowledge for nursing" (Jones and Borbasi 2004, p. 99). However, the term 'phenomenology', although used frequently in nursing scholarship, is accompanied by confusion surrounding its nature. Firstly, it is not only a research method employed frequently by qualitative researchers, it is also a philosophy. Secondly, there are as many styles of phenomenology as there are phenomenologists (Spiegelberg 1982). There are a number of schools of phenomenology, and even though they all have some commonalities, they also have distinct features (Dowling 2007). Adding possible confusion is the interchange of terminology surrounding phenomenology, for instance, Gadamer's writings are referred to as both interpretive phenomenology and philosophical hermeneutics (Dowling 2004b). Furthermore, for this study, which espouses to adopt feminist interviewing and reflexivity from a feminist standpoint, it was necessary to explicate how such a hybrid view fitted into the heading of phenomenology. A primary concern was to clarify how the philosophical view of phenomenology, which is considered anti-feminist, as a result of its arguments of essentialism, could be philosophically accommodated in the study. The answer to this question may lie, in part, in the dual identities assumed by phenomenology as it is currently known today, that is, as a philosophy and a research approach. Moreover, while the philosophy of phenomenology is essential to its method, it would appear that an approach to phenomenology assumed dominance in this study.

It is important to acknowledge that feminist discourse has for the most part overlooked phenomenology. Fisher (2000), however, argues that the feminist charges of essentialism, universalism and absolutism of phenomenology can be removed by a careful and strong examination of what phenomenology actually, in fact, sets out to do. Moreover, feminist arguments against phenomenology would appear to suggest that there is only one type of phenomenology, whereas in fact there are many. Furthermore, the type of phenomenology that emerged from the United States over the past two decades, and labelled 'new' phenomenology would appear to fit with feminist views. Indeed, Fisher (2000) comments that post-structuralist, deconstructive, or post-modern perspectives have all informed and/or identified with feminist theory in North America, and have arguably been influenced by phenomenology. Furthermore, feminist argument that phenomenology is 'theory-bound' is interesting. Such a view reflects, perhaps, a view of phenomenology that only encompasses the philosophy of Husserl and not later phenomenological philosophies, such as that of Gadamer, where socio-political context is acknowledged. Moreover, Gadamer's phenomenology could not be viewed as essentialist as it fits into the constructivist paradigm, and considers culture, while the researcher is viewed as co-creator of the data.

Of importance too, is how feminist interviewing was utilised in this study. In order to ask patients and nurses about their interactions with each other, it was decided that the most suitable method of data collection was feminist interviewing, which is conversational in nature and simultaneously acknowledges the interview as a therapeutic opportunity (Birch and Miller 2000). Similarly, for Gadamer, since the principal aim of a conversation is to allow immersion in the subject matter, "a conversation between researcher and participant is a suitable method of achieving understanding of a phenomenon of interest" (Fleming, Gaidys and Robb 2003, p. 117). In addition, Gadamer views the research interview as a dialogue between researcher and participant where "they open up to each other...they try to understand each other's messages and want to assess their own views and points of departure" (Haggman-Laitila 1999, p, 13). Like feminist research then, the dialogue becomes a shared project. Moreover, intimacy between study participants and researcher is espoused in feminist research (Birch and Miller 2000) and with phenomenology, the researcher is the instrument (van Manen 1984), which suggests intimacy in the interview process.

This notion of the researcher as instrument is also feminist in orientation and suggests that a relationship must be built with study participants, in order for the phenomenon under investigation to be explicated. Furthermore, a diffusion of power between study participants and researcher is paramount in feminist research. Similarly, with hermeneutic understanding, the researcher "does not attempt to see through the eyes of the participants to understand the phenomenon of interest. Instead they work together to reach a shared understanding" (Fleming, Gaidys and Robb 2003, p. 117). Furthermore, Gadamerian phenomenology is also called "alethic hermeneutics" (from the Greek aletheia, or uncoveredness) (Alvesson and Skoldberg 2000) which "dissolves the polarity between subject and object ...characterised instead by a disclosive structure" (p. 57). In addition, the interview as a therapeutic opportunity, as in feminist research, entails repeat interviewing in order to "promote reflection" (Birch and Miller 2000, p. 196). Similarly, Gadamerian phenomenology assumes that "understanding depends on the particular historic situation, it is essential to speak two or three times to participants" (Fleming, Gaidys and 2003, p. 118). Finally, as mentioned earlier, Gadamer asserts that pre-judgements or prejudices have a special importance in interpretation and strongly affect one's understanding; a view which resulted in an identification of my own personal pre-understandings on the topic of nurse-patient intimacy. Banchetti-Robino (2000), in a critique of feminist phenomenology, argues that, before any phenomenological investigation begins, a description of the phenomena as it is experienced by the investigator and, thus, as it is manifested to the investigative consciousness must be undertaken. This explicit acknowledgement of me as co-creator of the research data also clearly necessitated a feminist approach to reflexivity for this study.

There are many approaches to reflexivity in qualitative research (Dowling 2006b). The approach adopted in this study acknowledges the centrality of reflexivity to feminist research. Reflexivity is vital in feminist research and acknowledges that the researcher identifies with study participants. This open acknowledgement of my influence on the study fits with a feminist view of research where the notion of value neutrality is challenged (Koch and Harrington 1998), and bias is not viewed as a position that distorts study findings, but is a resource (Olesen 1994). Moreover, in keeping with Oakley's (1981) view of the feminist interview utilised in this study, the reflexive approach chosen fits with the suggestion that engagement rather than detachment is necessary of the qualitative researcher (Sandelowski 1986).

Reflexivity in feminism is a "performed politics" (Marcus 1994, p.569), and current discussion on reflexivity in feminist research emphasises the power differentials within the various stages of the research process (Mauthner and Doucet 2003). The reciprocal nature of the researcher-participant relationship is evident in this 'positioning'. This view of reflexivity addresses the researcher as a unique person.

Feminist researchers have epistemological concerns at their centre, and the notion of value neutrality is challenged (Koch and Harrington 1998). This view is central to the approach taken in this study. Reflexivity and intersubjectivity are married in feminist research. Through reciprocal sharing of knowing, the researcher, and those being researched, become collaborators in the research project. The researcher and informants become partners in the research endeavour, and the researcher utilises their own experiences and reflections in order to illuminate important meaning (Schutz 1994).

Of relevance to this decision too, is that Gadamer's work, when fused with the philosophy of Jurgen Habermas, is known as 'critical hermeneutics'. Habermas's view resides in the critical paradigm, which regards knowledge as active and entrenched in a socio-political context and, like feminist research, rejects the notion that there can be 'objective' knowledge. Moreover, Gadamer's Hermeneutic "criticises the legitimacy" of scientific methods (Fleming, Gaidys and Robb 2003, p. 115), similar to the efforts of feminist researchers (Nielsen 1990).

Although the work of Gadamer offers valuable direction regarding the development of a deeper understanding of texts, he does not offer either a methodology or a method for developing such deeper insights (Fleming, Gaidys and Robb 2003). Nevertheless, while Gadamer argues that the task of philosophical hermeneutics is not the systematic collection and analysis of data, but the illumination of the ordinary process of understanding (Habermas, 1990), he also expresses the opinion that in order to reach understanding, methodological direction through a systematic approach is required (Fleming, Gaidys and Robb 2003). Additionally, the main arguments of philosophical hermeneutics are accepted as a research paradigm within the social sciences (Habermas 1990). The other methodological influence in this study is the work of Alvesson and Skoldberg (2000) regarding reflexive interpretation, which argues that analysis and interpretation are intimately related. Moreover, with reflexive interpretation, the researcher asks questions of the text that arise from their pre-understandings, which are transformed in the process.

The two central positions advanced by Gadamer are: (a) prejudgement-one's preconceptions or prejudices or horizon of meaning that is part of our linguistic experience and that make understanding possible, and (b) universality-the persons who express themselves and the persons who understand are connected by a common human consciousness, which makes understanding possible (Ray 1994).

Gadamer (1989) argues that to understand does not mean an individual understands better (for instance, because of clearer thoughts on the subject being understood); rather, an individual understands differently. Gadamer (1989) also argues that the detachment of our fruitful prejudices that facilitate understanding from our prejudices that obstruct our understanding occurs in the process of understanding itself (Gadamer 1989). Therefore, in his version of phenomenology, understanding is derived from personal involvement by the researcher in reciprocal processes of interpretation that are inextricably related with one's being-in-the-world (Spence 2001). Inquiry using Gadamerian hermeneutics, becomes dialogue rather than individual phenomenology and interpretation permeates every activity, with the researcher considering social, cultural and gender implications (Koch 1999).

Gadamer places a stronger emphasis on language than Heidegger, and affirms the position of the researcher in the hermeneutic circle (Koch 1996). He describes the hermeneutic circle as the fusing of horizons, which is circular in process, similar to the *alethic* hermeneutic circle embraced by Heidegger, mentioned above. Gadamer (1989, p. 268) asserts that in order to understanding the meaning of something held by another, we must not attach blindly to our own fore-meaning. He argues that we remain 'open' to, and also embrace the meaning held by the other person or text with our own meanings. What is essential throughout this process is that we are aware of our biases in order for the text to portray its uniqueness against our own fore-meanings (Gadamer 1989). Therefore, the hermeneutic process becomes a dialogical method whereby the horizon of the interpreter and the thing being studied are combined together. This view of Gadamer placing more emphasis on language than Heidegger may explain why some believe Gadamer's phenomenology to be pure hermeneutics and not phenomenology as defined by Heidegger.

Gadamer's (1989) view of the hermeneutic circle brings it a step forward from that of Heidegger, and researchers inspired by his work, therefore, should ensure that feedback and further discussion takes place with study participants (Fleming, Gaidys and Robb 2003). This dialogue with study participants can be achieved by the employment of repeat interviewing with study participants, providing the opportunity for discussion of interpretations gleaned from earlier interviews. Therefore, the hermeneutic process becomes a dialogical method whereby the horizon of the interpreter and the phenomenon being studied are combined together. This latter point is central to the approach taken in this study since it illustrates why Gadamer's work has been able to be utilised by feminist research.

Ethical Issues

Ethical approval was granted from the three hospitals offering oncology services chosen for the study, before the interviews began. A consideration to the principle of beneficence resulted in much reading on the therapeutic nature of the qualitative interview (for instance, Birch and Miller 2000). It was viewed important to reflect on the opinion that the qualitative researcher may, because of this perceived therapeutic benefit, overlook the risk of non-maleficence in qualitative research (Richards and Schwartz 2002).

The principle of non-maleficence was also examined, and the possible risks for study participants of emotional distress was one considered carefully. Therefore, contact was established with a health service psychologist before beginning the study, should her services be required for any nurse following their interview with me. With regard to patients, I discussed with each nurse manager the need for me to inform them if I felt that any patient required follow-up and they would arrange psychological support, as considered appropriate. Debriefing was also undertaken with all study participants. With nurses, at the end of each interview, I asked them how they felt being interviewed. With patients, I also asked them how they felt being interviewed, but I also talked with them for some time (ten minutes to one hour) after the tape was turned off to assess how they were feeling and to ensure that they felt comfortable having shared some of their thoughts with me. Like Colbourne (2004) (in Colbourne and Sque 2004), I also had a fear that I might unwittingly inflict harm (particularly emotional harm) on the study participants. Staying to talk with patients after the tape was turned off fits with what Colbourne and Sque (2004) call the researcher as 'professional friend' which allows the researcher resolve such fears.

With regard to maintaining the participants' autonomy, efforts aimed at this included offering them enough information about the study and also ensuring that they knew clearly that they could leave the study at any time they wished. An attempt to address this principle was made in my information leaflet that accompanied the study. However, I was cognisant of Flinders' (1992) argument that it is often difficult for the qualitative researcher to inform the study participants of the necessary level of information when "they do not know the twists and turns their work is likely to take" (Flinders 1992, p. 103).

Process consent was also undertaken during the study with repeat interviewing of nurses, which involved discussing and clarifying the issue of informed consent again with each nurse. Furthermore, each study participant was assigned a number rather than a pseudonym. Moreover, serious consideration must be given to the safe storage of data, and this was achieved by the use of a locked cupboard for all the tapes used in the study.

Underlying the ethical approach taken in this study was an ethic of care evolved from the work of Gilligan (1982), which, when compared against traditional approaches to ethics, is very strongly feminist (Glass and Cluxton 2004). An ethic of care approach to this study is evident in the intersubjectivity achieved between me, as researcher, and the study participants. I shared aspects of my life with all study participants as I considered appropriate and, in keeping with a feminist view of the researcher-participant relationship, reciprocity was embraced. This reciprocity, in turn, resulted in engagement with each study participant, which consequently enhanced communication processes before, during and after interviews in the study. Moreover, an ethics of care is predicated on interdependence, mutuality and recognition of context in addition to such moral emotions as empathy and compassion (Hudson 1999). This approach is particularly appropriate to this study of nurse-patient intimacy in light also of the view of Beauchamp and Childress (1998) who remind us that feminist thought places value on emotion, attachment and interdependence.

Rigour

Criteria for the assessment of validity of conclusions reached from qualitative analysis have always been the centre of much debate, and continues in many fields (Edge and Richards 1998, Chamberlain 2000, Barker 2003). The views of Hammersley and Atkinson (1983) are most relevant to this discussion of what constitutes as rigour in a qualitative study such as this. In their discussion of 'ethnographic authority', they assert that because the researcher was there (in the field), it is the researcher's interpretations that should prevail. However, it must be acknowledged that Lee and Fielding (2004) warn that some disagree with such a view. Moreover, the diversity of qualitative methodologies contributes to the difficulty in demonstrating their value and intellectual honesty, which may result in the danger that only those qualitative methodologies that appear most compatible with the criteria of traditional qualitative research will be accepted (Yardley 2000). Therefore, a study such as this, by virtue of its adoption of feminist tenets in a phenomenological approach, may be at risk of criticism for not adhering to the rules of rigour. However, the integral role of reflexivity expressed in the study aims to overcome such criticism.

With this in mind, rigour in qualitative research does not mean that all the data was collected exactly the same way or that analysis was closely controlled. It means that all the decisions made were done thoughtfully, alternatives considered and ramifications measured (Steeves 2000a). This view is related to 'dependability', which involves leaving a decision trail by discussing explicitly decisions taken about the theoretical, methodological and analytic choices throughout the study (Koch 1998). Moreover, because the data for this study is the participants' narratives, an inherent difficulty with reliability arises. Narrative studies do not have formal methods of reliability (Polkinghorne 1988), instead, they "rely on the details of their procedures for procuring the best possible information, which evokes a sense of trustworthiness for the validity of the information used for study" (Eberhart and Pieper 1994, p. 46).

The suggestion of Eberhart and Pieper (1994), is also useful to this discussion, since they propose the following as examples for the procurement of reliable information in hermeneutic research: selection of an appropriate sample, a structure for capturing the phenomenon under investigation, including a preliminary research question, direction for information to be relayed in the interview to be given to participants prior to the interview, and multiple interviews with participants to clarify information in the text and expand on the original narrative that was collected. They also suggest that the transcription of the audiotaped interviews into a written text should be carefully checked against the audiotape to ensure the language in the text accurately reflects the verbal description of the experience (Eberhart and Pieper 1994). All of these suggestions were adhered to in this study.

Another attempt to display evidence of trustworthiness is the adoption of member checks (Long and Johnson 2000). This is recommended by many authors of qualitative research, such as, Cutliffe and McKenna (1999), and requires the enlisting of the assistance of colleagues to help with verification of the study results. However, there are inherent philosophical difficulties with this strategy, as there is a unique interpretive relationship between each qualitative researcher and the data, which may result in the auditor not necessarily uncovering the primary researcher's findings (Sandwlowski 1998). This is especially so if the primary researcher has been involved in all stages of the research process and the auditor joins the study at the end (Cutliffe and McKenna 2004), as is the case with this study.

Moreover, Cutliffe and McKenna (2004) caution that the primary researcher and auditor are "philosophically and methodologically polarized" (p. 131) and, therefore, it is difficult to imagine them reaching the same findings and interpretations, and they conclude that this notion of confirmability is driven by positivist tenets. In addition, de Witt and Ploeg (2006) argue that confirmability and credibility, as explicated by Sandelowski (1986), are "inappropriate generic qualitative criteria for expressing rigour in interpretive phenomenological studies" (p. 222). Nevertheless, member checks were considered appropriate for this study. The view that two individuals arriving at the same interpretation of a text does not mean that subjectivity is eliminated, as argued by Yardley (2000), was adopted here. The inclusion of member checks is to further demonstrate that "care, thoroughness and professionalism" (Chamberlain 2000, p. 291) was adopted for the study. Therefore, an academic colleague, familiar with phenomenological research undertook member checks of a sample of transcripts from both nurses and patients. Her feedback to me reflected a similar interpretation from the data, but with the use of different words.

However, to be even more specific regarding 'criteria' for an interpretive phenomenological study such as this, the view of de Witt and Ploeg (2006) is most relevant. They propose what they term a "new framework of rigour" specific to interpretive phenomenology consisting of five expressions: balanced integration, openness, concreteness, resonance and actualisation (de Witt and Ploeg 2006, p. 215). With regard to the first expression, balanced integration, this study has adopted a comprehensive explication of its methodological philosophical underpinnings. The second expression of 'openness' has been displayed by "a systematic, explicit process of accounting for the multiple decisions made throughout the interpretive phenomenological study process" (de Witt and Ploeg 2006, p. 225). The third expression is reflected in the study findings by its readers recognising "concreteness" when they read the study findings (de Witt and Ploeg 2006, p. 225). Resonance is the experiential or felt effect on the reader in the process of reading the study findings (van Manen 1997). Finally, the fifth expression of 'actualization' represents the continuous interpretation by readers of a interpretive phenomenological study in the future, and "no formal mechanism presently exists within the research community" for its recording (de Witt and Ploeg 2006, p. 226).

Sampling

A discussion on sampling in hermeneutic research can be organised in one of three frames: the experience of place, the experiences of events in time, and ways of talking about experiences. However, most hermeneutical phenomenological researchers are interested in all three at the same time and would argue that no single phenomenon can be understood in isolation (Steeves 2000b).

This framework of Steeves (2000b) is inspired by the work of Merleau-Ponty (1962) and Gadamer (1989). Steeves (2000b) argues that the rationale for utilising their work rests in Merleau-Ponty's view that people are first and foremost a body of space and Gadamer's interest in interpretation, which further supports its relevance to this study.

In the context of this study, intimacy cannot be understood without an understanding of the place or context where the nurse-patient interaction occurs. The informants for this study were recruited from three centres offering oncology care in one Irish Health Service Executive area. The first unit where data collection took place was in a nurse-led oncology unit (Site A), which offers a satellite service to the Supra-Oncology regional centre (Site B). The second centre where data collection was collected was at the area's Supra-oncology centre (Site B) offering out-patient chemotherapy, in-patient chemotherapy, radiotherapy, and surgical oncology services. The third centre (Site C), situated in another county, like Site A was nurse-led.

Steeves (2000b) argues that how people experience events over time is of immense interest to hermeneutic phenomenological researchers. In following the philosophical views of Gadamer, I had planned also to repeat interview patients. However, this plan was abandoned early in the study, as the realities of repeat interviewing surfaced. The main reason for not pursuing this strategy of interviewing was due to my experiences in at Site A. Patients' physical and mental conditions had often altered considerably when I went to re-interview them. This issue of changes in patients' conditions is also reported by McIlfatrick (2003) and Birch and Miller (2000).

The issue of experiencing events over time is central to cancer patients' experiences. However, despite interviewing patients on various aspects of the cancer trajectory, for instance, patients on early and later rounds of chemotherapy treatment regimens, a prevailing sense of optimism and hopefulness persistently emerged.

Steeves (2000b) argues that the informants are interviewed to "understand the tradition or way of talking about experience. The way people talk about a certain topic is the source of and the reposititory of interpretations of the world. The individual uses these interpretations in a unique way to understand his or her experience" (pp. 54-55). This theme of 'talking about experience' very much relates to the theme above of 'experiencing events over time', as optimism was a key feature of my interviews with patients.

The sampling strategies adopted included elements of both purposive and opportunistic with patients, and purposive and theoretical with nurses. Purposeful/theoretical sampling attempts to select research participants according to criteria determined by the purpose, but also is guided by the unfolding theorising (Tuckett 2005). Furthermore, since the data collection for this study took place over a ten month period, ongoing sampling was an element of this study and is a strategy that supports emerging ideas about ideas (Tuckett

2005). In addition, sampling in qualitative research is a process within which sampling criteria may change as the study unfolds (Tuckett 2005). Finally, the study began with an indeterminate sample size of participants and continued until it was felt that saturation had been reached.

The sampling began as one of purposive in so far as the sample was all cancer patients and cancer nurses. However, theoretical sampling with nurses became evident about mid-way through the study. I actively sought nurses in Clinical Nurse Specialist [CNS] roles, for instance, breast care nurses, as my earlier interviews with nurses in day oncology units suggested that these CNSs might have had greater opportunities for intimacy with patients. Moreover, these nurse specialists play a central role in offering emotional and psychological support to cancer patients (Corner 2002, Skilbeck and Payne 2003). This mixture of sampling is evidence of the method slurring (Baker et al. 1992) or pluralism (Johnson, Long and White 2001) with grounded theory that occurred in this study. This mixed sampling strategy also reflects the experience of being a qualitative researcher, where assuming a role of bricoleur emerges.

The voices of women feature strongly in the study, since the sample consisted of mainly women. It was not the intention of this study to focus mostly on the experience of women, however, all of the nurses interviewed were women and I only encountered one male nurse in one of the study sites. Eighteen of the patients interviewed were women, reflecting the number of breast cancer patients attending the day care services.

Interviewing

The data collection method for this study was feminist interviewing. In-depth interviewing, as that used in feminist methodology, is the predominant method of data collection in phenomenological research (Wimpenny and Gass 2000). However, it is important to point out that interviewing is often viewed as a generic method without consideration paid to how it is to be used in a particular methodology (Wimpenny and Gass 2000). According to Price (2002), interviews are influenced by philosophical considerations such as the role of the researcher in the interview process and the role of the interview in the research study. He further argues that the research paradigm employed by the researcher is "at least as important as the contextual difficulties *of* conducting interviews in the field" (Price 2002, p. 274). This view is key to the interview strategy adopted in this study. I adopted feminist interviewing in a philosophical hermeneutic study within a constructivist paradigm.

I spent considerable time deciding what my opening question would be. van Manen (1990) argues that, in the conversational interview, it is important to realise that the interview process "needs to be disciplined by the fundamental question that promoted the need for the interview in the first place" (p. 67). However, intimacy is not a word used appropriately in the context of nurse-patient interactions. Indeed, Williams (2001a) reports that some nurses she interviewed in her study, exploring their perceptions and experiences of intimacy in their relationships with patients, expressed the view that intimacy was an inappropriate term to describe closeness in the bonding or closeness in the nurse-patient relationship. Also, my concept analysis revealed its surrogate terms to be 'sexuality' and 'sex', and, I was cognisant of the words of van Manen (2002) referring to Wittgenstein who has shown that "the meaning of any term is always conditional on the usage of that term within the social practices of the language games in which we are involved" (p. 270).

Therefore, my opening question to patients was "Could you tell me about your interactions with nurses who care for you". To nurses, I posed the following question: "Could you tell me about your interactions with patients you care for?" By using an open question like this, I didn't want to assume that intimacy, as I viewed it, was an aspect of their interactions. Moreover, using an open-ended opening question, the interviewees can choose for themselves which experiences and feelings are central to their past and present experiences. In addition, with an abstract concept, such as intimacy, by asking participants about their interactions with nurses/patients, it would identify for them a more "concrete, specific experience" (Kahn 2000a, p.63).

Moreover, I found Walsh's (1996) experience of asking nurses about their relationships with patients helpful. He reports that when he asked psychiatric nurses about their relationships with patients, they would look at him blankly or give a psychological treatise on the helping relationship. So instead, he asked about their 'encounters', similar to my approach of asking about interactions.

With unstructured interviewing, the interviewer refrains from using a definitive framework that leads the questions asked, but follows the participant's direction through their narrative in response to the opening question posed (Moyle 2002). This helps ensure that the narrative is that of the participant's perspective and not of the interviewer (Moyle 2002).

"The art of questioning is that of being able to go on asking questions, ie [sic] the art of thinking" (Gadamer 1975, p. 330). I found this advice useful, as I did the views of van Manen (1990), who advises that as the researcher interviews a person about a certain phenomenon, it is vital to "stay close" to the experience as lived (p. 67). He recommends, therefore, that when the person is asked about what an experience is like, the researcher should be concrete and ask the person to think of a specific instance, situation, person, or event. Then the whole experience is explored to its fullest. I attempted this strategy in many of my interviews and found it helpful as patients often found it difficult to articulate their experience of interactions with nurses caring for them. Moreover, I would then ask them to think of an experience or incident that stood out for them or that they clearly remembered.

Also, it is important to point out that a feminist view of interviewing stands apart from the traditional view of the interview. I concur with the opinion of Levesque-Lopman (2000) who suggests that calling what she does an 'interview' as a way of gathering material or doing research makes her feel uncomfortable in that it has several connotations in conventional social research, such as the hierarchy between the participants and the informant and it does not have the spontaneity and mutuality associated with ordinary conversations. In addition, the feminist approach to the research relationship is viewed as "a two-way movement of information", rather than the "one-way" movement, as in the interview (Borbasi, Jackson and Wilkes 2005, p. 499). Therefore, of all the interview styles proposed in qualitative research, the conversational one sits most comfortably with a feminist interview.

Moyle (2002) argues that a personal engagement between interviewer and participant is necessary in qualitative research. A feminist framework takes this view further by viewing the interview as one that builds connections and avoids alienation of the researcher from the participant (Levesque-Lopman 2000). Lindlof and Taylor (2002) also suggest that if the researcher uses "brief personal stories or anecdotes judiciously" during the interview, "a sense of reciprocity and goodwill often unfolds" (p. 90). However, such a view of feminist interviewing must not lose sight of the need for reflection on the risk of essentialized understanding when conducting research with women (McCormick, Kirkham and Hayes 1998). Moreover, Domosh (2003) argues that a "more fully reciprocal research relationship" is created when the personal knowledge of the research interviewee is examined by the feminist researcher with the same scrutiny they appoint on themselves (p. 110).

The interview as a therapeutic opportunity is raised by Birch and Miller (2000), who encourage a therapeutic setting "especially if we are trying to construct a social relationships of reciprocity, friendship, and shared understandings with the aim to uncover what is being felt at a deeper level" (p. 199). However, Bondi (2003) cautions that a therapeutic effect is a "side-effect" rather than the "core purpose" of the interview (p. 67). Such a therapeutic setting also requires interviewer self-disclosure as a way to engage participant's interest and "pave the way for a meaningful interview" (Lindolf and Taylor 2002, p. 190).

The hermeneutic interview tends to render interviewees into participants or collaborators of the research project (van Manen 1990). Similar to the conversational interview, the researcher can go back to the interviewee in order to continue dialogue about the ongoing verification of the interview transcripts. This approach was taken in the study, and all the nurses interviewed (n=23) were interviewed a second time. However, as mentioned earlier, the plan to re-interview patients was abandoned early in the study due to a deterioration in the patients' conditions.

Repeat interviewing, where the participants check out the interpretations is often called 'member checking' (Kahn 2000a), and assists in providing a credibility of the interpretation in both hermeneutic and feminist studies (Maynard 2004), and also helps to reduce "researcher bias" (Kahn 2000b, p.64). Repeat interviewing is a strategy employed in hermeneutic studies, where it is acknowledged that the understanding of researcher and participants changes over time (Fleming, Gaidys and Robb 2003), and considers interviewees as collaborators of the research project (van Manen 1990). This allows reflection on the text (transcripts) of previous interviews in order to aim for as much interpretive insight as possible, and determine the deeper meanings or themes of these experiences (van Manen 1990). Furthermore, in the follow-up interview, the themes identified in the transcript become "objects of reflection in follow-up hermeneutic conversations in which both the researcher and the interviewee collaborate" (van Manen 1990, p.99). The interviewer is unavoidably implicated in creating meanings that reside within respondents (Manning 1967). In addition, although repeat interviewing is espoused as "therapeutic" in its potential, it can also be regarded as "unnecessary harassment" (Richards and Schwartz 2000, p. 138). This was certainly a possibility if I had persisted in repeat interviewing patients.

Interviewing patients was challenging because of the pre-and-post emotional work with all patients. This involved spending up to half an hour before the interview hearing the patient's story, and up to one hour after each interview, ensuring that the patient felt comfortable having been interviewed. However, listening to patients' stories was often a very tiring experience for me. Krishnasamy and Plant (1998) and Moyle (2002) also reports similar interviewing experiences.

Of relevance also, are the power relations between the interviewee and the researcher (McDowell 1992, Bondi 2003, Monk, Manning and Denman 2003). The impact of power and authority on the interview process was therefore, a factor I remained cognisant of throughout, and one that feminist geographers argue should be acknowledged (McDowell 1992). Paying due attention to issues of conflict of interest in the research relationship are essential to the maintenance of trust in the unequal power researcher-study participant relationship (Ferguson, Myrick and Yonge 2006). Nevertheless, it is argued that there are many influences "unknown and/or outside our awareness", on the feminist researcher's relationship with the interviewee (Bondi 2003, p. 73).

Data Analysis

Maynard (2004) suggests that it "seems strange" that feminists have not focused on the issue of data analysis as explicitly as they have on other issues (p. 131). She suggests that this may be because early feminist work on research was highly critical of the emphasis on technique, and also that many feminists (and others) do not consider analysis and interpretation as separate stages, but an ongoing aspect of research (Maynard 2004). The reflexive interpretation (Alvesson and Skoldberg 2000) adopted for this study, therefore, fits with a feminist view of analysis and interpretation, which argues that they are intertwined.

Chamberlain (2000) cautions that some qualitative research reports resort to exactly what quantitative researchers do; listing off headings and failing to convey the experience adequately to the reader. She further argues that interpretation of the data is much more useful than mere description as the researcher tries to connect the themes and account for their interrelationships (Chamberlain 2000). Nevertheless, a useful description of what the character of a theme should convey is suggested by van Manen (1990) as the experience of focus, of meaning, of point, that is not an object encountered at certain points in a text. It is also the form that captures the phenomenon one is trying to understand and, at best, a simplification.

My analysis and interpretation of the data evolved to reflect a reflexive interpretative methodology, where listening to the text is considered the core of interpretation (Frank 2006). The view of Alvesson and Skoldberg (2000) was most helpful in this process. They propose four aspects in relation to interpretation in hermeneutic research. The first is termed the 'pattern of interpretation', which, they argue, should be internally consistent, but also externally consistent with other interpretations in the same field. The pattern is developed by the researcher engaging in "dialogue with the text" (Alvesson and Skoldberg, p. 61). This dialogue begins with the interpreter's preconceptions which undergo transformation during the process. The pattern should ultimately reveal "a deeper understanding of the text, beyond what is immediately bestowed by reading above the common-sense level" (Alvesson and Skoldberg 2000, p. 61). Within this process, I adopted the view of van Manen (1990) who argues that "Phenomenological analysis can be understood as the *structures of experience*" (van Manen 1990, p.79). He asserts that the first task in illuminating the 'structures of experience' is to transcribe the interview data verbatim. Following this, an elective or highlighting approach was adopted, which involves reading the text several times and asking: "What statement(s) or phrase(s) seem particularly essential or revealing about the phenomenon or experience being described?" (van Manen, 1990, p.92).

However, despite the direction on reflexive interpretation provided by Alvesson and Skoldberg (2000) discussed above, the need to also be guided by a structured approach to data analysis was viewed essential. Moreover, the discussion earlier regarding the reluctance of hermeneutic phenomenology to focus on specific steps in the analysis process has not prevented the development of many methods of data analysis for phenomenological studies that can be followed in a systematic fashion (van Kaam 1969, Colaizzi 1978, Hycner 1985, van Manen 1990, Moustakas 1994). Two common features are evident in these approaches, these being, the division of the text into units, knitting together of meanings to reveal a general description of the experience, and all aspects of the text considered initially of equal value (Priest 2002).

Of all the data analysis frameworks reviewed, van Manen's (1990) and Colaizzi's (1978) were chosen to guide the process of uncovering themes from the study narratives. This decision was made because van Manen's activities of data analysis proposes describing the phenomenon through the art of writing and re-writing, as was adopted in this study.

Moreover, his activities for analysis adopts a fusion of the objectivist hermeneutic circle (part-whole) and the alethic hermeneutic circle (pre-understanding- understanding) as they acknowledge the experience of a phenomenon in a whole experience and also the researcher's role in the research process (Dowling 2007).

However, an explicit framework was required to reach the phase of describing the phenomenon, therefore, Colaizzi's procedural steps provided direction for this aspect of the process of analysis. This combination of van Manen's work with others in the field of phenomenology is not unusual. For instance, Jongudomkarn and West (2004) utilise Colaizzi's and van Manen's work in their phenomenological study. Moreover, others have utilised van Manen's phenomenology with Benner's paradigm cases (Fielden 2003, Hassouneh-Phillips 2003).

Utilising Colaizzi's procedural steps, eleven cluster themes in total were developed, as follows:

- First meeting
- Identification and empathy
- Patient characteristics
- Nurses' technical skills
- Reciprocity in self-disclosure
- Professional friend
- Homely atmosphere
- Satisfaction for the nurse
- Emotional effects of intimacy
- Peer support
- Patient comfort in feeling known

Exemplars were then identified from each coded cluster theme, which are defined as "bits of textual data in the language of the informant that capture essential meanings of themes" (Cohen, Kahn and Steeves 2000, p. 80).

An exhaustive description of the phenomenon of nurse-patient intimacy was then formulated, based upon the eleven theme clusters. The activity of writing and re-writing revealed a process of nurse-patient intimacy, with cluster themes being grouped into three main themes, as follows:

Theme 1: Developing intimacy	First meeting
	Identification and empathy
	Patient characteristics
	Nurses' technical skills
Theme 2: Experiencing intimacy	Reciprocity in self-disclosure
	Professional friend
	Homely atmosphere
Theme 3: Outcome of intimacy	Satisfaction for the nurse
	Emotional effects of intimacy
	Peer support
	Patient comfort in feeling known

A statement of the fundamental structure of nurse-patient intimacy was developed, revealing its process to involve three phases: developing intimacy, experiencing intimacy and the outcome of intimacy.

The final validating step was achieved by returning to each nurse participant and asking them about the phenomenon revealed in the first interview. This step was not achieved with the patient participants due to deterioration and changes in their condition. Not all phenomenological research adopts this final step (e.g., Miller 2003), which illustrates why Colaizzi's (1978) method is suitable for studies which employ a phenomenological method (e.g. Scannell-Desch 2005), and for those similar to this study, which are interpretive in orientation (Hodges, Keeley and Grier 2001, Fleming, Gaidys and Robb 2003, Perreault, Fothergill-Bourbannais and Fiset 2004).

Management of the large volume of interview transcripts accumulated during the ten months of interviewing was helped by the utilisation of the qualitative package, ATLAS. Ti. ATLAS.ti is an example of a code-based theory builder (Lindlof and Taylor 2002), which does not build theory but supports the researchers theory-building efforts (Weitzman 2000). Many qualitative research observers raise concerns that such programs contain implicit theories of analysis that direct the researcher's thinking and may decontextualise the coding process (Lindlof and Taylor 2002). However, such a package cannot automatically result in interpretation of the text (Muhr 2004). Its strength lies in its ability to store the inputted memos and creation of codes, and offer transparency in how the analysis process proceeded.

In keeping with the art of writing in the phenomenological tradition, the study findings are presenting in interconnecting themes using a fictive narrative approach (Steeves 2000a) to assist in maintaining context.

A fictive narrative approach is a form of case study, discussed by Steeves (2000a), as an appropriate format for the presentation of data in a hermeneutic phenomenological research study, as it is closely related to the notion of narrative. However, the fictive narrative approach is different from the narrative itself so the findings need to be presented in an understandable format to the reader (Steeves 2000a). This approach has been adopted in the presentation of nurses' and patients' narratives. In the case of nurses' narratives, it is represented in mingling narratives from the first and second interviews together to assist in making the narrative as understandable as possible for the reader. A fictive narrative approach is less evident in the patient narratives as repeat interviewing did not occur.

Although not labelling their approach 'fictive narrative', Jones and Borbasi (2004) write about the "woven text", which appears similar to the fictive narrative discussed above (p. 94). Moreover, Watson (2000) describes a style of writing termed "ethnographic fiction science" which is further described as "research writing", and supports the view that such a writing style is appropriate given the researcher's close involvement in their research and the need to shape their data (p. 89). This ethnographic fiction bridges the two genres of social science and creative writing and engages the reader in the way that creative fiction does (Watson 2000). Moreover, Geelen and Taylor (2001) employ what they term the literary/ethnographic methods of impressionistic tales (proposed by John van Mannen) to illuminate the mood and reveal the researcher's methodological brushstrokes. These views reflect the qualitative researcher as *bricoleur* mentioned earlier: "The product of the *bricoleur's* labour is a bricolage, a complex, dense, reflexive, collage-like creation that represents the researcher's images, understandings, and interpretations of the world or phenomenon under analysis. This bricolage will connect the parts to the whole, stressing the meaningful relationships that operate in the situations and social worlds studied" (Denzin and Lincoln 1994, p. 3).

What is, presented therefore, is a dialogue of an "intersection" (Koch 1998, p.1189) of the horizon of the study participants, along with my interpretation of their narratives.

Developing Intimacy

First Meeting

The first meeting is best described as an encounter that sows the seeds for the relationship to follow. The principle focus on this first encounter between the oncology nurse and oncology patient is patient education aimed to enhance his/her self-care for the long treatment journey ahead. However, an underlying focus of this first meeting is also the nurse's assessment of the patient's reaction to his/her cancer diagnosis as this influences how much or how little the nurse will reveal to the patient during this first meeting.

Moreover, it is vital to remember that when the oncology nurse and oncology patient meet for this first time, it is a time of great stress for patients. They have been either diagnosed recently with cancer, or diagnosed with a recurrence of their disease and their personal calendar (their plans, hopes and dreams) has been abruptly interrupted. Furthermore, this first meeting can also be stressful for some nurses, especially if they are new to the oncology setting.

The nurses interviewed viewed this first meeting as essential to subsequent interactions with the patient, as illustrated in their comments below. The narrative to follow strongly suggests that the seeds of intimacy between oncology nurses and their patients is cultivated at this first encounter.

Nurse 4 "I think a lot of it stems from when we do the education sessions at the start, when you meet them for the first time, before they start the chemo, and we educate them, and it can take up to an hour to do the education, but you get to chat a lot as well during it, and I think you're definitely a lot closer to those patients, that they know you a lot better, and you know them more than some of the other staff, and you'll find then, when they come into the unit, or if they ring up even, they might specifically ask for me, and I think then that it's built on that then, that they know if they ask about something, that you'll tell them honestly".

Nurse 17 "That first meeting is probably the one where you'd probably spend the most time with patients… and you could spend an hour, you could spend two hours, you could spend three hours maybe with them……you would definitely form the beginning of a like a good relationship with them, and it's at the meeting really that …it depends from that meeting really how you get on with them from there on. It's like first impressions and all that, and how they …like if they get a good feeling for you, which is the most important thing really. You really have to sort of build up an element of trust, and if you don't get it at that first meeting, you're not going to get it".

Although the focus of this first meeting is the provision of information, the nurse and patient appraise each other and this sets the tone for future interactions. The patient's role in how the relationship develops, following the first encounter, is also significant. This is evident in the nurses' expressions of patients' personal characteristics in their narratives. Patient characteristics, therefore, also contribute significantly to how the nurse responds, and many nurses talked about 'clicking' with some patients, and not 'clicking' with others. This emergence of 'clicking' with certain patients is evident in the following narratives. The views expressed suggest a spontaneous and intuitive response by nurses, to patients.

Nurse 7 "She's [patient] a very interesting woman to talk to. I suppose ….one of the first encounters I had with her, I nearly spent two hours talking to her, where she had a very interesting background…"

Nurse 4 "You kind of click with some patients a bit more than others. So you get on better with some patients more than you do with others, who would be very open".

Nurse 3 "I think you get into an ease with the person and you can tell if you have a relationship with them…you might have met this person on the first day, and you do bond…"

Nurse 9 "You either click with somebody or you don't. That's what I would find. …it wouldn't really matter whether they were ill or not. If you click with them, you click with them, and it does make things easier…"

The first meeting between the oncology nurse and their patient, therefore, is critical to how their relationship develops. Another crucial process which unfolds during the first meeting, is that of identification. This process begins with a mutual search for something in common, and must occur in order for the encounter to develop into one that has the potential to foster an intimate relationship.

Identification and Empathy

The term, 'identification', in this context, is the process revealed in the nurses' narratives, whereby the nurse identifies something in the patient that triggers the encounter to move to another level, prompting empathy on the part of the nurse. The empathic response, in turn, propels the nurse's caring response and the intensity of the encounter, and subsequent intimacy.

The nurses' narratives reveal the association between the 'clicking' outlined earlier, and the actual identification. The 'clicking' referred to earlier seals this identification process. This is evident in the following two nurses' narratives, where the use of the terms 'clicking' and 'identify with' are used.

> Nurse 4 "...there was a girl in recently and I kind of clicked with her as she's the same age as myself, has young kids as well... I think you'll always meet up with some patients that are you'll click with, and a lot of the time it's probably similar lifestyles to yourself".

> Nurse 15 "I suppose it's human relations really that...just...I suppose there are just patients that you just click with, and there's ...I feel myself I'm pretty much not bad at clicking with a large number of patients, but there's always people that you will really identify with, I guess some of it must be identification, you know...you're identifying...".

> Nurse 22 "I suppose there are people I get a bond with because I suppose I have kids, and I suppose I just feel that if I was in the same situation, how I'd cope".

Identification, therefore, is a critical antecedent to nurse-patient intimacy. When nurses identify something in common with the patient, an accelerated empathic response follows which results in the development of intimacy. Similarly, for some patients interviewed, there was something about the nurse that prompted them to engage or not with them. This is apparent in the following narrative.

> Pt 10 "...from the very day I met her [Nurse 7], back...straight away I knew that she was somebody I could talk to. And I knew she'd be honest with me from day one. There was no beating about the bush, like, you know? She would be honest. If I asked a straight question, I got a straight answer. And I feel I could talk to her about anything, you know? Apart from illness, personal things, if I needed to".

Subsequent to the process of identification, is the emergence of nurses' empathy for patients, which subsequently fuels nurses' experience of intimacy. Nurses described empathy for the patient as a feeling of being at their 'level' and an awareness of how they are feeling. Suggestions of 'clicking' and identification and also evident in the following nurse's narrative.

Nurse 2 "Well I think you have to be at the one level with them. That you're not thinking, not a step above that you're like you're talking with them, you know as if you were. Like empathy maybe like you were...as if picture yourself in their shoes. How you'd like to be treated... I think that would go a long way".

The Process of Empathy

The study narratives reveal that the first nurse-patient encounter begins a process of identification by the nurse that results in empathy for the patient. Similarly, Crigger (2001) reports that student nurses in her qualitative study identified "similarities between themselves and the client"(p. 619), which was categorised as an antecedent to what Noddings (1984) terms 'engrossment'. Moreover, identification is also a feature of nurses' "special relationships with [cancer] patients" in a study of psychosocial care reported by Roberts and Snowball (1999).

Identification is described as, "to involve a growing sensitivity to the 'movement' within" another person (Smyth 1996, p. 935), and is highlighted as a characteristic of empathy (Rogers 1975, Rawnsley 1980, Smyth 1996). In a similar vein, Scott (1995) discusses empathy in the context of constructive caring as imaginatively identifying with the patient that requires working of the imagination, "which are unbounded by rules or laws, because beginning with preconceptions is likely to be damaging" (p. 1199). This view bears a resemblance to the work of Scheler (1874-1928) (1992) on identification. In an analysis of the writings of Scheler, Campbell (1984) discusses empathy and identification in the context of caring in the helping professions. Scheler (1992) describes emotional identification as an "infection" to illustrate its limiting capacity and argues that identification is something that is not rational or deliberate but a letting-go of self, and childlike in nature (p. 50). The reference to childlike is important to this discussion. The nurse's empathy for the patient must be naïve in nature so that the patient is viewed as a unique being and his/her experience of illness is also viewed as unique to them. Moreover, this view would suggest that identification fits with the description of the 'lifeworld' *(Lebenswelt)* proposed by Husserl (1970). The 'lifeworld', is one where individuals experience pre-reflexively, without resorting to interpretations.

The work of phenomenologist Edith Stein contributes a pertinent perspective to a discussion of this study's findings. Stein's conceptualisation of empathy, *Einfuhlung,* is a radical one based on recognising a lived experience, occurring on three levels. Moreover, her view of empathy seems 'active' in contrast to that of another phenomenologist, Emmanuel Levinas (1905-1995), in that Stein (1917/1970), suggests that I go out of myself and encounter the other, through "the emergence of the experience" (p. 11), whereas Levinas suggests that the other initiates the relationship. Moran (2000), on Levinas, describes this as "the other presents him-or herself to me. I am called on to respond to that claim" (p. 348). Stein's conceptualisation of empathy is, therefore, useful in explaining the empathy explicated in this study. Moreover, the differentiation between her view of empathy and that of Levinas could be compared to the difference between Kohlberg and Gilligan on moral decision-making.

Stein's (1917/1970) three "grades or modalities" in the "accomplishment" of empathy are "(p. 1) the emergence of the experience, (2) the fulfilling explication, and (3) the comprehensive objectification of the explained experience" (p. 11). Davis (2003) uses the term 'level' to describe these grades and explains that level 1 is a cognitive process whereby there is an attempt to enter into another's feelings and to put ourselves in their place. This first level of empathy requires the ability to use imagination and reflects the art of empathy (Davis 2003). By reading the facial expressions or other signals, we attempt to obtain an idea of the person's emotional and mental state. This represents a determined aspiration to enter into the feelings of another and an attempt to position ourselves in another's place (Davis 1990). Stein (1917/1970), describes this as, "When it [empathy] arises before me all at once, it faces me as an object (such as the sadness I "read in another's face"), but when I enquire into its implied tendencies (try to bring another's mood to clear givenness to myself), the content, having pulled me into it, is no longer really an object" (p. 10). Davis (2003) uses the term *self-transposal*, one proposed by Spiegelberg (1982), to describe this first level. This description is also similar to that of caring by Noddings (1984) who argues that "all caring involves engrossment" (p. 17) which results in the carer investing full attention in the one being cared for and is characterised by a "move away from the self" (p. 16), and suggests the primacy of ethical comportment in relationships with the other.

Level 2 is one that follows closely after the first and is a gut feeling of identification following a shift from intellect to emotion. Davis (2003) calls this second phase a "crossing over" (p. 269) , a term derived from the work of Buber (1955/2002). Level 2 involves an attempt to clarify the person's emotional state and a sudden feeling of being in the person's place (Davis 1990). The empathiser feels that s/he is identifying with the other, but it occurs as "a parallel experience" (Maatta 2006, p.6). This second level moves from one of intellect to emotional understanding and a deeper awareness of the other. The connection with the other is experienced so earnestly that identification results and "for that moment it is as if they are one" (Maatta 2006, p. 6). This second phase appears similar to the view of Noddings' (1984), on engrossment mentioned earlier. Noddings (1984) considers the term "engrossment" is more suitable than "empathy" in ethical caring (p. 30). Rather than "put myself in the others shoes", Noddings argues that engrossment means, "I set aside my temptation to analyse and to plan. I do not project; I receive the other into myself, and I see and feel with the other. I become duality" (p. 30). Similarly, descriptions of mutuality concur with this second level of empathy, since it requires empathy and "is characterised by the interpretation of the experience of self with other" (Gaydos 2003, p. 41).

The final stage is a movement described as a "reaching out to the other" in an effort to reinforce the reality that this was happening to the other person and not themselves, resolving into "a deep fellow feeling for the other person, or sympathy" (Davis 2003, p. 269). Level three, a form of self-recovery, is represented by a cessation of this feeling of affinity and the empathiser becomes themselves again. "Sympathizing with the sense of affinity that just arose, we stand side by side with the person again" (Maatta 2006, p. 6). Nurse theorist, Joyce Travelbee (1971) also views sympathy as "a step beyond empathy" (p. 141). However, Travelbee considers sympathy as active in orientation, with a "*desire to alleviate distress, absent in empathy*" (Travelbee's emphasis, p.142), as opposed to the "neutral process" of empathy (Travelbee 1971, p.143).

Travelbee (1971) also suggests a similar process in her view of nursing as a process. She describes the first phase of the process of nursing as the original encounter, following which the phases of emerging identities, empathy, sympathy and rapport result. Travelbee (1971) too, like Stein, differentiates between identification and empathy. She describes identification as: "an unconscious process and a mental mechanism wherein an individual strives to be like another…it is an unconscious imitation process" (Travelbee 1971, p.132), and argues that the person is unaware of identification when it occurs. However, she differs from Stein in her assertion that "empathy is a conscious process. One knows, if, and when, empathy is occurring" (Travelbee 1971, p.137). Nevertheless, as illustrated above, Travelbee (1971) similar to Stein (1917/1970) suggests that empathy is an antecedent to sympathy, and "the sympathetic person takes action to relieve the distress of another" (p.144). Travelbee's view of empathy is, therefore, curiously similar in orientation to that of Stein. However it is not evident if her work has been influenced by the writings of Stein, since she makes no explicit reference to such influence in her book (Travelbee 1971).

The nurses in this study vividly described their emotions for patients they felt close to. Acknowledging emotions is, therefore, necessary in order to allow the empathic processes to proceed. Others, too, describe emotions in the identification stage of the empathic process. One of the nurses in a study by Henderson (2001) talked about identification and how the patient's characteristics promotes this: "*So I think it's a characteristic that somehow touches you, and whether it comes from within you or reminds you of someone else, that you care about, that's probably where a lot of it comes from*" (Henderson 2001, p. 134). The symbiotic nature of identification is related eloquently by another study respondent reported by Henderson: "*That sort of dancing between you and the patient or client where you're feeding off each other and it's backwards and forwards and you're picking up the cues from each other. You know it's real, almost like a tango or something, you learn each other's moves- that can't occur* [if you're not emotionally engaged]" (Henderson 2001, 134). Moreover, she reports that nurses' responses to specific patients are possibly mediated by previous personal or professional experiences (Henderson 2001). This can be explained by the words of Stein (1917/1970) who describes "reflexive sympathy" as one "where my original experience returns to me as an empathized one" (p. 18).

It is also reported how student nurses described, in their journals of clinical practice experience, that "the act of identifying and empathizing with patients appeared natural and immediate" (Lemonidou et al., 2004, p. 125), and that the students' "thoughts and actions were driven by their emotions and by compassion" (Lemonidou et al., 2004, p. 131). This further suggests the role of emotions in mobilising moral action in nurse caring. Moreover, it also suggests the impulsiveness of empathy, and its ability to 'just happen'. The work of Scheler (1992) on identification supports this notion. He argues that irrespective of the type of identification, it is "always automatic, never a choice or of mechanical association" (p. 66). Moreover, the "unconscious dimensions" of identification influence the development of interactions with others "beyond our conscious awareness" (Bondi 2003, p. 68). This impulsive emotion, therefore, seems vital to caring endeavours. The interviews with nurses in my study suggests that a passion for caring endures over many years of nursing and the satisfaction from caring fuels nurses' caring actions. Emotions and empathy, therefore, play a reciprocal role in caring in nursing.

Returning to the description of 'clicking' with patients described by nurses in my study, Stein's theory argues that empathy is given "after the fact" in that it cannot be made happen but "catches us in its process" (White 1997, p.254). This is termed the "Z factor, an unspecified relational quality" (van Manen 2002, p.279) that cannot be described. This could explain the use of the term 'clicking' by many participants in this study. Moreover, "clicking" was also used by patients in a study reported by Fostbinder (1994, p. 1088) to describe the process of getting to know nurses. The word 'click' also means to 'be on the same wavelength', which suggests an identification. Furthermore, it is a word which suggests something instantaneous and something that 'just happens'. Moreover, the antecedents of intimacy occur by chance (Kadner 1994).

Patient Characteristics in the Development of Nurse-Patient Intimacy

The patient's personal characteristics trigger the nurse's response to them. Most of the nurses interviewed expressed their admiration for patients who displayed a positive outlook regarding their illness and its treatment, and were attracted to engage with such patients.

Most of the patients referred to by the nurses interviewed, were considered positive and optimistic in their approach to their illness and its treatment. Moreover, my interviews with patients reflect the optimism generally communicated by cancer patients.

When patients were optimistic and hopeful in outlook, nurses reciprocated with similar sentiments of optimism, and some patients commented on this. The narratives from Patients 4, 12 and 21 below, suggest the value patients place on the optimism displayed by nurses.

> Pt 21 "...if you had any worries like that, they [nurses] always were optimistic, which I found extremely important. To have hope, and I found that extremely important that they would boost your confidence as much as possible. Now, I know they can't make false claims or whatever, but just to hear one word of optimism, or you know that you're going to make it, or something that would boost... I found that important to me...".

> Pt 12 "She [Nurse 16] said 'I'm going to help you, I'm going to give you the confidence. Whether it's true or not, at the end of the day the treatment is going to work for you, and that you're going to come through this'. And as far as possible, I felt that they did that, without making false claims at the same time".

> Pt 4 "I remember, I sat up the morning I came in and I said '*** [Nurse 3], will it work?'. 'It will work' she said. ' I feel it in my bones' she said, 'It's going to work' [laughs]. That meant an awful lot. You know".

Similar to nurses' views of most oncology patients being optimistic in outlook, most nurses interviewed also talked about patients' fighting spirit. This admiration for patients is also evident in the following nurses' narratives:

> Nurse 5 "Our patients are lovely really, I don't know what it is, but since I've started in Oncology, I have to say that they give me strength as well, because they are so brave, and so strong, and very positive, and it works both ways. But, in general, generally the patients, I really have to say I admire them, they are really, really, really strong..., I think they are just brilliant. They just cope very, very well and get on with their lives, and are very, very sensible about it all, and I just find that very admirable, and I would hope if I was ever diagnosed, that I would have the same strength to cope".

Nurse 7 "A good 80% of the people I meet just have a great outlook on it. You know, they seem to be in control, or able to manage their family life, their personal life, their treatment part of it, and the whole lot in such a way that a good bit of the time, it doesn't affect what goes on for them outside the hospital walls... I mean coping-wise I suppose, I would find that they're very easy .....you know, that they cope well, a lot of them, and I don't know how you'd describe it really ....to me, they'd be special, and I can't describe that ...".

Nurse 18 "...These people are just amazing, they're just brilliant, and these people would take any treatment available, anything! If you told them to drink the patient's beside them blood, it will make you better, they'd do it, because they are just so eager, and they just want to live, and I just find that amazing".

Nurse 16 "I've one woman who's terminal and like ...but she's just so positive, and that's her frame of mind, and anything she can do, and anything to help another person, she does it, and I suppose I admire her for that".

The narratives described above, clearly suggest that the patient's personal characteristics influence the nurse's response to them. It is evident from the nurses interviewed, that they are drawn toward patients who are optimistic in outlook. However, patients displaying what nurses perceive as a negative outlook are described as difficult to develop intimate relationships with. The difficulties nurses experience in forming relationships with such patients are displayed in the following narratives, which suggest various emotions experienced by nurses in their interactions with these patients.

Nurse 10 "I find it frustrating if a patient won't, won't open up or won't..., puts a barrier against us..."

Nurse 1 "You mightn't ask the questions or you mightn't kind of be, leave yourself open to get into a kind of a two-way long heavy conversation with them, you know , when they'd be kinda looking at things in a negative way. ...Well I suppose you learn, I suppose you learn to side-step too".

Nurse 3 "We had a patient, a woman that had a very; I don't mean a poor outlook now, really kind of 'took to the bed' kind of attitude and that was... I actually find; I find it a little bit difficult to deal with people...It was **so** hard to communicate with her".

Evident in the narratives just described, is the influence of the perceived patient's negativity on the nurse's response to them. Similarly, patients who assume a detached position are also described by the nurses interviewed, as difficult to engage with. Moreover, some nurses interviewed expressed their frustration with such patients as they often experience adverse effects of treatment through not communicating their response to treatment with nurses. This frustration was expressed by Nurse 1, who described how a "bad relationship" results when a patient does not "tell you how they are actually feeling, how they are coping with chemotherapy and if they are having any adverse reactions". Nurse 14 also expresses her difficulty in nursing patients she describes as "depressed", below.

Nurse 14 "I find I get nervous if you're asking questions and somebody's just looking at you, and you're getting through to nothing at all. That makes me very nervous...To be honest, I find people that are very depressed and *don't* want to be helped, I find that very hard. Or somebody who might have problems but won't tell you about them. And then a few days later you're dragging things out, and then they'll tell you. And they're going "But I've had that for weeks"...I find it very hard".

Similarly, other nurses' narratives suggest the detached patient as one who 'shuts down' and just wants to get through their treatment journey in a position of denial.

> Nurse 2 "You know if they're listening or if they're not hearing anything. Sometimes they've just shut off and they don't want to know anything".

> Nurse 5 "He just likes to get in here, get his treatment on time, and he's very particular about... he knows what his treatment involves, and it's a very, very complicated treatment, and he knows when he's having this, and when it finishes, and really he just wants to get on with it, and move on, and move out".

> Nurse 8 "They shut down. They put up this wall against you, and they just don't want to let you in, and you don't want to push yourself on them...So you have to walk away, you have to...".

Despite the majority of nurses interviewed expressing difficulties in their relationships with patients perceived as negative or depressed, some nurses relayed an acceptance of patients described as detached. Interestingly, all these nurses worked in the same unit.

Role of Patient Characteristics in the Development of Nurse-Patient Intimacy

Returning to the view of Stein, an emotional response to the patient must first occur for the three levels of empathy to evolve. My study has revealed that a patient's personal characteristics either facilitates or hinders this emotional response. The findings reported by Shattell (2005) provide some interesting evidence to support such a conclusion. Shattell (2005) reports that patients are aware of how their response to the nurse affects the response they receive. One patient offered the following view:

> "As a patient...your attitude can affect the attitude of the people that are giving you care. If you are grumpy, maybe they won't try to be extra chatty with you because they know you're not going to chat back. But if you're showing them that hey, I'm interested in what you're saying, then maybe they'll be a little more chatty with you, or not even saying that they wouldn't be helpful with people that aren't as friendly, but maybe they were checking in a little bit more because they felt like, hey you know, she's a nice person, let's just see how she's doing while I'm walking past the door...If you come across nice, friendly, then people will be more likely to be that way to you" (29-year-old woman) (p. 215). This comment also suggests the perceived power relations between nurses and patients, where, for the patient, "negotiation is in pursuit of the service they require" (Johnson 1997, p. 110).

Baillie (1996) also reports from her phenomenological study with surgical nurses that empathic feelings are difficult for nurses to generate when the patient is difficult to know or communicate with, or displays lack of trust. Moreover, the nurses revealed that some patients may not want the nurse to get to know them, which results in difficulty for the empathic response for the nurse (Baillie 1996). Yegdich (1999) argues that this finding suggests that the "patient must do something for nurses" if they themselves are to be empathised, and that patients "need to empathise with nurses" (p. 89). Patients clearly play a key role in the development of a therapeutic relationship with nurses. Similar to the experience of nurses I interviewed, Aranda and Street (1999) cite the experience of a nurse Jane, who believed her relationship with a patient was "ineffective and nontherapeutic because it was not the kind of helping relationship she valued" (p. 81). The patient actively refused to be a "good patient" because her attitude was: "just do it [treatment] and don't talk to me" (Aranda and Street 1999, p. 81).

Most of the nurses I interviewed passionately expressed their admiration for patients who were positive in outlook. These positive patients were possibly perceived as more hopeful than others, and nurses, subsequently more readily approached closer relationships with such patients. Conversely, patients described as difficult to get to know are less likely to develop close relationships with nurses. It is highly suggestive, therefore, that patients' characteristics have a major impact on the nature of the nurse-patient relationship. Aranda and Street (2001), who, in the process of group narratives with nurses, reveal that nurses explore their choices to engage with patients as not simply a personal one, but also as influenced by the patient.

Roth (1972), a sociologist and a tuberculosis patient, coined the term 'negotiating social worth' for the process of social labelling. Shattell (2005) concludes that this theory explains the process patients' engaged in (being nice and friendly to nurses) as they were aware of the difference between 'good' and 'bad' patients. Shattell (2005) therefore asserts that patients are active participants in the building of nurse-patient relationships and use these relationships to build their power.

Being Positive and Showing Optimism

Being positive and showing optimism seemed paramount to the both patients and nurses I interviewed. Such expressions suggest that hopefulness and being positive are strongly connected. Other studies report similar findings. Nurses have been found to equate cancer patients' hope and acceptance as being positive (O'Baugh et al., 2003). In addition, McIlfatrick (2003) reports that many of the oncology patients in her study commented on their need to maintain a positive attitude towards treatment and the future, and that this behaviour was encouraged and endorsed by health care professionals.

The findings from my study suggest that most oncology nurses enjoy intimacy with patients who are positive, hopeful, and benefit from the use of humour in their interactions. This finding is supported elsewhere, where the characteristics of the patient is viewed as a promoting factor in the building of the nurse-patient relationship. For instance, Baer and Lowery (1987) report that student nurses liked best to care for cheerful and communicative patients who were accepting of their illness and the nursing care offered, and they conclude, therefore, that the characteristics of patient communication are essential variables in the nurse-patient relationship. Fosbinder (1994), also, agrees, arguing that the patient's interpersonal competence has an important influence on nurse-patient communication. Moreover, the findings of Allan (2001) also suggest that intimate nurse-patient relationships occur because of patient action rather than being initiated by the nurse. The findings from my study, therefore, confirm the view of Pettegrew and Turkat, (1986) who argue that "patients may have a far greater impact on and responsibility to the health-care relationship" than often revealed in research (p. 391).

The positive and accepting attitude displayed by most cancer patients to their illness could be explained by the view of Jarrett and Payne (2000) who argue that the cancer patient engages in "self comparison" which results in him/her feeling luckier than other cancer patients and, therefore, viewing his/her own situation is a more optimistic way (p. 85). They subsequently conclude that this process contributes to the positive façade that is part of the cancer patient role (Jarrett and Payne, 2000). However, others question if this positive approach is the best choice for all persons with cancer, which may be a huge burden for patients to bear (de Raeve 1997, Rittenberg 1995). Wilkinson and Kitzinger (2000) argue that people say they are positive in order to fit in with what is socially acceptable. This is not surprising, since cancer patients often equate hopelessness as a negative attitude (Wilkes, O'Baugh and Luke 2003).

Jarrett and Payne (2000) suggest that a "positive façade is probably part of the role of the 'cancer patient'" (p. 85). Moreover, O'Baugh et al., (2003) argues that nurses' perceptions of 'being positive' could be interpreted as being very demanding on patients, as it expects patients to be happy, fight their cancer and be compliant with treatment. Being compliant with treatment fits with the process of what Johnson (1997) describes as "acquiescing" or "going along with the wishes of others in the context of social labelling" (p. 176). Patients may fear to appear negative for fear of rejection by staff, and this may especially be the case if the staff find taking care of the positive patient easier (Gray and Doan, 1990). However, the potential consequences of such a positive stance results in the denial of the person's negative feelings, and health care professionals should consider more fully the potential implications of endorsing positive thinking (de Raeve, 1997).

Moreover, Schou and Hewision (1999) report that patients feel they need to be seen to be "bearing up well" (p. 151). "The illness and treatment calendars seemed to call forth a public display of 'coping well' from many patients…to be uncomplaining, to be grateful, to *show* gratitude, and to reward the attentions of others with bravery and an 'upbeat' presentation of oneself in daily contacts with community members and close others. …"(Schou and Hewison 1999, 151). Schou and Hewison (1999) further argue that the cancer experience in illness and treatment is both public and private, in which the patient is constantly "under surveillance" and which demands justification by both patients and professionals of resources used (p. 152).

The interview text has revealed that some patients choose to remain detached from the nurses' attempts to get to know them. Schou and Hewison (1999) highlight that the patient who does not "cope" well is described as "deviant" by some psycho oncology literature and this "deviance" is a failure to "cope" well, arising from personality characteristics of the patient" (p. 157). The interview text also suggests that some cancer patients who assume a detached stance appear to not want an intimate relationship with nurses. Rather, their relationship falls into the category of clinical, as defined by Morse (1991). Empathic feelings are difficult to generate when the patient is difficult to know or to communicate with (Yegdich 1999). Perhaps such patients are overwhelmed by their illness and its treatment due to a sense of hopelessness, and withdrawal is their coping response. Withdrawal may be due to their illness experience, for instance, the loss of control over their lives may result in their inability to relate to the nurse (Morse 1991). Moreover, feelings of detachment are a symptom evident in post-traumatic stress disorder, now acknowledged to be also caused by a diagnosis of cancer (Furlong and O'Toole 2006).

This distancing or avoidance can make demoralisation worse for the patient (Clarke and Kissane 2002). However, in an attempt to explain nurses' reactions to such patients, O'Baugh et al. (2003) conclude that nurses may not feel competent in dealing with patients who do not display a positive outlook. However, Morse (1991) argues that if a nurse "perseveres with helping a difficult patient", the patient may gain insight about their illness and decide to trust the nurse (p. 463). Campbell (1984) further argues that the "unpopular" patient presents the greatest challenge to nursing, and companionship means "staying with the 'difficult' person, at least for a time" (p. 50). This companionship was evident in the relationships recounted by some of the nurses interviewed, particularly in the narratives of Nurses 15, 16 and 18.

Nurses' Technical Skills

Another theme identified in the development of nurse-patient intimacy, is the patient's appraisal of the oncology nurse's technical skills. Nurses' technical skills was alluded to by both nurses and patients interviewed as a contributing factor to the success of their relationship. When the patient trusted the nurse's competence with regard to their technical skills, they wanted that nurse to care for them. Some patients alluded to their appraisal of nurses' technical ability.

> Pt 3 "There's one particular nurse in oncology, one particular girl I would have great time for, in oncology. She's not actually one of the more senior ones…Just even when I was going in for the chemo. I just liked to see her come to put in the needle. She just seemed to have a better you know".

The possibility of patients becoming reliant on a particular nurse is evident in the following narrative.

> Pt 13 "Well I suppose the ones that found it easier to put the needle in my arm were the ones that I [laughs] identified with. And now, em, I suppose, they now realise they get *** the phlebotomist to come up and do me so obviously I'm not an easy candidate…I mean, I suppose the best was *** [Nurse]. I would look for *** to be here, but unfortunately [laughs], my skin and ***, eventfully as time went on and he was excellent. And I would love to see *** here and that's I mean, you know you kinda do worry".

Patient 5 singled out the skills of Nurse 3 and talked enthusiastically to me about her patience in approaching venous access.

> Pt 5 "You have all those little fears, and you know, what's it going to be like, and first of all, we always had a problem of getting blood, we always had a problem, and indeed, some of the doctors just gave up on me, they just couldn't get it. But, one particular nurse, *** [Nurse 3], she's absolutely brilliant, she just takes her time, and there's no rush or hurry, if she has to give ten minutes or fifteen minutes getting the tube in, she just sits there, and waits until she gets the vein, so I have no problem. So, that to me, was a huge bonus for me… that was very

important, because I had been...in most places, they'd all given up on my veins, but this particular lady, ***[Nurse 3], she's absolutely brilliant, just the time she spends just getting the vein for me..."

Interestingly, during my first interview with Nurse 3, she identified Patient 5 as a patient she had a close relationship with. This closeness, according to Nurse 3, was helped by the "comfortable" nature of their relationship, as a consequence of this patient's confidence in her technical skills.

> Nurse 3 "I find it that, for example, now ***[Patient 5], I'm comfortable with *** and I know she's comfortable with me because she'd say to me, and I know she actually means it, because I think it actually stems from what I actually said about the cannula, because that's a big thing for *** [Patient 5] , and I know...whether, it's just that I spend more time or something...I don't know. When she came in first, I spent ages for looking for veins. .... she had problems, and people had given up on her...she was really stressed about it the first day she came in, so I just said 'Right, I'm going to sit here now', and I must have been at it 20 minutes, half an hour, and I just said 'Now, you have three', I found three, so I'm only going to need one today, and then got it the first time, and I think that's what's...that day she suddenly, you know...so, each time she's come in, I've actually dealt with her an awful lot, I've dealt with her most days".

Similar to the view of Nurse 3 above, other nurses I interviewed also acknowledged that patients considered nurses' technical kills important to the development of their relationship with them. These nurses suggested in their narratives that some patients became "hooked" on nurses who could cannulate competently. This is evident in the views below.

> Nurse 4 "...some patients then I think, when someone cannulates them, and gets first time, they just think, probably in their mind 'I must look for her again, she did it ...' 'she had no problem getting it the last time', so they definitely would look for different people to cannulate them, or...and then I think when you have a bad experience with some patient, you are reluctant to go back to them".

> Nurse 3 "...there's always some patient that will just feel like I want so and so to do me now because she always gets me whereas I don't want that one coming near me now because she doesn't. And that happens. I think that might strain a relationship a little bit..."

> Nurse 23 "...you take them to the unit and they have their treatment and it kind of...that fades a bit, they can get hooked on the girls in the unit then, and...'oh, she's good at cannulation now' ..'oh, oh, watch her now'. I know, I can see it! And I can hear it..."

Others, too, discuss the connection between technical competence and caring (Bertero 1999, Kleiman 2004). Radwin (2000) also highlights this issue of nurses' experiential knowledge and technical competence as being viewed as important by cancer patients. Moreover, Halldorsdottir and Hamrin (1997) report that competence is one of the themes emerging from interviews with cancer patients as caring behaviours. Finally, a connection between caring for (physical care) and caring about (relationship and commitment) are considered intimately connected (de Raeve 2002).

To summarise so far, the study narratives presented illustrate that the personal characteristics of the patient are a major antecedent to intimacy in nurse-patient relationships in oncology. During the first encounter between the nurse and patient, an appraisal of each other occurs. Nurses identify with patients who may remind them of a family member and/or displays optimism in outlook, and empathy follows, which promotes intimacy. Patients' appraise nurses' technical competence and approach to hopefulness, and they 'click' with some nurses, probably as a result of an identification process similar to that of nurses.

The resulting intimacy between the oncology nurse and patient displays the attribute of self-disclosure in the context of normal, everyday talk, peppered with humour. In addition, the context of this intimacy, in light of patients' difficulties in communicating with their families, must be acknowledged.

Experiencing Intimacy

Reciprocity in Self-Disclosure

The act of self-disclosure was discussed by many nurses interviewed, and most of these nurses considered their self-disclosure to patients as a means of dissolving any power perceived over the patient, and a means of simultaneously empowering the patient. This attempt to balance power is evident in the following narratives.

> Nurse 4 "I don't mind telling patients a certain amount of things about myself, or showing them photographs, or that kind of thing. It doesn't bother me, I wouldn't be that private that I wouldn't like to talk about anything. I think it's important to share a bit with them, because they share an awful lot with us, I mean we know everything about them in some ways, so it's nice to kind of give back a little to them as well......it shows the patients, I suppose that you know, you've a certain kind of trust in them as well, if you can talk about family things, and it makes it all a bit more on a personal level, I think as well."

> Nurse 8 "I mean here are the patients here and they are telling you all their problems, and they don't know anything about you. Sometimes if you give an example of something that may have happened, obviously you don't let them too close, or to tell them everything that is going on in your life... You see, that's what I feel that if they're telling you a bit of your problems, that it's ok to sometimes...obviously not to let them into you like, but like to say 'well, that happened to me', or that might have happened to somebody I know like. You can always open up a little to them as well like, and I think that's good too like as well, because they get to know you as well, on a personal basis, without getting to know everything about you, but you do have to open up to them as well like you know".

> Nurse 3 "They're giving their all to it so, it's nice to feel that there's someone there as well that's giving a little back, can develop a bond".

Some disclosure of personal information was viewed as important to the quality of the nurse-patient relationship by all the nurses interviewed.

> Nurse 15 "It's all sort of part of forming that relationship. I think it helps hugely in giving them little things that they can...because people do see, no matter how we look at this, there is always...we're the medicals, we're the nurses, we're the doctors, people in uniforms, people in coats, in whatever, there is...that automatically brings a barrier, as you know, and somehow

then, that little link with normality, yeah, she's a mother too, she's this, that, the other, she's just like me. I don't know what it is, but it actually… I think it really helps the bond… Of course I would share little aspects of my life with patients, because I think that they feel; that that's really important to them…so I actually think that's important; that they see us much more, at their level, that we're human".

Nurses' disclosure of personal details helped to shed their 'professional face' from patients, and some patients interviewed expressed an appreciation for this type of relationship. This is suggested in the views of Patient 7 below.

Pt 7 "I also like the fact that you can talk to them as human beings, you can get to know them quite well, even with all the change, the nurses".

Patients clearly play a role in initiating the process whereby nurses disclose personal details about themselves. This is suggested in the following patient narratives .

Pt 10 "I like to get to know them and them to get to know me. And I do try and get their names…I mean that you can have this contact and form a trust with them to know, and they will tell you things about themselves and you in turn will tell them things about yourself. And you form a relationship with them".

Pt 15 "…you can make very free with the nurses, that's what I feel. I think it's up to a person [patient] themselves. Some people would come in and they'd be afraid to speak to the nurses".

Patients' characteristics clearly influence the extent to which nurses will engage with them.

Nurse 1 "The patient that doesn't engage with you - they won't ask, and they don't want to talk to you, so they'll, they're not going to know anything about you because you don't really have this two-way conversation with them".

The disclosure discussed by nurses interviewed was mostly of a conversational nature, or 'superficial talk'. This form of conversation appears to serve the purpose of normalising an abnormal situation. This view is clearly expressed by Nurse 23 below, who shared with me how she tells patients about her daily events.

Nurse 23 "I wouldn't be telling them everything now I'm telling you about my husband, or three kids, or that, but like …I'd be afraid I'd smother, and I'd be 'I know, I'd be exactly the same', definitely smothering would be a big thing to me, and I think it kind of normalises …now, it wouldn't be faked by me. Well, there's things that I'd certainly agree with them on, and that I'd share with them. Like they'd say 'what drives me daft when I come home is my husband has a big dinner in front of me, and I'm not fit for it', and you know, you can say that feeling, and the guilt that you'd have because you …because sometimes like I'd have my dinner here, and then I'd go home, and *** [husband] might be home ahead of me, and he'd have it ready, and I'd be 'oh Lord! He's after going to all this trouble".

Similarly, Nurse 20 shared with patients her wedding plans, and labelled this disclosure as "public knowledge", and Nurse 4 shared her experience of giving birth for the first time, with her patients.

This superficial talk between nurses and patients is peppered with humour. Patients interviewed talked to me about how humour was common-place in their interactions with nurses. The normalisation of the situation is also evident below, where Patient 26 describes the "great fun" and "great chat" with less emphasis on the patients' illness.

> Pt 26 "Oh yeah, very light-hearted. That's what I'm trying to say about coming in, and the chairs and everybody everywhere. It's not talking about your sickness, or it's not; you get away from your sickness sometimes because it's great fun and great chat, and we all have got to know each other and different things, you know. It's like, if constipation comes up, you can kind of have a laugh about it, you know. Instead of thinking, Oh God, you know".

The value patients place on humour in oncology settings in vividly captured by the narrative below:

> Pt 23 "I mean you can joke along with them [nurses], you know, and; in the case that they can throw a joke at you, or see a funny side to something, or whatever, and it makes, it takes that edge off things. You don't feel 'oh God, I'm going in for treatment!' If everyone, you know, they're young nurses and what have you, they have that serious side, and the happy-go-lucky side sort of thing, which is important too".

The presence of this conversational, superficial talk, however, also serves another function. It assists in developing a comfortable rapport between the nurse and patient which subsequently opens the potential to tackle more sensitive issues. This is suggested in the narrative of Nurse 23 below, where a conversation that began with humour, moved quickly to talk of death.

> Nurse 23 "I remember a lady, I was giving her drugs and she said to me 'do you know, I think I'll get cremated', and I was going to say 'I think I'll stop giving you this right now if that's what you're thinking!' but I didn't, I just said 'is that what you're thinking, Mary?' 'I am' - and I said 'why?'. 'Oh!' she said 'I'd hate to be out there on a cold night, I love the heat!' and I was thinking 'well you certainly do love the heat if you're going to be ...'. But I think I'll get cremated too, because I would, I was saying that to her, and we talked about cremation then. I also think you have to share some of yourself".

Many nurses expressed the view that patients needed to be able to confide in them, since they could not disclose their true feelings to their family.

> Nurse 23 "They get relief maybe speaking to professionals about their illness, because they're trying to protect the ones at home by saying 'I'm fine', and I think that when it comes to us then, I think they want to let everything out".

> Nurse 18 "Sometimes, they can release a lot of information to us that they don't want to worry other family members...because they're too close to them, but also you'd know from an emotional response that it would be like a void, it would be a tense release of emotion - they could be like hysterically crying...

Nurse 20 "Sometimes they want someone to talk to, because they come in on their own a lot of the time, I suppose that you often find that their families can't talk to them. They'd tell you more. We'd have some patients that you'd know they wouldn't tell their families a lot, but they'd tell us".

Nurse 14 "...they don't want their family members to know...like they have awful fears too, and they feel they're trying to protect their own family from".

Nurse 15 "People so need that at times of diagnosis, and at times of treatment, because they're protecting their families, and then families can smother them and crowd them, and of course there's huge support that's very necessary as well, but just at times, the only time they can be truly real is when they're just allowed to be ...when people aren't propping them up, or ...do you know what I mean?".

Revealed in the narratives provided above, is that the attribute of self-disclosure in nurse-patient intimacy in oncology reflects a need for both nurses and patients to sustain some normality under very abnormal conditions. Moreover, it is essential for patients' support since they often feel unable to communicate with their families in the same way that they do with nurses caring for them.

The sharing of personal information has been found to help develop a trusting relationship between the nurse and patient. Disclosure on the part of the patient is dependent on the nurse-patient relationship being one that is non-threatening (Reynolds and Scott 2000). By the nurse revealing something about her self first, the patient may feel less threatened and then reciprocate. It could be argued, therefore, that the nurse plays a significant role in the development of trust in the nurse by the patient.

Levels of Disclosure

Nurses' disclosure revealed in my interviews with them suggests that it is mostly related to social conversation. Kleiman (2004) reports such communication to involve a naïve attitude and a welcoming demeanour and labels this 'chitchat' (superficial talk). This finding of superficial conversations between oncology nurses and patients is also evident in a study of nurse-patient communication whilst chemotherapy is being administered, reported by Dennison (1995), and also in a study involving both in and out-patient radiotherapy and chemotherapy patients (Jarrett and Payne 2000). Moreover, Hunt (1991) reports that much of the verbal conversation between terminally ill patients and nurses is social in nature. However, such social conversation should not be underestimated in the role it plays in intimacy. O'Brien (1999) suggests, following his ethnographic study, that psychiatric nurses use a conversational style in their interactions with patients in order to put patients at ease. Moreover, the ability to foster a relaxed atmosphere is reported by cancer patients as the most important personal characteristic of nurses (Bailey and Wilkinson 1998).

Ersser (1991) and Taylor (1994) reveal that patients appreciate nurses spending time with them and enjoy their company. Williams (2001a) concludes that intimacy is reflected in psychological and emotional closeness. Moreover, Kralik, Koch and Wotton (1997) report that nurses who are friendly and warm display engagement behaviour. Therefore, disclosure has many levels, and superficial talk, although appearing casual in nature, should not be considered of lesser relevance with regard to intimacy. Such supposedly superficial social interactions as has been revealed by both nurse and patient interviews in this study, allows patients a welcome opportunity to discard their sick role and forget about their cancer for momentary shades of time. The need for relief from the daily suffering experienced by cancer patients is evident, where they describe a cascade of losses over the course of their cancer trajectory (Gregory 1994). Moreover, superficial revelations by the nurse can often show his/her human self with patients subsequently accepting the nurse as being human and not performing a role (Kralik, Koch and Wotton 1997). Such a view has surfaced strongly in my study with many nurses striving to show their human side and patients revealing their comfort experiencing this approach. Moreover, patients report that superficial talk helped them know staff, which contributed "to their experience of emotional comfort" (Williams and Irurita 2004, p. 812). One study participant revealed: "*I mean for a nurse to turn around and have a joke with you or talk to you for just a few minutes, that means so much, you feel that you're wanted here*" (Patient: Williams and Irurita 2004, p.812).

Different levels of disclosure in nurse-patient intimacy is reported by Williams (2001a). The building relationship level was the exchange of superficial information, such as family (Williams 2001a). This exchange of superficial information has been previously described by May (1991) as "primary involvement" (p. 555). Similar to the findings presented in my study, Williams (2001a) also reports that superficial disclosure opens the door for disclosure on a deeper level. The use of social conversation by patients is reported by Shattell (2005) as a method of getting nurses to like them. Moreover, Maher (2003) reports that nurses experience a sense of power in being made to feel special by patients. One study participant revealed, "*when you walk into a room and…somebody would say, 'howaya M, you were off for a few days were you?' That's a nice feeling, that's a powerful feeling*" (p. 85). Maher (2003) also reports the levels of disclosure revealed by patients to nurses. Her phenomenological study which involved interviews with nurses (n=10) revealed a spectrum of nurses' knowledge of patients, from being aware of patients' preferences in relation to minor needs, to being privy to sensitive personal information.

Another interesting finding from my study is nurses' revelations that they measure their disclosure by not disclosing too much and being selective in what they feel is appropriate to disclose. This strategy is reported elsewhere. A participant in a study reported by Maher (2003) revealed that "*you have to draw the line between you* [nurse and patient] *…something like that might go to your disadvantage you know in the sense that you can be taken for granted*" (p. 85). Such expressions of disclosure by nurses reflects the description of engagement/detachment continuum suggested by Henderson (2001) to explain the process of nurses' relationships with patients, depending on the response to different patients or circumstances. This involvement with patients at different levels is also reported elsewhere, and suggests that nurses naturally become very close to some patients in circumstances of intense patient need, and less intense at other times (Rittman *et al.* 1997). Campbell (1984) also refers to the "delicately balanced relationship" of personal involvement and argues that with "either an absence or an excess of professional detachment" affects the companionship (p. 50). Similar to this, is the description of "being a chameleon" as described by Aranda and Street (1999) when nurses used ways to "reveal or conceal aspects of themselves depending on the situation" (pp. 76-76).

It is important to acknowledge also that the employment of self-disclosure by oncology patients is influenced often by their inability to openly disclose to their family members. A cancer diagnosis can result in isolation from family (Rustoen and Hanestad 1998). Oncology nurses, therefore, can provide a means by which cancer patients can disclose their feelings.

Professional Friend

Many of the nurses interviewed alluded to a type of professional friendship with patients. This permits the development of intimacy, but at a distance; somewhat like 'disinterested love' discussed by Meehan (2003). This is evident in the following narratives:

> Nurse 16 "But she's [patient] very positive and we have a very special relationship. Now it doesn't go beyond professional, but there's a very close relationship there".

> Nurse 3 "I think in oncology because you get to know people so much better you develop more a friendly, not a, it's professional but you do develop this friendly interaction as well".

A number of nurses employed the use of the term 'journey' in conveying their role as professional friend to patients. For these nurses, being a professional friend meant taking a journey with the patient, and being there as a support.

> Nurse 5 "...to be able to help them go through that journey, and to be able to answer their question, and to be able to meet their needs, and to explore their needs together, and that's what I think is important for the patient, and for the nurse to work well together, to have open communication, to have an easy access to...for both people to travel that journey properly together".

> Nurse 13 "You meet them early on in diagnosis, and you kind of go through the journey with them as they come and go for their treatments".

> Nurse 16 "I just want to make it a *good* journey for them. And I do tell them, I say, I will do anything, and my colleagues, to make this better for you."
> Nurse 19 "I know that we're cannulating them, we're giving the chemo, but we're helping them, and you know, I have a voice, and I give them my number and my name, and they can ring if they've any problems. I feel that we're helping, I'm helping, we're all doing it, helping them along the road, and that we're making their journey a little bit easier, and that they're not as frightened, and that they've somebody out there that they can ring and talk to. It probably sounds a bit corny".

For Nurse 8, the role of professional friend was about 'being there' for the patient, expressed keenly in the following narrative.

> Nurse 8 "I would like to think I am their friend, and that they can depend on me. I mean we give our telephone numbers out and I mean when I'm not here at the weekend, they would be ringing me like. I'd always have my messages when I come in on Monday like... You want to catch up with them, you want to be their friend, you want them to be able to trust you, to have confidence in you, to be able to open up..."

Similarly, Nurses 16 and 18 also relay in the following narratives, how they consider 'being there' for the patient essential to their role.

> Nurse 16 "She [patient] needs reassurance. She needs to link in and she says: "Do you think I'll get through this ***? Do you think I'll get through it?" and I'd say ***, Look what you've been through already? Look back and reflect. And look where you're at." And that's what she needs for her to keep going".

> Nurse 18 "...they would find perhaps that when they come into you, that they can void all of their concerns, and all their worries, and they can go out pretty much strong, and semi-intact again to deal with their family".

The empowering nature of the professional friend role is beautifully described by Nurse 16 in the following narrative, where she expresses her belief in helping patients "get control back in their lives".

> Nurse 16 "I always feel like if I can really get control back in their lives... because they've lost their total power. They've had surgery if they had surgery. Everything is taken away from them. They feel like they're nobody. And I really believe: educate them, reinforce education. Empower them. Give them simple language that they understand. And usually I won't leave a patient and I'll tell them. What I normally do is I'll meet them, follow up by phone the next day, and when they ask questions, I reinforce it all the time. So you're building that bond, you're building a journey, but I don't think there's any patient, so far, that I've met that I haven't got that with. I know that when I meet them, I make an impact on them. I'm not going out to do that, but I do want to make their journey a little bit better, because I know from my life experiences, what I went through at that time. And nothing prepares you for cancer".

An examination of nurses' professional friend role reveals that it involves a type of love and acts to support the patient on his/her cancer journey. One of the first references to the nurse as a professional friend to patients is made by Campbell (1984), who argues that such a type of friendship requires a form of love to exist, which he labels "skilled companionship" (p. 935). However, the term was adopted by Trygstad (1986) to describe oncology nurse-patient relationships. Moreover, the terms 'friendliness' and 'friendships' have also been used in the context of nurse-patient relationships in oncology (Turner 1999, Geanellos 2002).

Campbell (1984) argues that a way of understanding the "love as caring" in nursing may be found by an exploration of companionship (p.49): "Nursing is a companionship which helps the person onwards" (Campbell 1984, p. 50). He asserts that companionship between the nurse and patient often arises from a chance meeting and is terminated when the joint purpose which kept the companions together is severed. He further adds that, "the good companion is someone who shares freely, but does not impose, allowing others to make their *own* journey" (Campbell 1984, p. 49).

Use of the term 'friendship' to describe nurses' caring relationships with cancer patients is also revealed elsewhere (Roberts and Snowball 1999, Turner 1999). The nurses working in an oncology setting in a study reported by Roberts and Snowball (1999) describe their relationships with patients "in terms of friendships" (p. 44). Similarly, Turner (1999) reports that cancer nurses (n=40), in her grounded theory study, described two forms of friendships with their patients. The first was coded as "befriending clients" and was expressed as a temporary alliance in which the nurse used the hand of friendship to assist the patient through a difficult period, was therapeutic to the patient and associated with "a positive, beneficial type of involvement". The other type, by contrast, was labelled "being a friend" and indicated a more intense permanent type of friendship and was often associated with over-involvement, and is "essentially dysfunctional" (Turner 1999, p. 156). Interestingly, others suggest that the nurse-patient relationship cannot be described as one of friendship (Caroline 1993, Bignold, Cribb and Ball 1995). This is argued based on the view that such a relationship lacks reciprocity and personal exchange, and that use of the term 'befriending' is suggested as more appropriate (Bignold, Cribb and Ball 1995).

Nurses I interviewed described the journey they accompanied patients on. Moreover, oncology nurses (n=15), in a qualitative study reported by Wengstrom and Ekedahl (2006) also viewed themselves as "accompanying the patient on their walk through life" (p. 23). Interestingly, Ellyn Bushkin, a nurse who also had breast cancer, expresses the view that no other nursing speciality recognises the balance needed between the physical and emotional aspects of illness in the same way as it is approached in oncology nursing (Bushkin 1995).

The words of nurse philosopher Sally Gadow illustrate the impact of nursing on patients' illness journey: "If nursing is a world where we live, rather than a service we provide, then they [patients] and we together constitute it, inhabit it, each depending upon the other to share local knowledge about where safe passage may be found" (Gadow 1995, p. 212). Gadow's (1980) conception of existential advocacy, therefore, is appropriate to this discussion, as patients do require assistance in understanding the meaning of their illness for their life, and reaching decisions with regard to possibilities that foster well-being (Bishop and Scudder 2003). This is no more certain than for patients diagnosed with cancer.

Humour in Professional Friendship

The interview text has also revealed that the professional friendship between the nurse and patient is also represented by the use of humour. Humour, in the form of 'light-hearted' death talk, is also reported by Langley-Evans and Payne (1997) in an ethnographic investigation of a palliative care day unit in England. Bolton (2000) also reports the use of humour by gynaecology nurses to ease tension or lighten the situation. Bolton (2000) suggests that the nurses offer humour as a gift in the context of Hochschild's (1983) conception of 'emotion work' as a gift.

Moreover, it is argued that humour in the nurse-patient relationship builds trust and rapport (Astedt-Kurki 2001). Similarly, Kralik, Koch and Wotton (1997) report the "engaged" nurse was authentically her/himself and was normally happy and smiling, utilising humour in their approach to patients (p. 401). They assert that such an approach to the patient makes the patient "feel special because the nurse has made the effort to acknowledge her as an individual" (Kralik, Koch and Wotton 1997, p. 401).

The employment of humour in oncology has also been revealed elsewhere. Jarrett and Payne (2000) report that nurses attempt to move the tone of nurse-patient communication to a more positive tone by sometimes "turning it into a joke" (p. 86), and Savage (1995) views humour as "a *means* of offering care" (p. 52). Lawler (1991) also reports how nurses use humour as a technique to help themselves and their patients manage difficult encounters in an attempt to minimise the size of the problem.

I consider the humour I see between oncology nurses and patients as 'flirting', since it appears to be utilised as a strategy to connect the relationship. Savage (1995) reports that humour between staff and patients is used as "a way of building or even accelerating the development of relationships towards intimacy or 'closeness'" (p. 78). Furthermore, she reports that nurses liked when patients began to tease them, as they interpreted this as a "positive comment on the patient's morale and on the nurse-patient relationship" (Savage 1995, p. 79). The nurses in Savage's (1995) study expressed their use of humour as a way to break down barriers, which Savage suggests "could be used to bring about change within social relationships" (p. 76). The nurses I interviewed, however, took, their use of humour in their interactions with patients for granted. Nevertheless, many of the patients I interviewed commented on the humour prevailing in their interactions with nurses and were initially surprised that so much light-hearted exchange was part of their caring experience in a cancer setting.

Savage (1995) suggests that nurses use humour to "lighten" the atmosphere (p. 76). Moreover, it is reported that nurses use humour to deal with difficult clinical situations (Beck 1997). This could also provide an explanation for the humour employed in intimate nurse-patient relationships in this study, where the relationship subsists in a climate fraught with uncertainty. Savage (1995) notes that relationships marked by joking are "often characterised by a combination of friendliness and antagonism and tend to occur in situations, where, for some reason, there is ambiguity" (p. 74). Ambiguity is certainly a key feature of life in cancer care settings, and humour in such a climate is perhaps "another of the soul's weapons in the fight for self-preservation" (Frankl 1959, p. 42).

The role of humour in developing the professional friend role is also evident. It is also reported elsewhere that patients enjoy being treated as a friend and when the nurse spends time with a patient enjoying simple conversation, it expresses affection and genuine liking of the patient as a person (Kralik, Koch and Wotton 1997). Others have also reported that using humour and developing a friendship with the patient makes patients feel cared for (Ersser 1991, Taylor 1994). Moreover, as highlighted earlier, Shattell (2005) found that patients described building relationships with nurses as fundamental to seeking nursing care (p. 213). Study participants spoke of deliberately "building friendships" and described forming relationships with nurses by making friends, using nurses' first names, taking an interest in them, making them laugh and making them feel liked (p. 213).

Use of First Names in Friendship

The friendships between nurses and patients are evident in the use of first names by both throughout the interviews. Buresh and Gordon (2000) discuss how, in the past, nurses were discouraged from using their first names with patients, a practice that has since past. They cite the views of nursing historian Joan Lynaugh, who asserts that, by using their first names nurses are doing so "in the hope of showing the patient that they are on their side, that they are equals, on a par with, in the same shoes as the patient", and that, "nurses generally are not seeking 'respect' from their patients, but some kind of identification with them" (Buresh and

Gordon 2000, p. 52). This point further suggests that empathy is displayed to patients in various ways by nurses.

However, Buresh and Gordon (2000) highlight that Lynaugh sees a problem with this use of first names by nurses, since, she argues, that it conceals the power and authority nurses actually have and misconstrues what patients need most and want from nurses. Lynaugh asserts that, "patients don't want a friend, they want a nurse with knowledge and skill. A really good nurse will establish the context for a relationship" (Buresh and Gordon 2000, p. 52). Such a view suggests that nurses solely determine their relationships with patients, which, in itself, is an open acknowledgement of the power nurses may have over patients. This is clearly not the case, and patients' characteristics, as has been revealed in earlier discussions, plays a key role in how nurses respond. Moreover, Buresh and Gordon (2000) point out that many nurses initiate reciprocal first-name interactions with patients to ease patients' fears, let down defences and ease communication. They argue that the ability to establish closeness within a professional context is "one of the great qualities that nurses bring to patient care" (p. 54).

Maher (2003) reports that the power for nurses of being known may be in its role of protecting nurses from feeling like "anonymous, interchangeable caregivers" (p. 85). This conclusion supports the finding in my study that suggests that patients become intimate with many nurses simultaneously. Moreover, a participant in Shattell's (2005) study reported: "*You build relationship differently...with the older* [nurses], *I would talk about the hospital and what a great hospital it was and even try to word it to produce positive conversation...I'd try to talk to them about that kind of stuff, and* [say] *"remember the farmers' market and remember..." you know, talk to them about that kind of thing. And then the young ones, I'd ask them why they majored in nursing and with the shortage and that I was encouraging my daughters to do it. Just bullshit, total bullshit*" (52-year-old woman) (p. 213).

Similar to Paley's (2002) view, where he posits that nurse theorists have striven for moral supremacy over the medical profession in their writings on caring, Buresh and Gordon (2000) also question if nurses' use of first names has similar motives. They ask if nurses use first names "to create and protect one area where they clearly can claim superiority in any doctor-nurse comparison or competition- the ability to establish intimacy with patients" (Buresh and Gordon 2000, p. 52). They continue their argument by asserting that nurses may feel in their struggle for recognition that they cannot win the knowledge competition with doctors but can easily win the "intimacy competition" (p. 52). However, they also ask if intimacy resides in a name or title, or does it reside in genuine attentiveness and empathy (Buresh and Gordon 2002). Such a question raises the issue of whether intimacy and empathy are indeed co-dependent concepts.

Homely Atmosphere

It is important to emphasise that the role of professional friend to cancer patients is nurtured in the context of where care is given to these patients. All three oncology sites sampled in this study, were viewed by patients there as warm and friendly environments, where humour was an aspect of the experience of care. The friendly atmosphere prevailing in these units is expressed in the following narratives.

> Pt 29 "Just as soon as you go in there's a great sense of "Hiya." "Hi, how are you today?" "Any news?" ... the girls [nurses] are so... oh, they're so... and we have the craic with them, and it's as jolly a place as you could spend a few hours... No dwelling on how you are, or are you well... they'll ask you if you're well all right, how you feel, but there's no sense of you know, all day long, as long as you are there. You know, cancer isn't mentioned and I like that. We know we have it. That's enough. Just, you know, have a bit of jolliness and a bit of fun. And try and divert away from that altogether...We want normality. The Thursday is a day we find *hard* enough to come in, and spend the day here without listening to this all day long. And we don't hear it here. And we don't, we could be in a beauty salon for all we know."

> Pt 19 "Well they make you feel at ease, you know. You just feel you're among friends... family, actually. They really are, I find. That's my opinion anyway. They're wonderful like, you know... when you walk in you just feel as if you've come into a friend's house".

> Pt 15 "Once I got in here [unit], and I met those girls [nurses], and the welcome I got. They treat you as if they knew you for years... I've no inhibitions about coming in here at all. I do, I like it, and I look forward to it ....as I say, I look forward to it, and to having a bit of craic".

> Pt 17 "Oh, it's lovely - it's a lovely atmosphere in there, like it's a joke a second, do you know what I mean... You're coming into a completely natural atmosphere every day like, you come in and nothing is a problem. ".

> Nurse 6 "...if you're having a bit of fun with one patient, the other patients would be all laughing, and you know, it's just a bit of humour, and it's good, it's good for the patients. You cannot focus 100% of the time on the disease and the chemotherapy and, you just have to be aware that humour is important."

The friendships between the oncology nurses and patients was reflected particularly in patients' descriptions of the friendly atmosphere they experienced. The description by Patient 29 of the unit being like a "beauty parlour" reflects the view of a participant in a study reported by Wilkes, O'Baugh and Luke (2003) who equated the oncology treatment facility to going shopping; "If you go to into a shop to buy something, and someone is there and they have a sad look on their face and you don't get a word out, so they are so negative in their attitude, it has a terrific effect on you. You don't go back to the shop" (p.415). Similar comments were made by cancer patients in a study by Schou and Hewison (1999) who report the comments of the following patient about going to the clinic for treatment: "it's like going to the supermarket, they make it so easy." (p. 124) Other studies too, reveal the therapeutic outcomes of friendliness (Ersser 1991, Fosbinder 1994, Williams and Irurita 1998).

Like the findings reported in my study, patients in the study reported by Wilkes, O'Baugh and Luke (2003) reveal that the attitude of staff in the oncology unit make a difference and supported the patients' positive attitude. Savage (1995), too, reports that patients related to the ward staff as 'family' and perceived the ward as 'home'. Similarly, Schou and Hewison (1999) report patients' view of their cancer treatment centre exuding a homely atmosphere (p. 35). One patient commented on how the nurse in charge introduced herself as "Lily" and described that "...*everything seemed, you know, homey and, you know, different to the old cold idea of, you're here to get done...*" (p. 35). Another patient commented that the unit was like "*...a little family, a little, you know just generally chatting, before you go and a cup of tea afterwards, puts you in the right frame of mind*" (Schou and Hewison 1999, p. 37). The 'everydayness' of the unit was also mentioned by patients interviewed in one of the centres where the study took place (Schou and Hewison 1999, p. 38).

This homely atmosphere was particularly evident in Site C. The nurses' office was situated at the other end of the open plan treatment area, where they answered the 'phone, wrote notes and had coffee breaks. The door was always open, so patients could easily overhear nurses' social conversations. Tea for patients and visitors was made in the same area, since there was not a separate kitchen. Like Savage's (1995) study, the nurses "thought that the absence of a specific space for nurses fostered 'involvement' with patients" (p. 91).

Outcome of Intimacy

The employment of social conversation emerged strongly in my interviews with nurses and patients and suggests that nurses assumed the role of professional friend to their patients. Nurses' role of professional friend in their intimate relationships with patients, brings with it satisfaction and also possible intense emotional consequences. The consequence of nurse-patient intimacy in oncology care is therefore like a two-sided coin for nurses. They feel a sense of satisfaction, which sustains their caring efforts. However, simultaneously, they make efforts to achieve and maintain a comfortable emotional distance from patients for fear of over-involvement. For patients, the consequences of intimacy are less clear. Many patients I interviewed equated caring as intimacy, and they talked about feeling known by the nurses and they implied a sense of comfort in this knowledge.

Satisfaction for the Nurse

Most of the nurses interviewed expressed a sense of personal satisfaction as a result of their intimacy with patients.

> Nurse 21 "Patients are much more likely to tell you their tale of woe, and I don't mind that, and I think that's good and I think that's a brilliant part of nursing..."

> Nurse 8 "And I love when patients open up to me, you know, even though I know we're not counsellors, but like when you walk out of the room, and they say 'I feel so much better', at least you know you have done your job...Oh, I love it, I love it. You know, to know that you've helped them in some way, ...I love the connection with patients. "

The satisfaction gained by nurses is beautifully described in the following narrative from Nurse 10, where she expresses the personal gains from intimacy with patients.

Nurse 10 "I mean it's what can make it very rewarding for you. I mean that you can have this contact and form a trust with them to know, and they will tell you things about themselves and you in turn will tell them things about yourself. And you form a relationship with them. I mean obviously you have to be careful how, how deep a relationship you form or what have you. But it is, well it makes you feel that sometimes that what you do is worthwhile if you're able to make contact with someone...when you have this connection, therefore someone can feel more at ease with you, they can talk more freely, and maybe feel better or feel that they can, by talking to you, or by having a chat, unleash their feelings with you, or feel comfortable with you, that if you can make things just that little bit easier, that little bit better or; then maybe, and they do very much value that, and that time that you can; and they think sometimes that you know; because they often describe us as being angels or fantastic people, that you do this for them, I think sometimes they don't realise that we get something from it too, that we don't just sit there with a false smile on your face, or you don't sit and pretend that you do actually empathise with them, and they are very thankful for it, but the thing is, at the end of the day, if you do feel that you've made a little bit of a difference with them, you do feel; going home ok, well if; that it was worthwhile being there today".

The satisfaction gained also helps nurses in their caring role. This is expressed by Nurse 9, below, where she shares the view that patients are "easier to look after", and Nurse 5, who finds she can do her job "effectively" when she has an "open relationship" with patients.

Nurse 9 "It does bring me satisfaction in that I find them easier to look after, and I think you're more likely as well to know a little bit more about what's going on with them, and they're more likely to reveal stuff to you. When they feel they know you, they trust you, they like you, and vice versa. So it does make things easier".

Nurse 5 "It helps me to do my job effectively, that we can have an open relationship, that the patient would feel free to ask me about anything really".

For some nurses interviewed, the satisfaction they gained from this intimacy with oncology patients had clearly an existential quality for them, and impacted on their personal views of life. Nurse 23, in the following narrative, expresses reveals that she finds herself "humbled in their [patients] presence", and left questioning her "integrity" and "outlook on life".

Nurse 23 "Well, I just, I think health is such a wonderful commodity, and how we take it so much for granted...I just find I'm humbled in their presence, because I just think gosh, you are so great dealing with this, how would I be? I think I'd be a lunatic. Maybe I wouldn't. I don't know. They just make you question your own morals and your own; I suppose morals is the wrong word to use, but your own integrity, and your own outlook on life. I think every meeting is unique, and you learn from them. You learn not to be cross when you go home because they never unpacked the dishwasher and put in cocoa on top of it, because it's really so minute. You learn how much you love someone when you see someone trying to say goodbye here. It's sad sometimes, but if you take each encounter as learning, and I mean...like, I sometimes...you nearly get strength from their weakness, if you know what I mean by that, that my God like, you would be in awe of them! As I say, each patient is an encounter, and long after they're gone, sometimes... I saw in a book one day 'long after you had left, I heard your music in my soul', isn't that lovely?".

Similarly, Nurse 21 below, expresses how much nurses can "take" from their intimacy with patients.

> Nurse 21 "You get...to get the opportunity to kind of talk to people, and when you say, like I suppose when you talk to people, and you know they talk about priorities, and their family and stuff, like that's what I mean, I think it's something that you're taking...I don't think patients often realise how much you take away from that, and how much you might think about it when you go home, and look at your own children, and you know, I feel that like the experiences I get; like, you know, the good thing that happens when you're dealing with people here on an everyday basis, I think that sometimes patients maybe don't realise that they are giving you sort of so much back, and for like, for every one bad day, you have ten or twenty good days".

"The more I care for this person, the more I worry, and the more I worry, the stronger my desire to care" (van Manen 2002, p. 272).

Nurses I interviewed talked passionately about the satisfaction they gained from their intimate relationship with patients. Satisfaction for nurses from emotional engagement with patients is also reported elsewhere (Tippl 1995, Turner 1999, Henderson 2001, Williams 2001a). Moreover, although nurses admit that their emotional involvement with patients causes them the most anxiety, they also regard the emotional stresses as bringing the greatest potential for job satisfaction (Bolton 2000).

The positive outcome for nurses, as a result of experiencing involved relationships with cancer patients, is reported by Turner (1999) to result in job satisfaction and feeling valued. Cancer nurses' relationships with their patients provides for them a "deeply meaningful experience" (Bertero 1999, p. 417). Moreover, nurses state that they develop their sense of self-esteem and satisfaction from the patient in seeing the value of their presence for their patients (Bertero 1999). Noddings (1984) argues that human beings "want to care" (p. 7) and the desire to care is a principle motivating factor for those who choose nursing as a career (Roach 1987). Moreover, it is reported that oncology nurses enter cancer nursing due to a desire to care being strong and characterises the development of nurse identity by "setting the trend for the individual's outlook on life" (Wengstrom and Ekedahl 2006, p. 23).

The outlook on life of nurses I interviewed reflects an existential benefit. Some nurses I interviewed expressed thoughts existentialist in nature in their descriptions of what close relationships with patients meant to them. Such revelations suggest the reciprocity in close nurse-patient relationships, and reflects the reciprocal and interactive element of care whereby the nurse grows mentally and spiritually through caring for others (Watson 1988). The mutuality of intimacy in the nurse-patient relationships is further understood when existential advocacy is translated by Bishop and Scudder (2003) to mean that "it helps other persons *be* what they cannot *be* without helping, caring relationships with others" (p. 107). Although this comment refers to the patient in receipt of caring, it could also be applied to the nurse who gives the care. Such an assertion is supported by the findings of this study, where nurses described existential feelings derived from their close relationships with cancer patients. Similarly, Wengstrom and Ekedahl (2006) also report that oncology nurses' own quality of life is defined by their work, with quality of life encompassing the desire to be healthy and see their children grow up. This results in an awareness of living in the present and an appreciation of living life to the full.

Similar to nurses' views expressed in my study, nurses in the study reported by Wengstrom and Ekedahl (2006) report how cancer nursing influenced their belief system. The views of one respondent in this aforementioned study illustrate this: "*I look on life as a gift, it is incredible, incredible, almost every day...I am very content with life. I think I have got...there are a lot of things you can influence in life...it is important that you choose what you want to do...*" (Wengstrom and Ekedahl 2006, p. 23).

Campbell (1984) in a discussion on the existential benefit from the act of caring argues that, "it is often more blessed to care than to be cared for; and the ability to care is frequently made possible by the understanding and sensitivity of the needy person. Such reciprocity suffuses the relationship of caring with a spontaneity, with a sense of grace which enriches carer and cared-for alike" (p. 107). Such a view also relates to the view of caring as a shared endeavour evident in existential advocacy as proposed by Gadow (1980).

The view of reciprocity, emerging in this study therefore, is one that results in an existential feeling and not the mere behaviour of reciprocity of self-disclosure as I had interpreted in my initial concept analysis. Other researchers also report a similar finding. Savage (1995) reveals that nurses find personal satisfaction and their "morale was lifted" (p. 124) by the reciprocal nature of their relationships with patients, and "the concern expressed by patients for nurses' welfare represented a significant source of support" (p. 124). It is also reported by Appleton (1993) that both nurses and patients experience "a transcendent togetherness" (p. 896) from their intimate union that bond the patient with the nurse in friendship. Stein (1917/1970) also writes about the "significance of knowledge of foreign personality for 'knowledge of self'" (p. 105). She argues that through empathy with "persons of our type, what is "sleeping" in us is developed. By empathy with differently composed personal structures we become clear on what we are not, what we are more of or less than others" (p. 105).

Suggestions of transcendence signal a spiritual element to nurse-patient intimacy, and are clearly evident in the views of some nurses I interviewed, similar to that reported by Kendrick and Hughes (2002). Victor Frankl (1984) offers a useful perspective to this discussion, with his view that "self-actualisation is possible only as a side effect of self-transcendence" (p. 133). The revelations of nurses I interviewed, with regard to their self-transcendence through their relationships with patients, may be interpreted as reflecting the self-transcendence in patients. Through suffering, the experience of self-transcendence can emerge (Wayman and Gaydos 2003), and perhaps nurses' intimacy with patients results in a sharing of some of this experience. Patterson and Zderad (1975) use the term transcendence to describe patients rising above their difficulties with the assistance of nurses. Lauver (2000) asks, "when women create opportunities for human connection, are they engaging in sacred acts?". They could be, since, "in a transpersonal caring moment, both nurse and patient are healed" (Wayman and Gaydos 2005, p. 264).

Despite the satisfaction oncology nurses experience as a result of their intimacy with oncology patients, the potential for intense emotional effects is also evident in their narratives.

Emotional Effects of Intimacy

Some nurses expressed the emotional pain that can result when a patient they experienced intimacy with, dies.

Nurse 7 "It's a difficult job, yeah, not physically. I mean people say 'God, you've a great job', it's a lovely job and everything, but emotionally, it can be very draining ... Very often as well, you see a run of people that you might be close to, and not getting well. Either there's ten of them doing very well, or there's five of them doing very badly, and if it's five that you're getting on very well with, it can be emotional, because it can be a couple of people in a row I suppose or whatever, and you do find that. You get kind of good runs, and you get your bad runs, and the bad runs are emotional".

Nurse 18 "It is difficult. I mean...but it's rewarding, but it can drain you a little as well though, particularly for me - personally I would often find if there were very young children involved, I'm not saying that you can quantify age, or quantify life, but I particularly personally find if there is a situation where they are crying about leaving a two-year old behind, I find that absolutely horrendously difficult to deal with, because I would find it hard to listen to that person without reacting myself, without even crying, because I just...it's just a horrendous situation for them to be faced with".

Nurse 16 "I remember in in-patients at one stage, we had five or six teenagers, and we sang with them on Christmas Eve, we sang Christmas carols, and by New Year's there was about two of them, three of them who had died. And that was huge, and for not to cry for the family when that child died, and to hug a parent and say 'you know we loved them too', in a different way, because I suppose sometimes they look on us as their second family. Like we've patients that have been coming in here so long, and some of them say that we're like a second family, because they're in here so often".

During my interviews with nurses, it was clear that some patients elicited strong emotions from a number of nurses, simultaneously. For instance, Nurse 10 also talked about another patient who had died a few years earlier and left an "impact" of all of the nurses on the unit.

Nurse 10 "She would have been a hard person not to, to take to. I suppose, but I suppose as well, we're in such close contact with these people. I mean, that lady was here for six months... I mean, you know we worked here all of the time so we saw her; every week...you were involved with intimate parts of her life, whether you wanted to or not be you know. And, you know, there were lots of issues and different things going on and... but in saying that, you know, she was a wonderful person to have got to have known and, you know, it had an impact on all of us I think really".

The potential for emotional pain is clearly high in oncology care settings. It is not surprising, therefore, that most nurses revealed to me that they needed to be careful about getting too intimate with patients because of the possible emotional effects on them.

Nurse 5 "I have cried definitely, definitely I've cried with my patients, now not all the time certainly, but I know that that's ok, that's normal, and that's when a person, you know, when things have come become very close, and you have developed ...and you feel really, really strongly for the situation that they're in, and it's about understanding, but what I meant to say is that a nurse cannot cry …cannot be in a situation where they are crying all the time… I'm very aware of my own limitations or weaknesses, and I know that I cannot expose myself to too much distress or trauma, because that's not healthy, so I have to say 'ok, hold on, try and be reasonable about it, but it is important to protect oneself, because what good is a nurse who's going to break down in front of somebody. Isn't it true?"

Nurse 20 "I mean obviously you draw a line yourself, like; but there's no harm, I feel, in telling them certain things".

Nurse 4 "I'd never close myself off to patients or that but I think sometimes you have to, you have to draw the line and say that work is work and you give everything while you're there but then when you go home…Sometimes you don't have any choice, but I think you'd be just a little bit more aware of it, or more wary of getting in too deep with people".

Nurse 16 "Like that woman now with the … who was only young. Was 39 at the time, and was asking was she going to die… I didn't cry in front of her because I had to, had to set my boundaries…I suppose that's where you're professional and your job experiences, your life experiences, your experience with work…you know that you can't cross boundaries, do you know what I mean?".

Nurse 11 "I do have boundaries, it's very important that you set boundaries for yourself to protect yourself, because you cannot afford to kind of get personally and overly involved in anybody's life. If you set up boundaries or professional…the patient also knows where she stands with you in their relationship as well. It could be very difficult if somebody becomes overly dependent on you because of time constraints and workloads".

Similarly, the need to maintain a professional distance from patients is expressed in the following nurses' narratives, where being "careful" and keeping a "professional role" is stressed.

Nurse 1 "Well sometimes, you could be quite close to a patient…But at the same time it would always be on a professional level. You wouldn't be really close close".

Nurse 6 "You do just have to hold back a little bit…you have to maintain some kind of professional level".

Nurse 23 "I think it's trusting, I think it's good to be open, but not too open. Like you have to be careful as well".

Nurse 10 "I mean obviously you have to be careful how, how deep a relationship you form or what have you… Well, obviously sometimes you can get too, too emotionally involved with, and you find yourself getting upset with a patient that you become particularly fond of, dying or getting very ill or. You know, sometimes you get very involved with their families as well. Especially if people have children or whatever, or you know they're young or they are parents. So it's hard at times too to do that, draw that line, but you just have to be more [laughs] cautious… I do still get upset about people, but I would get upset as in have a bit of a cry, have a chat with someone about my feelings, but it wouldn't impact me any further than that. I haven't let things get to that sort of thing again. I do think as well I am more cautious in how I approach the whole …you know, I'll very much be involved with them, but I'm more protective of myself, do you know what I mean…I just try not to get just too involved. I suppose it's something you can't ….it's just sometimes hard to …but there are sometimes ways you can I suppose prevent yourself getting too involved in the whole thing, by not getting too knowledgeable about the whole family dynamics, and not getting too involved in taking on what is their journey at the end of the day".

The need to maintain professional distance was viewed by some nurses as a way of avoiding the risks of identifying too much with patients, which they equated as over-involvement. Two of the most experienced oncology nurses I interviewed, Nurses 12 and 15, also talked about the risk of over-involvement. The following narrative from Nurse 12 illustrates how she manages this risk.

> Nurse 12 "I make myself stand remote from it...when I'm talking to them, I'd be talking about the children, talking about whatever, but I suppose I'm never really...I probably don't let myself get totally into it. I don't...I mean how into it do you get? I just...I talk about it, I feel that I put it out of my mind then, but I can relate to them because if I thought about it, I'd get very upset. If I kept thinking about it, I'd get very upset".

Other nurses talked about switching off, by not thinking about work when off duty, as a way of managing their relationships with patients, as illustrated in the following narratives.

> Nurse 11 "...I suppose the hardest part sometimes is if you're not on duty, and you meet people outside of work, and I find that difficult because you have your own life to live, and you might be doing your shopping, and it's awkward if somebody starts a conversation off ...and you're not on duty, and it's very important that you have time out and away from the job as well".

> Nurse 18 " I think...you have to have that line, where you don't go home, and you're not affected for the full weekend. You really have to mind you as well, so any discussions that have to be done, you talk about at work... You couldn't, you wouldn't last a year in an oncology unit, if you were going around for a full weekend upset about people, you just can't do it, you just have to ...not programme yourself, but you just have to ....you do really have to, whatever is on your mind at work, discuss at work, but once 5 o'clock comes and you go out that door, you have to go into 'I'm not a nurse' mode, 'this is my life mode', you have to, for your own mental health, it's vital.".

Nurse 10 openly shared with me her decision to leave oncology nursing for a while and work in a different speciality, partly due to the death of a patient she had become very close to. The experience of Nurse 10 illustrates the potential risks for nurses of over-involvement with patients, and supports nurses' attempts to balance their intimacy with patients. "Caring puts the nurse in a position of risk and vulnerability, in the sense that it determines what will be stressful and what will be perceived as an appropriate coping strategy" (Wengstrom and Ededahl 2006, p. 20). This comment suggests that the more nurses experience intimacy with a patient, the more emotional risks they are exposed to. Moreover, cancer nursing has been shown to create more stress for nurses than other specialities (Corner 2002).

Emotional Labour

The work of sociologist, Hochschild (1983), on 'emotional labour', is one that has been applied to nursing (Smith 1992, Froggatt 1998), and also applies to this study. Many of the nurses I interviewed expressed the need to hide some of their emotions from patients. These revelations illustrate the 'emotion work' involved in nurse-patient relationships in oncology:

"Emotion work refers more broadly to the act of evoking or shaping, as well as suppressing, feeling in oneself" (Hochschild 1979, p. 266). For Hochschild (1983) emotional labour is the management of feelings and, "this labour requires one to induce or suppress feeling in order to sustain the outward countenance that produces the proper state of mind to others-in this case, the sense of being cared for in a convivial safe place. This kind of labour calls for a co-ordination of mind and feeling, and it sometimes draws on a source of self that we honour as deep and integral to our individuality" (p. 7).

Savage (1995) reports that nurses in her study were clearly skilled in facilitating close relationships with patients, but they were "not *necessarily* emotionally intense" (p. 124). Similarly, Maher (2003) reports that for some nurses in her study, the intimacy associated with knowing patients was charged with a sense of emotional overload and was experienced as a type of powerlessness related to a feeling of loss of control over one's professional self. Maher (2003) suggests that this reflects the 'emotional impasse stage' described by Ramos (1992), but not as acute.

Nurses' skills in their facilitation of intimacy with patients is similar to that of the nurse assuming the role of professional friend, described earlier. Savage concludes that what she observed was not so much nurses' emotional labour as that described by Smith (1992), but "their labour to determine the *context* of nursing care, a context that would facilitate a therapeutic outcome for the patient without great personal cost for the nurse" (p. 124). This conclusion mirrors the findings of this study also, where nurses had to 'work' on maintaining a 'disinterested love' for patients.

The nurses' narratives also clearly express a need to support themselves by attempts to manage their intimacy through means of an awareness of keeping some distance, where they felt appropriate.

Over-Involvement

"Although it can be painful, parting is an essential element in companionship. The other person journeys on - to life or to death" (Roach 1987, p.51). Although no nurses interviewed in this study used the term 'over-involved' explicitly, it was implied as a concern through their narratives in their descriptions of balancing distance and closeness with patients. Travelbee (1971) also gives an interesting perspective on what she terms "over-identification" which she argues is "not sympathy...rather failure to proceed beyond the phase of the original encounter" (pp. 144-145). She further argues that such nurses "are not concerned about others and tend to view them only as extensions of themselves" (Travelbee 1971, p.145). Similarly, Hess (2003) asserts that engagement between the nurse and patient is not synonymous with "becoming enmeshed in experiencing the patient's perspective", as such an entanglement can only result in the loss of the nurse's self (voice) in the shared relational narrative with the patient (p. 145). Moreover, Kristjansdottir (1992) proposes that role-taking could be a substitute for empathy in circumstances where the nurse requires to use distancing. This concern for nurses who work with oncology patients is also revealed in an ethnographic study reported by Roberts and Snowball (1999), where "emotional closeness was referred to as over-involvement" (p. 44).

Over-involvement is a relationship in which the patient and nurse mutually respect, trust and care for each other (Morse 1991). Morse's (1991) use of the term 'care' as an aspect of over-involvement suggests a need to avoid the patient investing emotionally in their relationship with the nurse. Moreover, use of the term 'over-involved' in describing such nurse-patient relationships is problematic and "it raises the question of who can or should decide whether or not a nurse is too involved" (Turner 1999, p. 155). Turner (1999), reporting on her findings of interviews in a grounded theory study with cancer nurses (n=40), provides a quote from one participant which expresses this very point: "*It's difficult to know when somebody is over involved because what for one nurse is a relationship that they can cope with may be over-involved for another nurse*" (155). However, it would appear that over-involvement occurs when the nurse experiences a type of 'burn-out', as evidenced in the experience expressed by Nurse 10, highlighted earlier. This view is supported by Henderson (2001) who reports that "too much" emotional engagement with patients is where the nurse becomes incapable of "doing the job" (p. 133).

Over-involvement clearly can result in negative consequences for nurses and may result in "emotional pain" for cancer nurses (Turner 1999, p. 157). Similar to the findings reported in this current study, Turner (1999) reports that cancer nurses can find themselves feeling extremely upset when a patient, known for some time, dies. One of the nurses in Turner's study reported wanting to leave oncology nursing following the death of a patient: "*at the time when I became too involved with a patient, when she died I felt like I never wanted to nurse another cancer patient again. It's that painful really*" (Turner 1999, p. 157). This latter comment parallels the views of Nurse 10 earlier. Over-involved relationships in oncology care also have possible negative consequences for patients. Turner (1999) reports that patients may become dependent on nurses and this can lead to problems when the nurse is off duty.

Over-involvement appears to equate with over-identification or excessive emotional identification with patients and puts nurses at risk of stress-related burn-out (Morse and Mitcham 1997). Moreover, Roberts and Snowball (1999) suggest the existence of "the problem of identification; feeling closer as a result of being a similar age" (p. 44), among nurses working in an oncology setting. An interesting finding to add to this discussion is reported by Mehrabian and Epstein (1972), who reveal that study participants who scored highly on emotional empathy are more likely than low scorers to be sensitive to rejection and to engage in approval-seeking and sociability behaviours. This suggests that nurses who may be co-dependent in nature may be more at risk of over-involvement with patients they care for. Similarly, Geanellos (2002) suggests that over-involvement may arise from a nurse's "inability to maintain a separate sense of self" in their relationships with patients. (p. 239).

Peer Support

All of the nurses I interviewed talked about the support they valued from their nursing colleagues when they experienced emotional effects of intimacy with their patients.

For instance, Nurse 6 talked about two of her colleagues calling to her house the night before our first interview. They had called to offer support as a patient they had all been intimate with, had died.

> Nurse 6 "...I know yesterday when that girl died, actually two of the girls called out to me last night, but they ....one of them put her arm around the other nurse, and said 'are you ok?', and one would be the older nurse, and the other would be the bit younger, and the other nurse started to cry, and they just went in and had a little cry, the two of them".

Similarly, my first interview with Nurse 9 was two days after a patient, who had developed an intimate relationship with many nurses on the unit, had died unexpectedly. She told me that many nurses were upset and when I asked her how they were coping with this patient's sudden death:

> Nurse 9 "There's a lot of chat going around between people, and there seems like in the last two days, there's been a lot of just sort of huddling in corners and just having general chit-chats whenever we've had time or whatever, and there's a meeting on today and it'll probably come up at that. So I think people are just talking to each other about it basically".

Forrest (1989) highlights the role of support in caring work. In order to manage emotions in their caring relationships, nurses need to support each other. Reynolds and Scott (2000) suggest that a lack of support from unsympathetic colleagues is a barrier to empathy in nursing. Moreover, nurses' willingness to engage in intimate relationships with patients often depends on the opportunities and encouragement within particular work settings to develop methods for coping with emotional situations (Henderson 2001).

All of the nurses I interviewed told me about the support they received from their colleagues, especially if a patient died. Nurses expressed the view that only the nurses who also knew the patient and experienced a close relationship with them would understand their feelings. Perhaps because the nurses display such empathy towards each other, they are given the strength to continue developing intimate relationships with patients. It would, therefore, appear that, through the caring nurses express for each other, they experience the strength to care deeper for their patients. Smith (1992) concurs with the view that it is the climate of the ward that determines the emotional tone for the staff, where staff feel supported, they have the freedom to care for each other and the patients. Interestingly, nurses in the study by Henderson (2001), mentioned earlier, were not from an oncology setting and some expressed the view that detachment was an important aspect of the therapeutic relationship. This further suggests that nurses who choose to work in oncology settings may value intimacy with patients perhaps more than generalist nurses and indeed may need such relationships with patients to fuel their caring endeavours.

It is argued that nurses require clinical support in the form of clinical supervision to manage their intimate relationships with patients (Smith 1992, Turner 1999, Jones 2001, Teasdale, Brocklehurst and Thom 2001). Moreover, clinical supervision contributes to reduce burnout among nurses (Severinsson and Borgenhammar 1997). However, the nurses I interviewed reported that they required acute, on the spot, support when a patient died, and this was sought from their colleagues. This finding is reflected in that reported in an ethnographic study of in-patient mental health nurses by Cleary and Freeman (2005), where they found that "teamwork and collegial relationships were considered part of the *nature of work*" (p. 495). Nevertheless, some of my interviews reveal that a number of nurses would benefit from more structured support in the form of regular, individual, clinical supervision to help them manage their intimate relationships with patients. The importance of clinical support is highlighted even further when one considers that many view the uniqueness of nursing to be based "upon the health enhancing use of personality and personal knowledge base, through the medium of nurse-patient relationships" (Antrobus 1997, p. 834). This would suggest that nursing is actualised chiefly through the nurse-patient relationship, which clearly suggests support for the nurse as paramount.

A consequence of intimacy for nurses is that of personal satisfaction but also emotional pain. In contrast, the patients' interview data suggest that a consequence of intimacy for them is a feeling of comfort in being known.

Patient Comfort in Feeling Known

Some of the patients interviewed relayed to me how they felt nurses knew them. This comfort is feeling known is illustrated in the following narratives:

> Pt 27 "They seem to get to know me, to recognise my personality straight away. And they seem to know when to crack a joke with me…They got to know, seemed to know me from the word go".

> Pt 10 "If I want to talk to her [Nurse 7] she'll talk to me. Now, they won't push themselves on you, you know. They won't. No, they're good. You know, and if you want to be left alone, they'll leave you alone. If you want to talk, they'll talk. And sometimes I might go that little bit further and make it better talk that you just need. Teardrops fall and then that's it. That kind of thing… If I was down now and if there was one that would come in there [pointing to the door], I'd know right away whether she'd be able to cope with me or not".

Similarly, Patient 28 expresses her comfort in feeling known by Nurse 18, below.

> Pt 28 "She [Nurse 18] mostly deals with me, and I think she's an exceptionally good girl. I would definitely approach her if, you know…she seems to understand me better, maybe, than the others and know more about me, like, or whatever do you know? Well I suppose it's that she's mostly been dealing with me. Some of the others might put in the needle and all that, but she knows everything about me, and she even remembers that that leg does swell up a bit, do you know, sometimes? And she remembers that, do you know! She keeps an eye on that, you know. You know, that she's interested in you, and that she knows your case, and she knows why you're here, and what your problem is, and all that…"

Positive Outcomes for Patient in Feeling Known

Turner (1999) reports that involved relationships between cancer nurses and their patients has positive consequences for patients in continuity of care, security/safety and trust, and nurses strive to know patients in order to care for them better (de Raeve 1996). Williams and Irurita (2004) similarly report that patients "perceived that they received a higher quality of care from hospital staff who knew them" and the outcome was "feeling secure" (p. 810). Baillie (1996) also reports that nurses in her study revealed that "getting to know the patient and hearing his story was important to empathizing" (p. 1303). Moreover, Shattell (2005) reports that patients who felt they knew and trusted their nurses "felt more comfortable about their care" (p.214). This suggests that knowing the patient precedes the empathic response. However, my interpretation of the interview text of this study would not support this assertion. I have interpreted empathy as occurring rapidly and before the nurse 'knows' the patient. Moreover, Baillie (1996) reports that, "stress, lack of time, workload, and being busy" were barriers to empathy (p. 1304). However, these factors did not feature predominantly in my interviews with nurses, with only two nurses alluding to the issue of time being a barrier to their relationships with patients.

Knowing the patient means that the nurse knows the patient's typical responses and is, therefore, central to clinical judgement (Tanner et al., 1993, Finch 2004). The benefits for the oncology nurse of knowing their patient is significant. When cancer nurses know their patients, they can help them understand their cancer (Bertero 1999). Furthermore, knowing patients gives nurses a basis for effective planning of care (Billeter-Koponen and Freden 2005). Knowing the patient is also a reciprocal process whereby the patient engages in getting to know the nurse also (Jenny and Logan 1992). Similar to the findings reported in my study, Jenny and Logan (1992) report that patient characteristics, such as the patient's ability to co-operate influenced the knowing process.

In relation to nursing debate on the concept of knowing the patient, an interesting view of a dialectical concept of 'unknowing' is also proposed (Munhall 1993). Munhall (1993) argues that to engage in an "authentic encounter" it is important to assume a stance of unknowing which results in openness towards the other (p. 125). Being fixed in a state of knowing, she argues, results in a "state of closure". This highlights the need for nurses to be aware of the process of identification prior to empathy, as identified in my study. There is the risk that during encounters with patients where identification is difficult, the nurse may close him/herself off to the possibility of knowing this patient. Moreover, Munhall (1993) argues that in order to achieve a stance of 'unknowing' the nurse must hold his/own own beliefs in abeyance. This view mirrors that of Noddings (1984), highlighted earlier, in which she describes the process of "engrossment" characterised by a "move away from the self" (pp. 16-17), which, I argue, is similar to the identification phase of empathy described by Stein (1917/1970). Moreover, 'engrossment' (Noddings 1984), 'unknowing' (Munhall 1993), and 'identification' (Stein 1970) bear a striking resemblance to the act of phenomenological reduction, where the 'lifeworld' *(Lebenswelt)* is understood pre-reflectively (Husserl 1970). This is not surprising, since Edith Stein followed the work of Husserl closely and, as his assistant, edited Volume 11 of his work, *Ideas* (Stein 1970).

The patients I interviewed revealed that, in being known, they experienced individualised care. This finding is also supported by Larson (1984) who, in a study of cancer patients' (n=57) perceptions of caring, revealed that instrumental behaviours (those related to knowledge on giving treatment) ranked higher than expressed behaviour. This also reflects the view of Cameron (2002), who describes 'Nancy', a patient who just wanted most the presence of another person, information about her condition and competent physical care, and fits with Campbell's (1984) description of competence "as the state of having the knowledge, judgement, skills, energy, experience and motivation required to respond adequately to the demands of one's professional responsibilities" (p. 61).

In conclusion, the study narratives have explicated the process of nurse-patient intimacy in oncology care settings. This intimacy has been shown to be one based on a professional friendship. This friendship is given birth on the first meeting where both nurse and patient appraise each other. The characteristics of the patient promote the nurse's response to them, which highlights the influence the patient has on his/her relationship with nurses. Nurses, in turn, balance their intimacy with patients in order to avoid over-involvement, by assuming a level of distance and restraint in their disclosure.

Conclusion

This concluding discussion revisits some key issues arising from the study findings. In particular, because the role played by patient characteristics in the development of nurse-patient intimacy emerged strongly in the study findings, an examination of this finding from a social judgement perspective is required.

The study findings suggest that empathy and intimacy are two sides of the same coin. Empathy is intimately associated with the concept of 'closeness', and simultaneously requires closeness (Baillie 1996). Yegdich (1999), however, questions this conclusion and asks: "Can 'closeness' be sustained as the key defining feature of empathy? After all, this study [Baillie's] found that closeness could reduce objectivity, affect commitment to other patients and cause personal stress to the nurse when their feelings were aroused." (p. 90). Yegdich (1999), however, in this argument appears to be focusing on the possible consequences of over-identification, rather than on closeness. Nevertheless, Kirk (2007) provides a convincing philosophical argument distinguishing empathy from intimacy.

This issue of balancing engagement and detachment surfaces repeatedly in the nursing literature on nurse-patient relationships. Campbell (1984) argues that "a *critical distance* is required between the helper and the person helped – too great a distance prevents the helper from responding to the other's need: too little a distance disables the helper from seeing the problem objectively and offering support from outside the situation" (p. 81). The role of identification and empathy in the balancing of engagement and distance is also a feature of this discussion. Campbell (1984) drawing on the work of Scheler's with regard to fellow-feeling (that is, empathy, identification, mutual feeling, vicarious feeling, emotional infection), argues that, "the professional who cannot participate in the other's feelings (empathy) is too distant to help: but where loss of self (in 'identification') occurs there is too much closeness for professional help" (p. 81).

The most appropriate term to use in describing nurses' attempts to achieve a balance on the intimacy continuum with patients is that of 'moderated love': "the subtle balance between involvement and detachment" (Campbell 1984, p. 126), which requires the self awareness to 'switch off'. Turner (1999) reports on the importance of nurses' self-awareness in managing involvement in their relationships with cancer patients. Moreover, Campbell (1984) argues that the professional "who learns to question his or own assumptive world, will be in a better position to give the expected comfort and to help the client grow beyond the assumptions of which help is sought and offered (pp. 96-97). Nurses 15 and 16 suggested much self-awareness, and were also two of the most experienced oncology nurses interviewed. Moreover, they expressed their ability to manage intimacy with their patients through self-awareness guiding their balancing on the intimacy continuum.

Nurses have been reported elsewhere to express profound disappointment in the failure of nurse education to address the emotional requirements of nursing work (Henderson 2001). However, Henderson (2001) questions whether the nurses are "getting the message" (p. 137), in other words, whether self awareness exists sufficiently during their educational preparation, to allow them to recognise its relevance until they enter practice. There is some validity in Henderson's suggestion. However, the findings of my study suggest that perhaps nurse educators should also pay due attention to promoting nurses' awareness of their identification and empathy with patients in the context of behavioural components such as communication skills.

Life experiences also result in nurses being better able to manage their relationships with patients. It is reported that nurses perceived experience as antecedent to the development of maturity, which helps them deal with demanding emotional situations in their practice (Tishelman et al., 2004). Similarly, Turner (1999) reports that her data strongly suggests that the more life experience a nurse has, the better able he/she is able to manage involvement with patients.

It is also reported elsewhere that nurses acutely perceive the risks in "getting too close to patients" (Tishelman et al., 2004, p.427). The nurses in the aforementioned study displayed self-awareness, since they were sometimes self-critical of their own personal ways of coping by saying that they "shut down emotionally and tended to avoid difficult situations" (p. 427). This expression of avoidance of difficult caring situations should be viewed positively, since, if a nurse has the heightened self-awareness to care for themselves, they are better placed to engage more intimately with patients.

Without self-awareness, nurses may not question their motives to care. A view of nurses' pursuits to care for others is that which considers caring as nurses' need to be needed and as co-dependent.

The Need to Be Needed

Campbell (1984) writes of reciprocity in the context of "the need to be needed" (p. 105). He argues that there are "subtle rewards" for the professional helper and that the choice of such career stems from some needs in the helper, such as satisfaction in such work. Wengstrom and Ekedahl (2006) also suggest that love is related to nurses' need to care, and, when this desire is satisfied, the nurse is content. Similarly, cancer nurses (n=10), in a phenomenological study by Bertero (1999), report that their self development and self-awareness is learnt through their experiences of being in interpersonal relationships with patients and their families. Henderson (2001) also reports that the private self and the self, which is a nurse, are constantly interacting and changing one another, and nurses' reasons for coming into nursing are influenced by their personal life experiences from childhood and beyond. Henderson (2001) concludes that "who [nurses] are as people cannot be easily be separated from who they are as professionals" (p. 135).

Caring as Co-Dependency

This aforementioned view suggests that nurses need to care for personal reasons. "The *need* to be helpful becomes an insistent *demand* to be perpetually rescuing people" (Campbell 1984: pp. 105-106) (his emphasis). Campbell (1984) also argues that "...rather paradoxically, ...the truly needy person in some helping relationships may well be the helper" (p. 106). This latter comment of Campbell relates to a parallel discussion raging in caring literature, which views those who care as being co-dependent.

The concept of co-dependency was first applied to the literature on addiction, but nurse authors have since applied it to the discipline of nursing and its activities. Most of the literature on co-dependency, as it applies to caring roles, is negative in outlook. However, Stafford (2001) highlights those theories that view it as a personal empowerment that can be best achieved by the power of connection with others. However, Martsolf (2002) argues that such an association is dangerous.

It is argued by some that nurses become nurses because of a need to care for others that arises from early family dysfunction (Shelly 1991). Kines (1999) equates caring too much and becoming over involved with patient, to co-dependency and argues that co-dependency is widespread among nurses. Nurses labelled as 'co-dependent' are described as nurses who need to feel they are doing something good, and the caring behaviours of nurses may actually be dysfunctional (Sherman et al., 1989). They describe persons with this 'disease' as being in self-denial and if they continue to do the right thing, they will be loved, appreciated and accepted (Sherman et al., 1989, p. 26). Co-dependency, in these theories, then, as it applies to caring in nursing, is defined as an addiction and results in an alienation of one's public self from one's private self (Sherman et al., 1989). Moreover, caring in nursing is viewed as "self-established exploitation" (Bowden 1997, p. 124). However, such a view equating caring as co-dependency, is not reflected in the views of nurses I interviewed. Nurses' expressions of their intimacy with patients clearly reflected a blending of their personal and professional selves. Moreover, it is argued that the behaviours expressed in co-dependency include empathy and altruism (Malloy and Berkery 1993). However, such a view does not correlate with the interpretation of empathy revealed in this study, where it is considered as less of a behaviour one can control and more of a emotion that 'just happens'. Nevertheless, it is clear that nurse-patient intimacy brings with it the risk of heightened emotional response for nurses, as revealed by the nurses in this study. However, the study narratives also reveal that nurses develop intimacy with patients considered 'optimistic' in outlook much more readily than those described as 'detached' or 'questioning'. Only a few nurses revealed their commitment to developing intimate relationships with such patients, a finding reflected in a grounded theory study by Yonge and Molzahn (2002), where they report on the practices of nurses (n=18) "who go beyond the usual scope of practice to demonstrate caring" (p. 399). This finding therefore requires a closer examination in the light of social judgement literature.

Social Judgement

The nurses' narratives clearly reveal the judgemental labelling of oncology patients. Those patients who displayed anxiety and continually questioning of the nursing staff are described as 'questioning', whereas the patients who kept a distance from nurses and choose not to develop an intimate relationship with nurses are described as 'detached'. Moreover, nurses' descriptions of patients as 'optimistic' is open to scrutiny since it suggests that oncology patients may feel pressurised to put on a face of hopefulness. This judgmental labelling can be examined with the lens of Social Judgment Theory.

Social judgment is considered to be a more suitable term to use when discussing 'good' and 'bad' patients (Johnson and Webb 1995). Moreover, Johnson and Webb (1995) also consider 'social judgement' to be preferable to the label of 'moral evaluation' (Roth 1972, May et al. 2004), as this latter term, "has meaning more akin to the systematic philosophical analysis or evaluation of ideas or actions" (Johnson and Webb 1995, p. 472).

The judgemental labelling of patients by both nurses and doctors has been highlighted in nursing for over three decades (Stockwell 1972, Kelly and May 1982, Fielding 1986, Wigton 1996, Mohr 1999), and has been shown to negatively effect nurse-patient relationships and the outcome of care (Carveth 1995, Erlen and Jones 1999). Johnson (1997) considers judgemental labelling from an interactionist perspective, and views it as "a process through which care is managed and which provides nurses with a strategy for coping with the emotional labour of care" (p. 1). However, Goffman's (1959) work on 'performance' also plays a role, in that patients' behaviour [performance] is monitored by nurses and subsequently influences their views of the patient. This process, is, for instance, evidence in an analysis of psychiatric nurses' file notes, where some nurses made entries that judged the patient's behaviour in a "value loaded...negative way" (Mohr 1999, p. 1056).

From the perspective of this study's findings, therefore, this view of social labelling proposed by Johnson (1997) suggests that oncology nurses strive to assume the role of professional friend to patients, in order to minimise patients' experience of adverse effects along their treatment trajectory. However, Johnson's (1997) view could also suggest that oncology nurses' need for fulfilment and reciprocity in their caring role is deprived when they encounter 'detached' patients. This would fit with Johnson's view of nurses deriving power from their pursuit of "associated satisfactions" (p. 110).

The patient described as 'detached' in this study, however, does not fit into the category of 'bad' patient described in the literature. The 'bad' patient is one who, among other traits, is "demanding and unreasonable" (Johnson 1997, p. 49). This description fits more comfortably with the 'questioning' patient described by only a few nurses interviewed. Moreover, the questioning patient may be perceived as demanding due to their challenging, but not necessarily unpleasant behaviour (Johnson and Webb 1995). The 'detached' patient described by nurses in this study correlates somewhat to Lorber's (1975) description of the deviant patient, positioned at the opposite end of the continuum from the patient identified as conforming, and fits into the description of the 'problem' patients who do not conform to nurses' expectations of institutionalised practice (McNamarra, Waddell and Colvin 1994). The 'detached' patient therefore, fits into Parson's (1951) theoretical discussion of the *sick role,* where patients should co-operate with medical staff in striving to get well. This assertion is made based on the nurses' narratives where they suggest these 'detached' patients to be negative in outlook, and such an outlook is deemed unfavourable to fighting a cancer diagnosis. Moreover, the 'detached' patient may be labelled 'bad' by virtue of their lack of need for support from nurses, or assuming independence. This latter point is very relevant and fits with the view of labelling patients negatively when such patients' behaviour confronts the nurse's role in using his/her skills in a therapeutic way (Kelly and May 1982). The nurses' narratives clearly suggest the frustrations experienced in nursing such patients. However, it is argued that most patients do not want nurses to "become their friends and confidantes", or to be privy to "every aspect of their lives" (Levine 2002, p. 2088). Moreover, nurses often emphasise communicative interventions that encourage patients to express feelings, when patients and their families appear to value instrumental communicative behaviours (Skilbeck and Payne 2003).

The 'detached' patients described by nurses in this study, very possibly were experiencing distress, and unable to articulate their fears. According to Masseé (2000), display of demoralisation and pessimism towards the future, social isolation, and withdrawal unto oneself, are features of distress. While a number of nurses I interviewed explicitly expressed a need to understand and accept the detached approach adopted by these patients, it could be argued that such a nursing response is too passive. Only Nurse 15 and Nurse 16 clearly suggested committed and successful attempts to establish intimacy with these patients. A need to understand the 'detached' patient is clearly evident. Some tentative assistance is provided by the work of English and Morse (1988). Following their interviews and observation of patients perceived as 'difficult' by nurses, they identify that these patients were experiencing a range of emotions, from loss of control and power, lack of independence, lack of communication and lack of control of treatment (English and Morse 1988). The inclusion of 'lack of communication' warrants closer scrutiny. It is possible that oncology patients described as 'detached' are so overwhelmed by their diagnosis that they perceive their inability to cope, with resulting distress (Ridner 2004). The 'detached' patient may then attempt to close themselves off from oncology nurses in order to maintain personal control and prevent an unleashing of emotions. Such patients may not feel they have any choice to react otherwise, and "are confined by the practicality of getting through the day in comfort rather than presenting a 'positive image'" (Johnson 1997, p. 98).

The experience of nurses' intimacy with patients described as 'detached' should be a concern for oncology nurses. It is possible that oncology nurses do not experience the process of empathy, beginning with identification, described earlier, with patients described as 'detached'. This assertion is made based on the findings of an Australian study where 150 student nurses ranked their degree of liking eleven specified categories of unpopular patients (Roberts 1984). Roberts (1984) reports that 76% of his study participants responded that they change their views of patients when given time to talk to them and when experiencing empathy for them. Moreover, it is argued that nurses must firstly develop a trusting relationship with distressed patients before employing interventions to relieve distress (Ridner 2004). This latter point appears relevant to this debate. This study clearly suggests the central role played by identification, the first phase of empathy, in developing intimacy. This process of identification was accelerated when nurses experienced something in common with the patient. What then is the possible consequence for patients who, for instance, are poles apart in a cultural and/or religious sense from oncology nurses, and the process of identification is not immediate or primordial? The importance of raising awareness and examination of this issue with oncology nurses is paramount. Nurses clearly have a responsibility to address this issue and engage in a committed process to connect with patients described as 'detached'. Failing to make such attempts affects the overall experience of care for these patients.

Social judgment also applies to the 'optimistic' patients in my study. It is argued that the social judgment of patients by health care professionals may also depend on the how much effort patients are prepared to undertake (Strauss *et al.* 1982). Patients optimistic in outlook may therefore be perceived by their carers as working hard to cope with their cancer. Such patients could be described as similar to those discussed by Shattell (2002, p.2005) who use humour, kindness and charismatic behaviour in order to be perceived as 'good' patients, and patients with "charisma or a sense of humour" with which they used to "bargain for their moral status", as described by Johnson (1997, p. 125). Interestingly also, is the suggestion that patients employ social judgement of other patients in such comments as: *"I think I'm a pretty easy patient because I'm easy to talk to...some of them* [patients] *in there weren't"* (Shattell 2005, p.214). Moreover, Shattell (2005) reports that study participants believed their response to the nurse, i.e. "nice, friendly, calm, compliant and easy to talk to" affected the care they received (p.214). This effort by patients is viewed by Johnson (1997) as "negotiation", who reports that "patients are very concerned on the whole to maintain a positive reputation, and that this in itself is something to bargain with" (p.127). Indeed, it is argued that "power is both the source and outcome of social judgment" (Johnson 1997, p.110).

Many view this positive approach adopted by patients as a huge burden for them to bear (de Raeve 1997, Rittenberg 1995, O'Baugh et al., 2003). Wilkinson and Kitzinger (2000) argue that people say they are positive in order to fit in with what is socially acceptable. Patients comply with nurses' desires in order to avoid unpopularity and cause 'trouble' (Waterworth and Luker 1990). However, adopting a positive approach and expressing hopefulness is viewed by Omar and Rosenbaum (1997) as maladaptive when the most likely outcome is unrealistic, not hopeful. They also suggest that such unrealistic hope results in patients being unable to prepare themselves for possible bad news (Omer and Rosenbaum 1997).

It is therefore argued that the study findings presented here point towards patients' characteristics (these being, 'optimistic', 'questioning' and 'detached'), as the catalyst to how nurses socially judge them. This view, however, is in opposition to that proposed by Johnson (1997) who argues that social labelling of patients is "socially constructed in relation to a complex web of powerful social influences" (p. 92). Nevertheless, Johnson (1997) describes the central role played in the assessment process undertaken by nurses, in nurses' social labelling of patients. This view mirrors the importance of the first meeting between the oncology nurse and his/her patient, explicated earlier.

Clearly, the importance of promoting oncology nurses' exploration of their judgments of patients cannot be ignored. This issue has far reaching consequences for oncology patients and open discussion of patients' efforts to be viewed as 'good' patients, as well as nurses' judgments on what is a 'bad' patient is required. Clinical supervision has the potential to offer such a forum, as it acts as a structured means to facilitate nurses' reflection on their practice.

Personal meanings of the term 'intimacy' vary hugely and, therefore, labelling a nurse-patient relationship as 'over involved' is problematic. Moreover, each nurse has a unique response to close relationships with patients (Turner 1999). Nursing literature reveals many descriptions of intimacy as it applies to the nurse-patient relationship, and all present it as a dichotomous set with detachment (Table 1). What is not clearly evident in the use of these dichotomous sets is that they exist on a continuum. Moreover, this study clearly suggests that nurses move along this continuum depending on their identification and empathy with a particular patient and depending on their own self-awareness in the relationship.

This study has revealed that intimacy is a concept important to oncology nursing. Nevertheless, the suitability of the term 'intimacy' to describe close nurse-patient relationships in oncology is questionable. This conclusion is reached because the antecedents of intimacy include the technical skills of the nurse and this, therefore, broadens the use of the term intimacy to fit more comfortably into the concept of caring. Moreover, the concept of intimacy has been revealed to be central to the nurses interviewed, but, for the patients, it has been interpreted as less essential to their overall experience of care in oncology care settings.

Table 1. Dichotomous sets of intimacy-detachment

Dichotomous set	Source
Detachment versus Intimacy	Graber and Mitcham (2004)
Intimacy versus Distance	Aranda and Street (2001)
Related versus Separate	Barnsteiner and Gillis-Donovan (1990)
Engagement versus Detachment	Carmack (1997) , Henderson (2001)
Being close versus Being distanced	Lindseth et al. (1994)
Closeness versus distance Involvement versus Detachment	Campbell (1984)
Involvement versus Non-involvement	Travelbee (1971)
Scientific (professional) distance versus personal involvement	Johnstone (1987)
Interconnectedness versus Detachment	Beckerman (1994)
Being authentic versus Being a chameleon	Aranda and Street (1999)

Finally, the hybrid nature of the methodological influences adopted in this study reflects the qualitative researcher adopting the role of *bricoleur*. The term *bricoleur* (Jill/Jack of all trades) was proposed by Denzin and Lincoln (1994) to reflect the characteristics of the qualitative researcher who had to be flexible, responsive and reflexive. This hybrid approach is not surprising since nursing gains its theoretical underpinnings from diverse philosophical and theoretical standpoints. This work, therefore, reflects 'fuzzy logic', the use of multiple truths to represent nursing's *Weltanschauung* (Im and Chee 2003). Gobbi (2005) similarly addresses the issue of nursing practice as "bricoleur activity" which uses "bits and pieces" (p. 117) from the domains of nursing, philosophy, psychology, education, sociology and anthropology.

I finish with the words of Frank (2006) on interpretive phenomenology, which is considered "first and foremost, a discipline of seeing and being, a way of deepening the perplexity and mystery of what is going on, especially who exists and in what relation to whom…interpretive phenomenology, in research as in applied clinical practice, enables new interpretations, which in turn enable new possibilities of action" (p. 114). The new possibility of action was my choice to include a feminist perspective. Furthermore, the symbiosis of interpretive phenomenology with feminist research insights, challenges what Thorne (1991) calls "our acceptance of the wisdom of methodological orthodoxy in qualitative nursing research" (p. 195). What has been achieved in this study is an example of what Thorne (1991) terms "methodological heterodoxy" and represents the "emergence of an unique process" (p. 195) to generate nursing knowledge.

References

Antrobus, S. (1997) Developing the nurse as a knowledge worker in health- learning the artistry of practice. *Journal of Advanced Nursing. 25,* 829-835.

Allan, H. (2001) A 'good enough' nurse: supporting patients in a fertility unit. *Nursing Inquiry. 8*(1), 51-60.

Alvesson, M. and Skoldberg, K. (2000) *Reflexive methodology. New vistas for qualitative research.* London, Sage Publications.

Appleton, C. (1993) The art of nursing: the experience of patients and nurses. *Journal of Advanced Nursing. 18*, 892-899.

Aranda, S. (2001) Silent voices, hidden practices: exploring undiscovered aspects of cancer nursing. *International Journal of Palliative Nursing.* 7(4), 178-185.

Aranda, S. and Street, A. (1999) Being authentic and being a chameleon: nurse-patient interaction revisited. *Nursing Inquiry. 6,* 75-82.

Aranda, S. and Street, A. (2001) From individual to group: use of narratives in a participatory research process. *Journal of Advanced Nursing. 33*(6), 791-797.

Astedt-Kurki, P. (2001) Humour between nurse and patient, and among staff: analysis of nurses' diaries. *Journal of Advanced Nursing. 35*, 452-458.

Baer, E.D. and Lowery, B.J. (1987) Patient and situational factors that affect nursing students' like or dislike of caring for patients. *Nursing Research. 35* (5), 298-302.

Bailey, K. and Wilkinson, S. (1998) Patients' views on nurses communication skills: a pilot study. *International Journal of Palliative Nursing. 4*(6), 300-305.

Baillie, L. (1996) A phenomenological study of the nature of empathy. *Journal of Advanced Nursing. 24*, 1300-1308.

Baker, C., Weust, J. and Noerager, P. (1992) Method slurring: the grounded theory/phenomenology example. *Journal of Advanced Nursing. 17*, 1355-1360.

Banchetti-Robino, M.P. (2000) F.J.J. Buytendijk on Women: A Phenomenological Critique. In, Fisher, L. and Embree, L. (Eds) *Feminist Phenomenology.* The Netherlands, Kluwer Academic Publishers, 83-101.

Barker, M. (2003) Assessing the 'quality' in qualitative research. *European Journal of Communication. 18*(3), 315-335.

Barker, P. (2001) The tidal model: the lived-experience in person-centred mental health nursing care. *Nursing Philosophy. 2*, 213-223.

Barnsteiner, J.H. and Gillis-Donovan, J. (1990) Being related and separate: A standard for therapeutic relationships. *Maternal-Child Nursing Journal. 15*, 223-228.

Beauchamp, T.L. and Childress, J.F. (1998) *Principles of Biomedical Ethics.* Oxford, Oxford University press.

Beck, C.T. (1997) Humour in nursing practice: a phenomenological study. *International Journal of Nursing Studies. 34*, 346-352.

Beckerman, A. (1994) A personal journal of caring through aesthetic knowing. *Advances in Nursing Science. 17*, 71-79.

Bertero, C. (1999) Caring for and about cancer patients: identifying the meaning of the phenomenon "caring" through narratives. *Cancer Nursing. 22*(6), 414-420.

Bignold, S., Cribb, A. and Ball, S. (1995) Befriending the family: An exploration of a nurse-patient relationship. *Health and Social Care in the Community. 3*, 173-180.

Billeter-Koponen, S. and Freden, L. (2005) Long-term stress, burnout and patient-nurse relations: qualitative interview study about nurses' experiences. *Scandinavian Journal of Caring Science. 19*, 20-27.

Birch, M. and Miller, T. (2000) Inviting intimacy: the interview as therapeutic opportunity. *International journal of social research methodology. 3* (3), 189-202.

Bishop, A.H. and Scudder, J.R. (2003) Gadow's contribution to our philosophical interpretation of nursing. *Nursing Philosophy. 4*, 104-110.

Bolton, S. (2000) Who cares? Offering emotion work as a 'gift' in the nursing labour process. *Journal of Advanced Nursing. 32*(3), 580-586.

Bond, S. (1983) Nurses' communication with cancer patients. In, Wilson-Barnett, J. (Editor) *Nursing research: Ten studies in patient care: Development in Nursing Research Volume 2.* London, Wiley, 57-81.

Bondi, L. (2003) Empathy and Identification: Conceptual resources for Feminist Fieldwork. *ACME: An International E-Journal for Critical Geographies. 2*(1), 64-111.

Booth, K., Maguire, P., Butterworth, T. and Hillier, V. (1996) Perceived professional support and the use of blocking behaviours by hospice nurses. *Journal of Advanced Nursing. 24*, 522-527.

Borbasi, S., Jackson, D. and Wilkes, L. (2005) Fieldwork in nursing research: positionality, practicalities and predicaments. *Journal of Advanced Nursing. 51*(5), 493-501.

Bowden, P. (1997) *Caring. Gender-sensitive ethics.* Routledge, London.

Bradshaw, A. (1995) What are nurses doing to patients? A review of theories of nursing past and present. *Journal of Clinical Nursing. 4*(2), 81-92.

Buber, M. (1955/2002) *Between Man and Man.* London, Routledge.

Buresh, B. and Gordon, S. (2000) (Foreword by Benner, P. Afterword by Jeans, M.E.) *From silence to voice.* Ithaca, Cornell University Press.

Bushkin, E. (1995) Signpost of survivorship. Mara Mogensen Flaherty Lectures: Excellence in the psychosocial care of the patient with cancer. *Oncology Nursing Forum. 22*(3), 537-543.

Cameron, B.L. (2002) The Nursing "How are you?", In, van Manen, M. (2002) (Ed) *Writing in the dark. Phenomenological studies in interpretive inquiry.* Althouse press: Ontario, 10-25.

Campbell, A.V. (1984) *Moderated love. A theology of professional care.* London, SPCK.

Carmack, B.J. (1997) Balancing engagement and detachment in caregiving. *Image: Journal of Nursing Scholarship. 29*(2), 139-143.

Caroline, H. (1993) Exploration of close friendship: A concept analysis. *Archives of Psychiatric Nursing. 7*(4), 236-243.

Carveth, J.A. (1995) Perceived patient deviance and avoidance by nurses. *Nursing Research. 44*(3), 173-178.

Chamberlain, K. (2000) Methodolatry and qualitative health research. *Journal of Health Psychology. 5*(3), 285-296.

Clarke, D.M. and Kissane, D.W. (2002) Demoralization: its phenomenology and importance. *Australian and New Zealand Journal of Psychiatry. 36*, 733-742.

Cleary, M. and Freeman, A. (2005) The cultural realities of clinical supervision in an acute inpatient mental health setting. *Issues in Mental Health Nursing. 26*, 489-505.

Cohen, M.Z., Kahn, D.L. and Steeves, R.H. (2000) How to analyze the data. In, Cohen, M.Z., Kahn, D.L. and Steeves, R.H. (Eds) *Hermeneutic phenomenological research. A practical guide for nurse researchers.* Thousand Oaks, Sage Publications, 71-83.

Colaizzi, P.E. (1978) Psychological research as the phenomenologist views it. In, Valle, R.S. and King, M. (Eds) *Existential-phenomenological alternatives for psychology.* New York, Oxford University Press, 48-71.

Colbourne. L, and Sque, M. (2004) Split personalities: role conflict between the nurse and the nurse researcher. *NTresearch.* 9(4), 297-304.

Corner, J. (2002) Nurses' experiences of cancer. European Journal of Cancer Care. 11(3), 193-199.

Crigger, N. (2001) Antecedent to engrossment in Nodding's theory of care. *Journal of Advanced Nursing. 35*(4), 616-623.

Cutliffe, J.R. and McKenna, H.P. (1999) Establishing the credibility of qualitative research findings: the plot thickens. *Journal of Advanced Nursing. 30*, 37-380.

Cutliffe, J.R. and McKenna, H.P. (2004) Expert qualitative researchers and the use of audit trails. *Journal of Advanced Nursing. 45*(2), 126-135.

Davis, C.M. (1990) What is empathy. And how can it be taught? *Physical Therapy. 70,* 707-711.

Davis, C.M. (2003) Empathy and Transcendence. *Topics in Geriatric Rehabilitation. 19*(4), 265-274.

Dennison, S. (1995) An exploration of the communication that takes place between nurses and patients whilst cancer chemotherapy is administered. *Journal of Clinical Nursing. 4,* 227-233.

Denny, K. and McGuigan, M. (1999) The value of the nurse-patient relationship in the care of cancer patients. *Nursing Standard. 13*(33), 45-47.

Denzin, N.K. and Lincoln, Y.S. (Eds) (1994) *Handbook of Qualitative Research.* London, Sage.

Department of Health (UK) (1995) *A policy framework of commissioning cancer services.* London, Department of Health.

de Raeve, L. (1996) Caring intensively. In, Greaves, D. and Upton, H. *Philosophical problems in health care.* Aldershot, Avebury, 9-22.

de Raeve, L. (1997) Positive thinking and moral oppression in cancer care. *European Journal of Cancer Care. 6*, 249-256.

de Raeve, L. (2002) Trust and trustworthiness in nurse-patient relationships. *Nursing Philosophy. 3*, 152-162.

de Witt, L. and Ploeg, J. (2006) Critical appraisal of rigour in interpretive phenomenological nursing research. *Journal of Advanced Nursing. 55*(2), 215-229.

Dignam, D. (1998) Understanding intimacy as experienced by breastfeeding women. *Health Care for Woman International. 16*(5), 477-485.

Domosh, M. (2003) Toward a more fully reciprocal feminist inquiry. *ACME: An International E-Journal for Critical Geographies. 2*(1), 107-111.

Dowling, M. (2003) A concept analysis of intimacy in nursing. *All Ireland Journal of Nursing and Midwifery. 2*(11), 40-46.

Dowling, M. (2004a) Exploring the relationship between caring, love and intimacy in nursing. *British Journal of Nursing. 13*(21), 1289-1292.

Dowling, M. (2004b) Hermeneutics: an exploration. *Nurse Researcher. 11*(4), 30-39.

Dowling, M. (2006a) The Sociology of intimacy in the nurse-patient relationship. *Nursing Standard. 20*(23), 48-54.

Dowling, M. (2006b) Approaches to reflexivity in qualitative research. *Nurse Researcher. 13* (3), 7-21.

Dowling, M. (2007) From Husserl to van Manen: A review of different phenomenological approaches, *International Journal of Nursing Studies. 44*(1), 131-142.

Eberhart, C and Pieper, B.B. (1994) Understanding Human action through narrative expression and Hermeneutic inquiry. In, Chinn, P. (Ed) *Advances in Methods of Inquiry for Nursing.* Maryland, Aspen publications, 41-58.

Edge, J. and Richards, K. (1998) May I see your warrant, please? Justifying outcomes in qualitative research. *Applied Linguistics. 19*(3), 334-356.

English, J. and Morse, J.M. (1988) The difficult elderly patient: adjustment or maladjustment? *International Journal of Nursing Studies. 25*(1), 23-39.

Erlen, J.A. and Jones, M. (1999) The patient no one liked. *Orthopaedic Nursing. 18*(4), 76-79.

Ersser, S. (1991) A search for the therapeutic dimensions of nurse-patient interaction. In, McMahon, R. and Pearson, A. (Eds.) *Nursing as Therapy.* London, Chapman and Hall, 43-83.

Ferguson, L.M., Myrick, F. and Yonge, O. (2006) Ethically involving students in faculty research. *Nurse Education Today. 26*, 705-711.

Fielden, J.M. (2003) Grief as a transformative experience: weaving through different lifeworlds after a loved one has completed suicide. *International Journal of Mental Health Nursing.* 12 (1), 74-85.

Fielding, P. (1986) *Attitudes revisited: an examination of student nurses' attitudes towards old people in hospital.* London, Royal College of Nursing.

Finch, L. (2004) Understanding patients' lived experiences: the interrelationship of rhetoric and hermeneutics. *Nursing Philosophy.* 5, 251-257.

Fisher, L. (2000) Phenomenology and feminism: perspectives on their relation. In Fisher, L. and Embree, L. (Eds) *Feminist Phenomenology.* the Netherlands, Kluwer Academic Publishers , 17-38.

Fleming,V., Gaidys, U. and Robb, Y. (2003) Hermeneutic research in nursing: developing a Gadamerian-based research method. *Nursing Inquiry.* 10(2), 113-120.

Flinders, D.J. (1992) In search of ethical guidance: constructing a basis for dialogue. *Qualitative Studies in Education.* 5(2), 101-115.

Forrest, D. (1989) The experience of caring. *Journal of Advanced Nursing.* 14, 815-823.

Fosbinder, D. (1994) Patient perceptions of nursing care: an emerging theory of interpersonal competence. *Journal of Advanced Nursing.* 20(6), 1085-1093.

Frank, A.W. (2006) Interpretive phenomenology, clinical ethics and research. *Health: An Interdisciplinary Journal for the Social Study of Health, Illness and Medicine.* 10(1), 113-116.

Frankl, V. (1959) *Man's search for meaning.* Boston, Beacon Press.

Frankl, V. (1984) *Man's search for meaning.* New York, Washington Square Press.

Froggatt, K. (1998) The place of metaphor and language in exploring nurses' emotional work. *Journal of Advanced Nursing.* 28(2), 332-328.

Furlong, E. and O'Toole, S. (2006) Psychological care for patients with cancer. In, Kearney, N. and Richardson, A. (Eds) *Nursing Patients with Cancer. Principles and Practice.* Edinburgh, Elsevier, Churchill Livingstone.717-737.

Gadamer, G.H. (1975) *Truth and Method.* London, Sheed and Ward.

Gadamer, G.H. (1989) *Truth and Method* (2nd ed) (Translation revised by Weinsheimer, J. and Marshall, D.G.). London, Sheed and Ward.

Gadow, S. (1980) Existential advocacy: philosophical foundation of nursing. In, Spicker, S.F. and Gadow, S. (Eds) *Nursing: Images and ideals. Opening Dialogue with the Humanities.* New York, Springer, 79-101.

Gadow, S. (1995) Narrative and exploration: towards a poetics of knowledge in nursing. *Nursing Inquiry.* 2, 211-214.

Gaydos, H.L.B. (2003) The cocreative aesthetic process: a new model for aesthetics in nursing. *International Journal for Human Caring.* 7(3), 40-44.

Geanellos, R. (2002) Exploring the therapeutic potential of friendliness and friendship in nurse-client relationships. *Contemporary Nurse.* 12, 235-245.

Geelan, D. and Taylor, P (2001) Writing our lived experience: Beyond the (Pale) Hermeneutic? *Electronic Journal of Science Education.* 5(4), *http://unr.edu/homepage/crowther/ejse/geelanetal.html.*

Gilligan, C. (1982) *In a different voice, Psychological theory and women's development,* Cambridge, MA, Harvard university press.

Glass, E. and Cluxton, D. (2004) Truth-telling. Ethical issues in clinical practice. *Journal of Hospice and Palliative Nursing.* 6(4), 232-242.

Gobbi, M. (2005) Nursing practice as bricoleur activity: a concept explored. *Nursing Inquiry.* 12(2), 117-125.

Goffman, E. (1959) *The presentation of self in everyday life.* New Jersey, Doubleday.

Graber, D.R. and Mitcham, M.D. (2004) Compassionate clinicians. Take patient care beyond the ordinary. *Holistic Nursing Practice.* 18(2), 87-94.

Gray, R.E. and Doan, B.D. (1990) Heroic self-healing and cancer: clinical issues for health professions. *Journal of Palliative Care.* 6, 32-41.

Gregory, D.M. (1994) *Narratives of suffering in the cancer experience.* Unpublished PhD Thesis. Arizona, University of Arizona.

Griffin, A.P. (1983) A philosophical analysis of caring in nursing. *Journal of Advanced Nursing.* 8, 289-295.

Gubrium, J. and Holstein, J.A. (2000) Analyzing interpretive practice. In, Denzin, N. and Lincoln, Y. (Eds) *Handbook of qualitative research* (2nd edition). Thousand Oaks, Sage, 87-508.

Habermas, J. (1990) *Moral Consciousness and Communicative Action* (translated by Lenhardt, C. and Nicholsen, S.). Cambridge, Polity Press.

Haggman-Laitila, A. (1999) The authenticity and ethics of phenomenological research: how to overcome the researcher's own views. *Nursing Ethics.* 6(1), 12-22.

Halldorsdottir, S. and Hamrin, E. (1997) Caring and uncaring encounters within nursing and health care from the cancer patient's perspective. *Cancer Nursing.* 20(2), 120-128.

Hammersley, M. and Atkinson, P. (1983) *Ethnography: Principles in practice.* London, Rougledge.

Hassouneh-Phillips, D. (2003) Strength and vulnerability: spirituality in abused American Muslim women's lives. *Issues in Mental Health Nursing.* 24, 681-694.

Henderson, A. (2001) Emotional labour and nursing: an under-appreciated aspect of caring work. *Nursing Inquiry.* 8(2), 130-138.

Hess, J. (2003) Gadow's relational narrative: an elaboration. *Nursing Philosophy.* 4(2), 137-147.

Hochschild, A.R. (1979) Emotion work, feeling rules, and social structure. *American Journal of Sociology.* 85, 551-575.

Hochschild, A.R. (1983) *The managed heart: Commercialization of human feeling:* Berkeley, University of California Press.

Hodges, H., Keeley, A. Grier, E. (2001) Masterworks of art and chronic illness experiences in the elderly. *Journal of Advanced Nursing.* 36(3), 389-398.

Holloway, I. and Wheeler, S. (1996) *Qualitative Research for Nurses.* Blackwell Science: London.

Hudson, S. (1999) Ethics of alternative paradigms: An exploration of options. *Graduate Research in Nursing. http://graduateresearch.com/hudson.htm* (12 pages).

Hunt, M. (1991) Being friendly and informal: reflected in nurses', terminally ill patients' and relatives' conversations at home. *Journal of Advanced Nursing.* 16, 929-938.

Husserl, E. (1970) The idea of Phenomenology. The Hague, Nijhoff.

Hycner, R.H. (1985) Some guidelines for the phenomenological analysis of interview data. *Human Studies. 8*, 279-303.

Im, E. and Chee, W. (2003) Fuzzy logic and nursing. *Nursing Philosophy.* 4, 53-60.

Jarrett, N. and Payne, S. (1995) A selective review of the literature on nurse-patient communication: has the patient's contribution been neglected? *Journal of Advanced Nursing. 22*, 72-78.

Jarrett, N. and Payne, S. (2000) Creating and maintaining 'optimism' in cancer care communication. *International Journal of Nursing Studies. 37*, 81-90.

Jenny, J. and Logan, J. (1992) Knowing the patient: one aspect of clinical knowledge. *Image: Journal of Nursing Scholarship. 24*(2), 254-258.

Johnson, M. and Webb, C. (1995) Rediscovering unpopular patients: the concept of social judgement. *Journal of Advanced Nursing. 21*, 466-475.

Johnson, M. (1997) *Nursing Power and Social Judgment.* Aldershot, Ashgate.

Johnson, M., Long, T. and White, A. (2001) Arguments for "British Pluralism" in qualitative health research. *Journal of Advanced Nursing. 33*(2), 243-249.

Johnstone, M.J. (1987) Professional ethics in nursing: a philosophical analysis. *The Australian Journal of Advanced Nursing. 4*(3), 12-21.

Jones, A. (2001) Some experiences of professional practice and beneficial changes derived from clinical supervision by community Macmillan nurses. *European Journal of Cancer Care. 10*, 21-30.

Jones, J. and Borbasi, S. (2004) Interpretive research: weaving a phenomenological text. In, Clare, J. and Hamilton, H. (Eds) *Writing research. Transforming data into text.* Edinburgh, Churchill Livingstone, 85-101.

Jongudomkarn, D. and West, B. (2004) Work life and psychological health: the experiences of Thai women in deprived communities. *Health care for women international.* 25, 527-542.

Kadner, K. (1994) Therapeutic intimacy in nursing. *Journal of Advanced Nursing. 19*, 215-218.

Kahn, D.L. (2000a) How to conduct research. In, Cohen, M.Z., Kahn, D.L. and Steeves, R.H. (Editors) *Hermeneutic Phenomenological Research. A practical guide for nurse researchers.* Thousand Oaks, Sage Publications, 59-70.

Kahn D.L. (2000b) Reducing bias. In, Cohen, M.Z., Kahn, D.L. and Steeves, R.H. (Eds) *Hermeneutic Phenomenological Research. A practical guide for nurse researchers.* Thousand Oaks, Sage Publications, 85-92.

Kelly, M.P. and May, D. (1982) Good and bad patients: a review of the literature and a theoretical critique. *Journal of Advanced Nursing. 7*, 147-156.

Kendrick, K. and Hughes, N. (2002) Spirituality: its dynamics and purpose in Nursing a person with a new diagnosis of cancer. In, Clarke, D., Flanagan, J. and Kendrick, K. (Editors). *Advancing Nursing Practice in Cancer and Palliative Care.* Hampshire, Palgrave Macmillan, 140-152.

Kines, M. (1999) The risks of caring too much. *Canadian Nurse. 95*, 27-30.

Kirk, T.W. (2007) Beyond empathy: clinical intimacy in nursing practice. *Nursing Philosophy. 8*, 233-243.

Kleiman S (2004) What is the nature of Nurse Practitioners' lived experiences of interacting with patients? *Journal of the American Academy of Nurse Practitioners. 16*(2), 263-269.

Koch, T. (1996) Implementation of a hermeneutic inquiry in nursing: philosophy, rigour and representation. *Journal of Advanced Nursing. 21*, 827-836.

Koch, T. (1998) Story telling: is it really research? *Journal of Advanced Nursing. 28*(6), 1182-1190.

Koch, T. (1999) An interpretive research process: revisiting phenomenological and hermeneutical approaches. *Nurse Researcher, 6*(3), 20-34.

Koch, T. and Harrington, A. (1998) Reconceptualizing rigour: the case for reflexivity. *Journal of Advanced Nursing. 28* (4), 882-890.

Kralik, D., Koch, T. and Wotton, K. (1997) Engagement and detachment: understanding patients' experiences with nursing. *Journal of Advanced Nursing. 26*, 399-407.

Krishnasamy, M. (1996) What do cancer patients identify as supportive and unsupportive behaviour of nurses? A pilot study. *European Journal of Cancer Care. 5*, 103-110.

Krishnasamy, M. and Plant, H. (1998) Developing nursing research with people. *International Journal of Nursing Studies. 35*, 79-84.

Kristjansdottir, G. (1992) Empathy: a therapeutic phenomenon in nursing care. *Journal of Clinical Nursing. 1*, 131-140.

Kruijver, I., Kerkstra, A., Bensing, J.M. and van de Wiel, H.B.M. (2000) Nurse-patient communication in cancer care. A review of the literature. *Cancer Nursing. 23*(1), 20-31.

Langley-Evans, A. and Payne, S. (1997) Light-hearted death talk in a palliative day care context. *Journal of Advanced Nursing. 26*, 1091-1097.

Larson, P.J. (1984) Important nurse care behaviours perceived by patients with cancer. *Oncology Nursing Forum. 11*, 46-50.

Larsson, G., Widmark, V., Lampic, C. von Essen, L. and Sjoden, P. (1998) Cancer patient and staff ratings of the importance of caring behaviours and their relations to patient anxiety and depression. *Journal of Advanced Nursing. 27*, 855-864.

Lauver, D.R. (2000) Commonalities in Women's Spirituality and Women's Health. *Advances in Nursing Science. 22*(3), 76-88.

Lawler, J. (1991) *Behind the screens: Nursing, somology, and the problems of the body.* Melbourne, Churchill Livingstone.

Lee, R.M. and Fielding, N.G. (2004) Tools for qualitative data analysis. In, Hardy, M. and Bryman, A. (Editors) *Handbook of Data Analysis*. London, Sage, 529-546.

Lemonidou, C., Papathanassoglou, E., Margarita, G., Patiraki, E. and Papadatou, D. (2004) Moral professional personhood: ethical reflections during initial clinical encounters in nursing education. *Nursing Ethics. 11*(2), 122-137.

Levesque-Lopman, L. (2000) Listen, and you will hear: reflections on interviewing from a feminist phenomenological perspective. In, Fisher, L. and Embree, L. (Eds) *Feminist Phenomenology.* the Netherlands, Kluwer Academic Publishers, 103-132.

Levine, C. (2002) The lost art of caring. *Journal of American Geriatrics Society. 50*(12), 2086-2088.

Lidz, V. (2000) Talcot Parsons. In, Ritzer, G. (Ed). *The Blackwell Companion to Major Social Theorists.* Massechusetts, Blackwell, 388-431.

Lindlof, T.R. and Taylor, B.C. (2002) *Qualitative communication research methods.* (2nd edition). Thousand Oaks, Sage Publications.

Lindseth, A., Marhaug, V., Norberg, A. and Uden, G. (1994) Registered nurses' and physicians' reflections on their narratives about ethically difficult care episodes. *Journal of Advanced Nursing. 20*, 245-250.

Linge, D.E. (1976) Editors Introduction. In, Linge, D. (Ed) *Hans Georg Gadamer. Philosophical Hermeneutics.* Berkeley, University of California Press.

Liu, J.E., Mok, E. and Wong, T. (2006) Caring in nursing: investigating the meaning of caring from the perspective of cancer patients in Beijing, China. *Journal of Clinical Nursing. 15*, 188-196.

Loftus, L.A. and McDowell, J. (2000) The lived experience of the Oncology clinical nurse specialist. *International Journal of Nursing Studies. 37*, 513-521.

Long, T. and Johnson, M. (2000) Rigor, reliability and validity in qualitative research. *Clinical Effectiveness in Nursing. 4*, 30-37.

Lorber, J. (1975) Good patients and problem patients; conformity and deviance in a general hospital. *Journal of Health and Social Behaviour. 16*, 213-225.

Maatta, S.M. (2006) Closeness and distance in the nurse-patient relationship. The relevance of Edith Stein's concept of empathy. *Nursing Philosophy. 7*, 3-10.

Macleod Clark, J. (1982) *Nurse-patient verbal interactions: an analysis of recorded conversations in selected surgical wards.* PhD thesis. London, Royal College of Nursing, Maguire, P., Roe, P., Goldberg, D., Jones, S., Hyde, C. and O'Dowd, T. (1978) The value of feedback in teaching interviewing skills to medical students. *Psychological Medicine. 8*, 695-704.

Maguire, P. (1985) Barriers to psychological care of the dying. *British Medical Journal. 291*, 1711-1713.

Maguire, P. (1995) Psychosocial interventions to reduce affective disorders in cancer patients: research priorities. *Psycho-Oncology. 4*, 113-119.

Maguire, P. and Faulkner, A. (1988) Improve the counselling skills for doctors and nurses in cancer. *British Medical Journal. 297*, 847-849.

Maher, A. (2003) *The essential structure of power and powerlessness as experienced by staff nurses in their practice on surgical units in a General Hospital.* Unpublished MSc thesis. London, Royal College of Nursing.

Malloy, G.B. and Berkery, A.C. (1993) Codependency: a feminist perspective. *Journal of Psychosocial nursing. 31*(4), 15-19.

Manning, P.L (1967) Problems in interpreting interview data. *Sociology and Social Research. 51*, 301-316.

Marcus, G.E. (1994) What comes (just) after 'post'? the case of ethnography. In Denzin, N. and Lincoln, Y. (Eds) *Handbook of Qualitative research.* London, Sage, 563-574.

Martsolf, D.S. (2002) Codependency, boundaries and professional nurse caring. Understanding similarities and differences in nursing practice. *Orthopaedic Nursing. 21*(6), 61-67.

Masseé, R. (2000) Qualitative and quantitative analyses of psychological distress: methodological complementarity and ontological incommensurability. *Qualitative Health Research. 10*, 411-423.

Massie, M.J. and Holland, J. (1989) Overview of normal reactions and prevalence of psychiatric disorders. In, Holland, J.C. and Rowland, J.H. (Eds) *Handbook of psychooncology: psychological care of the patient with cancer.* New York, Oxford University Press. 273-282.

Mauthner, N. and Doucet, A. (2003) Reflexive accounts and accounts of reflexivity in qualitative data analysis. *Sociology. 37*(3), 413-431.

May, C. (1990) Therapeutic reciprocity: a caring phenomenon. *Advances in Nursing Science. 13*, 49-59.

May, C. (1991) Affective neutrality and involvement in nurse-patient relationships: perceptions of appropriate behaviour among nurses in acute medical and surgical wards. *Journal of Advanced Nursing. 16*, 552-558.

May, C., Allison, G., Chapple, A., Chew-Graham, C., Dixon, C., Gask, L., Graham, R., Rogers, A. and Roland, M. (2004) Framing the doctor-patient relationship in chronic illness: a comparative study of general practitioners' accounts. *Sociology of Health and Illness. 26*(2), 135-158.

Mayer, D. (1986) Cancer patients' and families' perceptions of nurse caring behaviours. *Topics in Clinical Nursing.* 8 (1), 63-69.

Maynard, M. (2004) Feminist issues in data analysis. In, Hardy, M. and Bryman, A. (EdS) *Handbook of data analysis.* London, Sage Publications, 131-145.

McCance, T., McKenna, H. and Boore, J. (1997) Caring: dealing with a difficult concept. *International Journal of Nursing Studies. 34*(4), 241-248.

McCormick, J., Kirkham, S.R. and Hayes, V. (1998) Abstracting women: Essentialism in women's health research. *Health Care for Woman International.* 19(6), 495-504.

McDowell, L. (1992) Doing gender: feminism, feminists and research methods in human geography. *Transactions, Institute of British Geographers.* 17, 399-416.

McIlfatrick, S.J. (2003) *Exploring patients', caregivers' and nurses' experience of day hospital chemotherapy: a phenomenological study.* University of Ulster, Unpublished PhD thesis, Faculty of Life and Health Sciences.

McLeod, M. (1994) It's the little things that count: the hidden complexity of everyday nursing practice. *Journal of Clinical Nursing. 3*, 361-368.

McNamarra, B., Waddell, C. and Colvin, M. (1994) The institutionalisation of a good death. *Social Science and Medicine. 11*, 1501-1508.

Meehan, T. (2003) Careful nursing: a model for contemporary nursing practice. *Journal of Advanced Nursing. 44*(1), 99-107.

Mehrabian, A. and Epstein, A. (1972) A measure of emotional empathy. *Journal of Personality. 40*, 525-543.

Merleau-Ponty, M. (1945/1962) *Phenomenology of Perception.* (Translated by Smith, C.). Boston, Routledge and Kegan Paul.

Miller, S. (2003) Analysis of phenomenological data generated with children as research participants. *Nurse Researcher. 10*(4), 68-82.

Mohr, W.K. (1999) Deconstructing the language of psychiatric hospitalisation. *Journal of Advanced Nursing. 29*, 1052-1059.

Monk, J., Manning, P. and Denman, C. (2003) Working together: Feminist perspectives on collaborative research and action. *ACME: An International E-Journal for Critical Geographies.* 2(1), 91-106.

Moran, D. (2000) *Introduction to phenomenology.* London, Routledge.

Morse, J. (1991) Negotiating commitment and involvement in the nurse-patient relationship. *Journal of Advanced Nursing.* 16, 455-468.

Morse, J., Solberg, S., Neander, W., Bottorff, J. and Johnson, J. (1990) Concepts of caring and caring as a concept. *Advances in Nursing Science.* 13(1), 1-14.

Morse, J., Bottorff, J., Anderson, G., OBrien, B. and Solberg, S. (1992) Beyond empathy: expanding expressions of caring. *Journal of Advanced Nursing.* 17, 809-821.

Morse, J.M. and Mitcham, C. (1997) Compathy: the contagion of physical distress. *Journal of Advanced Nursing.* 26, 649-657.

Morton, R. (1996) Breaking bad news to patients with cancer. *Professional Nurse.* 11(10), 669-671.

Moustakas, C. (1994) *Phenomenological research methods.* Thousand Oaks, Sage Publications.

Moyle, W. (2002) Unstructured interviews: challenges when participants have a major depressive illness. *Journal of Advanced Nursing.* 39(3), 266-273.

Muhr, T. (2004) Atlas ti (2004) *User's manual for Atlas.ti V5.0* (2nd edition) Berlin, Atlas ti. Mullholland, J. (1997) Assimilating sociology: critical reflections on the 'Sociology in nursing' debate. *Journal of Advanced Nursing.* 25(4), 844-852.

Munhall, P.L. (1993) "Unknowing": toward another pattern of knowing in nursing. *Nursing Outlook.* 41(3), 125-128.

Nielsen, J.M. (1990) Introduction. In, Nielsen, J.M. (Ed) *Feminist Research Methods: Exemplary readings in the social sciences.* Westview Press, Boulder, Colorado, 1-37.

Noddings, N. (1984) *Caring, a feminine approach to ethics and morals.* Berkely, California, University of California Press.

Northouse, P.G. and Northouse, L.L. (1987) Communication and cancer: issues confronting patients, health professionals, and family members. *Journal of Psychosocial Oncology.* 5, 17-46.

Oakley, A. (1981) Interviewing women: a contradiction in terms. In, Roberts, H. (Ed). *Doing feminist research.* London, Routledge and Kegan Paul, 30-61.

O'Baugh, J., Wilkes, L.M., Luke, S. and George, A. (2003) 'Being positive': perception of patients with cancer and their nurses. *Journal of Advanced Nursing.* 44(3), 262-270.

O'Brien, J. (1999) Negotiating the relationship; Mental health nurses' perceptions of their practice. *Australian and New Zealand Journal of Mental Health Nursing.* 8, 153-161.

Olesen V (1994) Feminisms and models of qualitative research. In Denzin, N.K. and Lincoln, Y.S. (Eds) *Handbook of qualitative research.* Thousand Oaks, California, Sage, 158-174.

Omer, H. and Rosenbaum, R. (1997) Diseases of hope and the work of despair. *Psychotherapy.* 34(3), 225-232.

Ozdogan, M., Samur, M., Artac, M., Yildiz, M., Savas, B. and Bozcuk, H. (2006) Factors related to truth-telling practice of Physicians treating patients with cancer in Turkey. *Journal of Palliative Medicine.* 9(5), 1114-1119.

Paley, J. (2002) Caring as a slave morality: Nietzschean themes in nursing ethics. *Journal of Advanced Nursing. 40*(1), 25-35.

Parsons, T. (1951) *The Social System.* New York, Free Press.

Pascoe, E. (1996) The value to nursing research of Gadamer's Hermeneutic philosophy. *Journal of Advanced Nursing. 24*, 1309-1314.

Patterson, J. and Zderad, L. (1975) *Humanistic Nursing.* (2nd edition). New York, National League for Nursing.

Peplau, H.E. (1952) *Interpersonal Relations in Nursing.* New York, GP Putman and Sons.

Perreault, A., Fothergill-Bourbannais, F. and Fiset, V. (2004) The experience of family members caring for a dying loved one. *International Journal of Palliative Nursing. 10*(3), 133-144.

Pettegrew, L. and Turkat, I. (1986) How patients communicate about their illness. *Health Communication Research. 12*, 376-394.

Polkinghorne, D.E. (1988) *Narrative knowing and the human sciences.* Albany, NY: State university of New York.

Price, B. (2002) Laddered questions and qualitative data research interviews. *Journal of Advanced Nursing. 37*(3), 273-281.

Priest, H. (2002) An approach to the phenomenological analysis of data, *Nurse Researcher. 10*(2), 50-63.

Radwin, L. (2000) Oncology patients' perceptions of quality nursing care. *Research in nursing and health. 23*, 179-190.

Ramos, M.C. (1992) The nurse-patient relationship: theme and variations. *Journal of Advanced Nursing. 17*, 496-606.

Rawnsley, M.M. (1980) Toward a conceptual base for affective nursing. *Nursing Outlook. 28*(4), 244-247.

Ray, M.A. (1994) The richness of Phenomenology: Philosophic, Theoretic, and Methodologic concerns. In, Morse, J.M. (Ed) *Critical issues in qualitative research methods*. Thousand Oaks, Sage publications, 117-133.

Reiman, J.H. (1976) Privacy, intimacy, and personhood. *Philosophy and public affairs. 6*, 26-44.

Reynolds, W.J. and Scott, B. (2000) Do nurses and other professional helpers normally display much empathy? *Journal of Advanced Nursing. 31*(1), 226-234.

Richards, H.M. and Schwartz, L.J. (2002) Ethics of qualitative research: are there special issues for health services research? *Family Practice. 19*, 135-139.

Ridner, S. (2004) Psychological distress: concept analysis. *Journal of Advanced Nursing. 45*(5), 536-545.

Rittenberg, C.N. (1995) Positive thinking: An unfair burden for cancer patients? *Supportive Care in Cancer. 3*(1), 37-39.

Rittman, M., Paige, P., Rivera, J., Sutphin, L. and Godown, I. (1997) Phenomenological study of nurses caring for dying patients. *Cancer Nursing. 20*, 115-119.

Roach, S. (1987) *The Human Act of Caring: A blueprint for the Health professionals.* Ottowa, Ontario, Canadian Hospital Association.

Roberts, D. (1984) Non-verbal communication: popular and unpopular patients. In, Faulkner, A. (Ed) *Communication: recent advances in nursing series.* Edinburgh, Churchill Livingstone, 3-25.

Roberts, D. and Snowball, J. (1999) Psychosocial care in oncology nursing: a study of social knowledge. *Journal of Clinical Nursing. 8*, 39-47.

Rodgers, B.L. (1989) Concepts, analysis and the development of nursing knowledge: the evolutionary cycle. *Journal of Advanced Nursing.* 14, 330-335.

Rodgers, B.L. (1993) Concept analysis: An evolutionary view. In, Rodgers B.L. and Knafl, K. (Eds). *Concept development in nursing. Foundations, Techniques, and Applications.* Philadelphia, W.B. Saunders Company, 73-92.

Rogers, C.R. (1975) The necessary and sufficient conditions of therapeutic personality changes. *Journal of Consulting Psychology. 21*(4), 95-103.

Roth, J. (1972) Some contingencies of the moral evaluation and control of clientele. *American Journal of Sociology. 77*, 839-856.

Rustoen, T. and Hanestad, B.R. (1998) Nursing intervention to increase hope in cancer patients. *Journal of Clinical Nursing. 7*, 19-27.

Salvage, J. (1990) The theory and practice of the 'new' nursing. *Nursing Times.* Occasional paper. *86*(4), 42-45.

Sandelowski, M. (1986) The problem of rigour in qualitative research. *Advances in Nursing Science. 8* (3), 27-37.

Sandelowski, M. (1998) The call to experts in qualitative research. *Research in Nursing and Health. 21*, 467-471.

Savage, J. (1995) *Nursing Intimacy. An ethnographic approach to nurse-patient interaction.* London, Scutari Press.

Sawyer, H. (2000) Meeting the information needs of cancer patients. *Professional Nurse. 15*(4), 244-247.

Scannell-Desch, E.A. (2005) Prebereavement and postbereavement struggles and triumphs of midlife widows. *Journal of Hospice and Palliative Nursing. 7*(1), 15-22.

Scheler, M. (1992) *On feeling. Knowing, and valuing.* Selected Writings (Edited with an introduction by Harold J Bershady). Chicago, The University of Chicago Press.

Schou, K.C. and Hewison, J. (1999) *Experiencing Cancer.* Buckingham, Open University Press.

Schubert. P.E. (1989) *Mutual Connectedness: Holistic nursing practice under varying conditions of intimacy.* Unpublished PhD Thesis, San Francisco, University of California.

Schutz, S. (1994) Exploring the benefits of a subjective approach in qualitative nursing research. *Journal of Advanced Nursing. 20* (3), 412-417.

Scott, P.A. (1995) Care, attention and imaginative identification in nursing practice. *Journal of Advanced Nursing. 21*, 1196-1200.

Severinsson, E.I. and Borgenhammar, E.V. (1997) Expert views on clinical supervision: a study based on interviews. *Journal of Nursing Management. 5*(3), 175-183.

Shattell, M. (2002) "Eventually it'll be over". The dialectic between confinement and freedom in the phenomenal world of the hospitalized patient. In, Thomas, S. and Pollio,

H. (Eds) *Listening to patients: A phenomenological approach to nursing research and practice.* New York, Springer. 214-236.

Shattell, M. (2005) Nurse bait: strategies hospitalised patients use to entice nurses within the context of interpersonal relationship. *Issues in Mental Health Nursing. 26*, 205-223.

Shelly, J.A. (1991) Codependency and caring. *Journal of Christian Nursing. 8* (2), 3.

Sherman, J.B., Cardea, J.M., Gaskill, S.D. and Tynan, C.M. (1989) Caring: commitment to excellence or condemnation to conformity? *Journal of Psychosocial Nursing. 27*(8), 25-29.

Sigsworth, J. (1995) Feminist research: its relevance to nursing. *Journal of Advanced Nursing. 22* (5), 896-899.

Skilbeck, J. and Payne, S. (2003) Emotional support and the role of the Clinical Nurse Specialist in palliative care. *Journal of Advanced Nursing. 43*(5), 521-530.

Slevin, M.L. (1987) Talking about cancer: how much is too much? *British Journal of Hospital Medicine.* July, 56-59.

Smith, P. (1992) The *emotional labour of nursing: How nurses care.* Basingstoke, Macmillan.

Smyth, T. (1996) Reinstating the person in the professional: reflections on empathy and aesthetic experience. *Journal of Advanced Nursing. 24*, 932-937.

Spence, D. (2001) Hermeneutic notions illuminate cross-cultural nursing experiences. *Journal of Advanced Nursing. 35*(4), 624-630.

Spiegelberg, H. (1982) *The phenomenological movement.* Dordrecht, the Netherlands, Martinus Nijhoff.

Stafford, L. (2001) Is codependency a meaningful concept? *Issues in Mental Health Nursing. 22*, 273-286.

Stein, E. (1917/1970). *On the problem of empathy.* (Translated by Stein, W.) (2nd Edition). The Hague, Martinus Nijhoff.

Stein, W. (1970) Preface. Stein, E. (1917/1970). *On the problem of empathy.* (Translated by Stein, W.) (2nd Edition). The Hague, Martinus Nijhoff.

Steeves, R.H. (2000a) Writing the results. In, Cohen, M.Z., Kahn, D.L. and Steeves, R.H. (Editors) *Hermeneutic phenomenological research. A practical guide for nurse researchers.* Thousand Oaks, Sage Publications, 93-99.

Steeves, R.H. (2000b) Sampling. In, Cohen, M.Z., Kahn, D.L. and Steeves, R.H. (Eds) *Hermeneutic phenomenological research. A practical guide for nurse researchers.* Thousand Oaks, Sage Publications, 45-56.

Stockwell, F. (1972) *The Unpopular patient.* London, Royal College of Nursing.

Strauss, A.L., Fagerhaugh, S., Suczek, B. and Wiener, C. (1982) The work of hospitalised patients. *Social Science and Medicine. 16*, 977-986.

Suominen, T., Leini-Kilpi, H. and Laippala, P. (1995) Who provides support and how? *Cancer Nursing. 18*, 278-285.

Tanner, C.A., Benner, P., Chesla, C. and Gordon, D.R. (1993) The phenomenology of knowing the patient. *Image: Journal of Nursing Scholarship. 25*(4), 273-280.

Taylor, B. (1994) *Being Human. Ordinariness in Nursing.* Melbourne, Churchill Livingstone.

Teasdale, K., Brocklehurst, N. and Thom, N. (2001) Clinical supervision and support for nurses: an evaluation study. *Journal of Advanced Nursing. 33*, 216-225.

Thorne, S.E. (1991) Methodological orthodoxy in qualitative research: analysis of the issues. *Qualitative Health Research.* *1*(2), 178-199.

Timmerman, G.M. (1991) A concept analysis of Intimacy. *Issues in Mental Health Nursing.* *12*, 19-30.

Tippl, H. (1995) Significant relationships: Nurses caring for adolescents with cystic fibrosis. *Contemporary Nurse.* *4*(3), 123-128.

Tishelman, C., Bernhardson, B, Blomberg, K., Borjeson, S., Franklin, L., Johansson, E., Levealahti, H, Sahlberg-Blom, E. and Ternestedt, B. (2004) Complexity in caring for patients with advanced cancer. *Journal of Advanced Nursing.* *45*(4), 420-429.

Travelbee, J. (1971) *Interpersonal aspects of nursing.* Philadelphia, FA Davis.

Trygstad, L. (1986) Professional friends: The inclusion of the personal into the professional. *Cancer Nursing.* *9*(6), 326-332.

Tuckett, A. (2005) Qualitative research sampling: the very real complexities. *Nurse Researcher.* *12*(1), 47-61.

Turner, M. (1999) Involvement or over-involvement? Using grounded theory to explore the complexities of nurse-patient relationships. *European Journal of Oncology Nursing.* *3*(3), 153-160.

van Kaam, A.L. (1959) The nurse in the patients world. *American Journal of Nursing.* *59*(12),1710.

van Kaam, A.L. (1969) *Existential Foundations of Psychology.* New York, Doubleday.

van Manen, M. (1984) Practicing phenomenological writing. *Phenomenology and Pedagogy.* *2*(1), 36-69.

van Manen, M. (1990) *Researching the lived experience: Human science for an action sensitive pedagogy.* New York, SUNY.

van Manen, M. (1997) From meaning to method. *Qualitative Health Research. 7,* 345-369.

van Manen, M (2002) Care-as-worry, or "Don't worry, Be Happy". *Qualitative Health Research. 12*(2), 264-280.

von Essen, L. and Sjoden, P.O. (1991) The importance of nurse caring behaviours as perceived by Swedish hospital patients and nursing staff. *International Journal of Nursing Studies. 28*, 267-281.

Walsh, K. (1996) *Being a psychiatric nurse: shared humanity and the nurse patient encounter.* University of Adelaide, South Australia, Unpublished PhD thesis.

Waterworth, S. and Luker, K. (1990) Reluctant collaborators: do patients want to be involved in decisions regarding care? *Journal of Advanced Nursing. 15*, 971-996.

Watson, J. (1988) *Nursing: Human science and Human care. A theory of nursing.* New York, National League for Nursing.

Watson, T.J. (2000) Ethnographic fiction science: Making sense of managerial work and organisational research processes with Caroline and Terry. *Organization. 7*(3), 89-510.

Wayman, L.M. and Gaydos, H.L. (2005) Self-transcending through suffering. *Journal of Hospice and Palliative Nursing. 7*(5), 263-270.

Webster, M. (1981) Communicating with dying patients. *Nursing Times. 77*(23), 999-1002.

Weitzman, E.A. (2000) Software and qualitative research. In, Denzin, N. and Lincoln, Y. (Eds) *Handbook of Qualitative Research.* (2nd edition).Thousand Oaks, Sage Publications, 803-820.

Wengstrom, Y. and Ededahl, M. (2006) The art of professional development and caring in cancer nursing. *Nursing and Health Sciences. 8*, 20-26.

Wettergren, L. (1996) Psychosocial nursing: a new discipline in cancer care. *European Journal of Palliative Care. 1,* 6-8.

White, S.J. (1997) Empathy: a literature review and concept analysis. *Journal of Clinical Nursing. 6*, 253-257.

Wigton, R.S. (1996) Social judgement and medical judgement. *Thinking and Reasoning. 2*(2/3), 175-190.

Wilkinson, S. (1991) Factors which influence how nurses communicate with cancer patients. *Journal of Advanced Nursing. 16*, 677-688.

Wilkinson, S., Bailey, K., Aldridge, J. and Roberts, A. (1999) A longitudinal evaluation of a communication skills programme. *Palliative Medicine. 13*, 341-348.

Wilkinson, S. and Kitzinger, C. (2000) Thinking differently about thinking positive: A discursive approach to cancer patients' talk. *Social Sciences and Medicine. 50*, 797-811.

Wilkinson, S., Gambles, M. and Roberts, A. (2002) The essence of cancer care: the impact of training on nurses' ability to communicate effectively. *Journal of Advanced Nursing. 40*(6), 731-738.

Wilkes, L.M., O'Baugh, J. and Luke, S. (2003) Positive attitude in cancer: Patients' perspective. *Oncology Nursing Forum. 30*(3), 412-416.

Williams, A. (2001a) A study of practising nurses' perceptions and experiences of intimacy within the nurse-patient relationship. *Journal of Advanced Nursing. 35* (2), 188-196.

Williams, A. (2001b) A literature review on the concept of intimacy in nursing. *Journal of Advanced Nursing. 33*(5), 660-667.

Williams, A. and Irurita, V. (1998) Therapeutically conductive relationships between nurses and patients: An important component of quality nursing care. *Australian Journal of Advanced Nursing. 162*(2), 36-44.

Williams, A.M. and Irurita, V.F. (2004) Therapeutic and non-therapeutic interpersonal interactions: the patient's perspective. *Journal of Clinical Nursing. 13*, 806-815.

Wimpenny, P. and Gass, J. (2000) Interviewing in phenomenology and grounded theory: is there a difference. *Journal of Advanced Nursing. 31*(6), 1485-1492.

Wong, K.Y., Lee, W.M. and Mok, E. (2001) Educating nurses to care for the dying in Hong Kong: A problem based learning approach. *Cancer Nursing. 24*(2), 112-120.

Yardley, L. (2000) Dilemmas in qualitative health research. *Psychology and Health. 15*, 215-228.

Yegdich T (1999) On the phenomenology of empathy in nursing: empathy or sympathy? *Journal of Advanced Nursing. 30*(1), 83-93.

Yonge, O. and Molzahn, A. (2002) Exceptional non-traditional caring practices of nurses. *Scandinavian Journal of Caring Science. 16*, 399-405.

In: Trends in Nursing Research
Editors: Adam J. Ryan and Jack Doyle
ISBN 978-1-60456-642-0
© 2009 Nova Science Publishers, Inc.

Chapter 2

Hospitalized Patients' Expectations of Spiritual Care from Nurses

Lisa A. Davis
West Texas A&M University, Texas, USA

Abstract

Nurses are aware that the profession of nursing is holistic, that every action taken in the care of a patient has consequences, and they like to believe that those consequences have a positive impact on the patient and their family's ultimate health. For nurses, gaining an understanding of patients' expectations regarding spiritual care is essential to entering into a truly holistic, caring relationship with patients. The purpose of this phenomenolo-gical study was to explore the expectations patients have of nurses and how patients describe good nursing care. Specifically, questions were posed to reveal participants' perceptions of spiritual care provided by their nurses. Using Paterson's and Zderad's framework of humanistic nursing, 11 participants were interviewed. Data were analyzed using the Giorgi method of repetitive reflection. Findings suggested that participants appreciated nursing presence, being there, as having a positive influence on their health and well being, and elements of nursing presence were used to describe good nursing care. In fact, the spiritual element of nursing presence, being with, comprised the most defining characteristics of good nursing care, but, paradoxically, was not expected. Sharing of self by nurses was appreciated from the participants' perspective. All participants were able to define spirituality, most frequently in terms of religiosity; and religious elements of spirituality were not expected, nor welcomed, by most participants. Participants revealed that they perceived nurses to be busy, and this perceived lack of time was offered as a rationale for not expecting spiritual care.

Introduction

The hallmark of nursing as a profession is that of holism, a concern with not only the physical health of the client, but the mental and spiritual health as well (Burkhart, 1989; Carson, 1989; Dossey, 1998; Fontaine, 2000; Patterson & Zderad, 1988; Stuart, Deckro, & Mandle, 1989; Taylor, 2002; Travelbee, 1969; Watson, 1999). Furthermore, nursing care should address needs that may arise from these human dimensions of body, mind and spirit and recognize the impact that each dimension has on the others (Patterson, 1998; Taylor, 2002). Martha Rogers (1972) further stipulated that the mind, body and spirit are an irreducible whole, not to be treated separately, and all (mind, body and spirit) contribute to overall human health with dynamic interplay.

Watson (1999) recognized holism in her assertion that persons need to be cared for and to find harmony in life. Given that, nursing is charged with helping people gain " a higher degree of harmony within the mind, body and soul" (Watson, 1999, p. 10). Dossey (1998) stresses that not focusing clinical attention to the concepts of mind, body and spirit in patient care is unscientific. Attention to issues of values and purpose in life are just as important as attention to physical parameters such as blood pressure. According to Benner (1985), nurses cannot understand health and illness by merely studying the mind or the body, but rather by studying the person in context. The integrality of body, mind, and spirit is central to holistic practice, so much so, that Quinn (2000) refers to the dimensions as bodymindspirit. Watson and Smith's (2002) framework of transpersonal caring emphasizes the spiritual dimension by honoring both nurse and patient as embodied spirits. Indeed, Bensley (1991) suggests that not only are body, mind and spirit dimensions of health, the spiritual dimension is the coordinator, the element that unifies the other dimensions of health. There is considerable discussion in nursing literature of the relative value of the dimensions of holism, but it is clear that value is placed in the holistic care of patients. Yet, nurses report they rarely, if ever, provide spiritual care (Stranahan, 2001; Thomas et al, 2002). The questions then arise: Are nurses meeting the needs of patients? Are those needs perceived as being met by patients?

Purpose of Study

Nurses understand that while each person is a unique individual and responds individually to care, all humans are more alike than different and value comes from that common humanness (Patterson & Zderad, 1985). The purpose of this study was to explore the expectations patients have of nurses regarding the spiritual dimension of care and to identify how patients describe good nursing care. Philosophically, separating the spiritual dimension from the whole changes it. David Bohm (1996) refers to this as fragmentation – thought that divides. While the spiritual dimension is the concept of interest, it should be remembered that spirituality is part of a greater whole. As with dialogue, separation from the whole should not take on great importance. Rather, exploring the dimensions and understanding the integrality of the human experience is the ultimate goal. Nursing literature is replete with studies of nurses' perceptions of the meanings and constituents of spiritual care, while studies of patient perceptions of the meaning of spiritual care are few.

Rationale for the Study

Nurses are aware that every action taken in the care of a patient has consequences and like to believe that those consequences have a positive impact on the patient and their family's ultimate health. Nursing actions such as administering blood products, clinical decision-making, and compassion are executed and have meaning to the nurse, but understanding is not achieved by singular experience. A caring relationship requires mutual understanding. Establishing a relationship is much like maintaining a dialog. As indicated by Bohm (1996), dialog is more than an effort at exchanging knowledge in order to have common information, but rather so that two people are making something *in common* (p. 2). Just as having a knowledge base and speaking without acknowledging the listener and what he/she has to say is incomplete, establishing care without the acknowledgement and participation of the patient is not a fully developed relationship. Understanding patients' perceptions regarding the spiritual care they receive and the spiritual care they expect can enhance the caring relationship, and in so doing, add to the overall understanding of the human condition and the impact that nursing has on the overall health of patients who find themselves in nursing's care.

After reviewing spiritual care and caring, there existed a gap in understanding the essence of patient expectations regarding the spiritual dimension of nursing care. For nurses, gaining that understanding is essential to entering into a truly holistic caring relationship with patients. There were four research questions pertinent to the purpose of this study (Davis, 2005):

1. Are the explicit and implicit actions of nurses to address body, mind and spirit recognized by patients?
2. Are the actions of nurses to address spiritual health perceived by patients as fulfilling a patient expectation?
3. What actions by nurses are perceived as spiritual interventions by patients?
4. How do individuals define spiritual care?

Theoretical Framework

Nursing has a humanistic orientation, and the humanistic values are manifested in the artistic aspects of caring (Watson, 1985). Cumbie (2001) interprets humanistic nursing as more than the technically competent subject-object relationship of nurse to patient in which the nurse directs care for the benefit of the patient. Humanistic nursing involves more of a transaction between nurse and patient in which the nurse is cognizant of self and others through reflection on personal experiences. These various personal experiences allow the nurse to see the patient as more than a person with a medical diagnosis. A key element in humanistic nursing is the idea of presence; being open or available in a manner that the patient finds meaningful or comforting (Godkin, 2001); both 'being there' and 'being with' the patient (Patterson & Zderad, 1988; Nelms, 1996). As a result, the nurse and patient develop a trusting relationship that allows for the multidimensionality of nursing care.

Humanistic nursing (Patterson & Zderad, 1988) is concerned with the uniqueness of each human being. Each human being has a specific and individual history and experience, as well as a collective history and experience as a member of a community. Each human being has a different response to self, others and environment. Each human has value and perceives value in others. Therefore, human potential as well as human limitations are reflected by both the patient and the nurse. Both the nurse and the patient contribute to and gain from the relationship (Watson, 1985; Patterson & Zderad, 1988). Because the nurse-patient relationship is both transactional and interactional, both the nurse and the patient should perceive this existential quality.

Humanistic nursing is described in terms of being a dialogic phenomenon (Patterson & Zderad, 1988). It is expected that the nurse will be helpful to the patient in that the nurse actively attempts to meet the patient's needs. The patient then expects to be helped; to have needs met. The nurse is actively listening, observing, and assessing, and the patient is conveying cues, both verbally and nonverbally. However, the nurse and patient may differ in their perceptions of what those needs might be, how to meet them, and if, indeed, the needs have been met. Furthermore, that relationship can only be established when each participant, the nurse and the patient, perceive each other as unique individuals.

Although widely accepted, there is no consensus about the value of humanism as a framework for nursing and it has also been suggested that practicing humanistic care places the patient solely responsible for setting health care goals, thereby relieving the nurse from accountability for quality patient care (McKinnon, 1991). However, Travelbee (1969) suggested that establishing, maintaining and terminating the nurse patient relationship is the responsibility of the nurse. Moreover, McKinnon believes that humanistic nurses de-emphasize physical care and questions whether responsible choices can be made by the patient. Finally, being more subjective than objective, McKinnon believes that humanistic nursing theory does not attempt to validate the nursing process. This interpretation of humanism argues that humanism is not objective and therefore cannot be measured. True, humanism lends itself to phenomenologic study.

Because much of the nursing literature is vague, idealistic and inconsistent in applied definitions, Mulholland (1994) believes that the humanistic framework is inadequate to fully explicate the social, economic and political dynamics of the nurse-patient relationship. However, Mulholland believes the imprecise nature of humanism's ambiguity to be problematic rather than an outright indictment of humanism, suggesting more discourse on the ontologic and epistemologic foundations of humanism. This suggestion is certainly well-founded, nevertheless, I believed that, rather than a weakness, the strength of humanism as a framework was that the basis of humanism is not linearly prescriptive.

Phenomenology is a qualitative research methodology as well as a philosophical framework designed to explore human experiences from the standpoint of the everyday meaning ascribed to the lived experience by the individuals who experience them rather than theoretical meaning ascribed by an observer (Streubert & Carpenter, 1999; Van Mannen, 1990). Philosophically, phenomenology allows individuals to give voice to actual lived experiences and to their own beliefs and ideas to another individual with the intent of understanding the meaning of that lived experience. Meaning is found in the existential dialogic interplay between nurse and patient (Patterson & Zderad, 1988). Examining the implications of their meanings leads to better understanding of the phenomenon in question (Polkinghorne, 1988). The value of the dialogic experience is in its uniqueness. Each interplay between nurse and patient is important in developing the overall meaning of the experience. Patterson and Zderad (1988) espoused a necessity for a phenomenologic approach in humanistic nursing. Humanism encompasses:

> …not a simple cataloguing of qualities or counting of elements…it involves an openness to nursing phenomena, a spirit of receptivity, readiness for surprise, the courage to experience the unknown…This being-with (subjective, intuitive knowing and experiencing) and looking at (objective analyzing) the phenomenon all at once sparks a creative synthesis, a conceptualization from which emanates insightful description (p. 79).

Phenomenology is a description of an experience based on the ideas, beliefs, knowledge and context of the moment. These internal and external factors do not remain constant. Time or subsequent life events may color the individual's perceptions of an event. The complexity of intrinsic and extrinsic factors will always exist, therefore alternate descriptions of an event will always exist (Van der Zalm & Bergum, 2000). Because of the possibility of a multiplicity of perceptions, it is not possible to assign inference or meaning, or to explain the events of the lived experience of another, but the recounting of the event, one to another, the "being with" and intuitive knowing as described by Patterson and Zderad are important in the discovery process.

Van Manen (1990) states that phenomenology is a study of essences. The essence is revealed by studying the details of the events of lived experience. Van Manen adds that, from the phenomenological perspective, the facts of the lived experience are less important than the essence of the experience (what was it like, rather than what was). "The essence or nature of an experience has been adequately described in language if the description reawakens or shows us the lived quality and significance of the experience in a fuller or deeper manner"(p.10).

Assumptions

For purposes of this study, it was assumed that:

1. Nursing is holistic, therefore concerned with the overall health and well being of the patient, to include physical, mental and spiritual dimensions.
2. Spirituality is a dimension of health.
3. Health is not defined by physical, mental or spiritual well-being, but by the dynamic juxtaposition of each on the other.
4. Participants in the study will respond honestly.

Review of the Literature

Spirituality and purpose in life have been studied in conjunction with other concepts such as quality of life, stressful life events, general health, depression, death acceptance, goal seeking and religious orientation. The main source of literature for the constructs included professional journals in nursing, theology, psychology, occupational health, and sociology. Spirituality as an element of holism is accepted in nursing. There is a lack of consensus regarding the definition of spirituality, however, discovering purpose or meaning in life is a central issue of spirituality. A theoretical exploration of the concepts of holism, spirituality, purpose in life, caring, and spiritual care are presented. Second, quantitative studies related to aspects of spirituality are explored. Lastly, qualitative studies regarding patient satisfaction, patient expectations regarding spirituality and caring in general are considered.

Central to holistic care are spirituality and healing which L. Dossey and B. Dossey (1998) state "encompass a person's values, meaning and purpose in life. They reflect the human traits of caring, love, honesty, wisdom and imagination and they may reflect belief in a higher power, higher existence or a guiding spirit" (p. 46). Because nursing is holistic, it is problematic that descriptions of the components of spirituality are quite diverse, with little consensus toward meaning (Carson, 1989; Taylor, 2002). The intangible nature of spirituality is compounded by the reality that it is shaped by cultural components as well as the context in which it is interpreted. There is a challenge for nursing to define spirituality in such a way as to take into account the importance and relevance of the dimension of spirituality without it being taken out of context or losing clarity with regard to nursing (McSherry & Draper, 1998).

The root of the word, spirit is from Latin meaning "breathe" (Woolf, 1978). As both fundamental and essential as the act of breathing, Carson (1989) asserts that spirituality is what defines us all as unique individuals. Taylor (2002) defines spirituality as "an innate, universal aspect of being human ...[that] integrates, motivates, energizes and influences every aspect of a person's life (p. 5)." Goldberg (1998) identifies concepts such as meaning, presence, empathy, compassion, hope, love, religion, transcendence, touch and healing as aspects of spirituality important to nursing (as cited in Taylor, 2002). Davidhizar, Bechtel and Cosey (2000) add that the nursing intervention of presence, both "being there" in the physical sense and "being with" in the psychological and spiritual sense is the most essential nursing intervention.

Patients, when faced with illness, often question the fundamental meaning of their lives. A sense of purpose in life has been identified as the seminal indicator or outcome of spiritual health (Carson et al, 1992; Frankl, 1984). Frankl observed that purpose of life was a unique trait that had to be identified and fulfilled by each person individually.

Travelbee (1968) asserts that nursing is an interpersonal process in which the role of the nurse is to help the individual/family to find meaning in illness experiences. As did Frankl, Travelbee believed that humans are motivated by meaning, and the illness experience offers a unique opportunity for the nurse to both witness and assist the ill person and the family to discover meaning. Newman (1989) also acknowledges the interpersonal process, stating that human interaction is a spiritual component. It is unclear from the literature whether spiritual growth allows one to know his/her purpose in life or if purpose in life is what allows spiritual growth, but the two are inextricably intertwined.

Wright (1998) defines spirituality as that "dimension of a person that involves one's relationship with self, other, the natural order, and a higher power manifested through creative expressions, familiar rituals, meaningful work, and religious practices" (p.81). Espland (1999) adds that spiritual wellness is that part of the individual that gives purpose to life. Further, a lack of meaning can lead to spiritual distress, hopelessness and despair. Purpose in life involves a search for relationships and situations that provide a sense of worth and a reason for living.

Richards (1991) identifies faith as a belief system that helps the individual develop a purpose in life. However, spirituality is a broader concept than religion (O'Neill & Kenny, 1998; Sheldon, 2000). It may or may not incorporate religious rituals. In fact, nonreligious or atheistic individuals have the spiritual need to find meaning or purpose in life (Tanyi, 2002). Reed (1987) defined spirituality in terms of values and behaviors that relate to something greater than self. In addition, she identifies indicators of spirituality as engaging in prayer, having a meaning to life, contemplation, closeness to a higher being, sense of community and a sense of awareness. Ross (1994) identifies aspects of spirituality as being: purpose and fulfillment, hope or will to live, and faith in self, others and God. B. Howard and J. Howard (1996) suggest that one's occupation is a spiritual activity, stating that how individuals spend their time is a crucial part of their well-being. Prayer and meaning or purpose in life are identified as empirical indicators for appraising spirituality (Meraviglia, 1999).

Burkhart (1989) describes spirituality as a process and a sacred journey to find meaning in life. Furthermore, spiritual needs are the most fundamental requirement of the self. She offers the following descriptive characteristics of spirituality: Unfolding mystery, harmonious interconnectedness with self, others and a higher being, and inner strength or inner resources necessary for transcendence.

Spiritual Care

Nelms (1995) asserts that the origin of nursing is caring and that caring is its reason for being. Sourial (1997) differentiates between the technical services of care and the affective aspect of care and identifies an ethical imperative of nursing to care, incorporating technical and affective competence. She further identifies that caring is not the purview of nursing alone and therefore cannot be specific to nursing's role, however it does come within the purview of holism, which she identifies as a more comprehensive concept than caring.

Spiritual care is acknowledged in descriptions of nursing interventions, and although freely accepted, spiritual care, like spirituality, is not as easily described. During times of illness, pain, suffering and stress, people search for meaning, a spiritual quest that can lead to insight and healing, or fear and isolation (Fontaine, 2000; Travelbee, 1969; Carroll, 2001). Wright (1998) goes so far as to say that spiritual care is not only an integral aspect of nursing care, but to ignore spiritual care would be unethical on the part of the nurse. Ross (1994) reinforces that spiritual care is a nursing responsibility, not an optional extra, but adds that such care is hindered by a lack of a clear definition of spirituality and the absence of a conceptual framework from which to deliver such care. Reed (1992) adds that spirituality is foundational to nursing because it provides the basic characteristic of human-ness, and is essential to human well-being.

Quantitative studies of spirituality have been conducted largely with regard to religiosity. The concept of spirituality was studied using various Likert type scales and questionnaires. Richards (1991) studied 268 undergraduate students enrolled in general psychology courses at the University of Minnesota, who volunteered for the project. Using results of the Religious Orientation Scale, he divided the subjects into four groups: intrinsically religious, extrinsically religious, pro-religious, and anti-religious. Richards then used the Center for Epidemiology Studies Depression Scale, the Spiritual Well-being Scale and the Existential Well-Being Scale. Richards had hypothesized that non-religious students would exhibit more depression than religious students. Results did not bear this out. The implication is that spiritual dimensions are not limited to religiosity.

Giblin (1997) studied marital satisfaction with relation to marital spirituality. Subjects were 35 self-selected couples who belonged to marital support or prayer groups known to the author. Instruments used were all Likert style scales and included the Barrett-Lennard Relationship Inventory (RI), Spiritual Experience Index (SEI), Spiritual Well-being Scale (SWBS) and ENRICH, a multifaceted relationship functioning questionnaire. The author identified the subjects as predominantly Catholic, well educated, middle class and married for greater than 20 years, factors that would limit generalizability. Overall, results showed a significant correlation between ENRICH and SWBS and the mean score on RI and ENRICH were not significant. For husbands, spirituality was found to be directly related to marital relationships. For the wives, however, spirituality was separate from marital relationships. The author concluded that women are more oriented inward, introspective and oriented to developing and maintaining relationships.

In a 1987 study, Reed matched 300 adults into three groups: (1) non-terminally ill hospitalized, (2) terminally ill hospitalized, and (3) healthy non-hospitalized. Matching criteria included age, gender, years of education, and religious background. All subjects were from the same geographic area. All groups were administered the Spiritual Perspective Scale (SPS) in a structured interview setting. An Index of Well-Being was also administered to measure overall life satisfaction. Statistically significant differences were noted in SPS scores of the terminally ill hospitalized group compared to the non-terminally ill and healthy group combined; however no difference was found between non-terminally ill hospitalized and healthy non-hospitalized subjects. Findings supported the stated hypothesis that terminally ill hospitalized adults would indicate a greater spiritual perspective. The correlation between spiritual perspective and well being in the terminally ill group was weak, but significant. This relationship was not significant in the other two groups. It was also reported that a significantly larger number of terminally ill adults indicated a recent increase in spirituality than the other groups.

Touch is more than the procedure related contact of nurse and patient. It also includes that touch which conveys caring in the sense of 'being with' and connectedness, and as such, is an integral part of spiritual care. Mulaik, et al. (1991) studied patients' perceptions of touch in an exploratory study using a descriptive-comparative design. A convenience sample of 98 adults were administered the Patient Touch Questionnaire (PTQ), designed by the investigators, and the Interpersonal Behavior Survey (IBS). The PTQ had four subcategories: traditional touch, instrumental touch, optional touch and essential touch. Results indicated that patients see touch as indicative of caring and that touch by the nurses was important in care (93%). Some reported that touch also indicated control on the part of the nurse and should not be used often (59%). There was no indication on what type of touch (traditional, essential, optional or instrumental), or whether or not all touch was an indicator of control. The study indicated that more time was spent by nurses on instrumental touch such as giving medications, examining, etc. (frequency of about 6 events per day) than on optional touch, described as activities such as patting patients' hands or backrubs (frequency of less than one event per day).

Perception of Care

Latham (1996) investigated self-esteem as a predictor of perception of nursing care with 120 hospitalized adults using a combination of questionnaire completion and interview. The Krantz Health Opinion Survey (KHOS) was used to measure desire for control and Rosenberg's Self-Esteem Scale (SES) was used to estimate self-concept. Humanistic caring was measured by the Holistic Caring Inventory (HCI) resulting in four subscales of caring: physical, interpretive, spiritual, and sensitive, and the Supportive Nursing Behavior Checklist (SNBC). All were Likert scale questionnaires. Findings indicated that personal characteristics such as threat appraisal and coping techniques were important. In addition, younger patients visualized more coping alternatives and reported a higher valuing of nurse caring behaviors. Pain was also identified as a predictor of valuing nursing care. Overall, physical caring received a higher rating than spiritual caring. The author suggested that future research about personal characteristics of patients may lead to greater understanding of their perceptions of caring by nurses.

Holistic care involves not only patients themselves, but also family members. Eriksson (2001) studied relatives' of cancer patients perceptions of care received by their loved ones and developed a structured questionnaire for the study. A sample of 168 relatives from nine Finnish hospitals participated. Results indicated that the manner in which care was delivered was more important than the content of the care. The most important factor identified was professional skill, followed by safety, friendliness and professionalism. Relatives indicated they were more interested in information about the side effects of treatments and other aspects of care than they were in prognosis.

With regard to quality improvement based on patient perceptions of care and satisfaction, Drain (2001) sought to develop a survey instrument to evaluate patient experiences in order to improve quality of care. Findings indicated that perceptions of service affect perceptions of quality of care and that both satisfaction and quality of care perceptions should be evaluated to improve services to patients.

Qualitative Studies

Spirituality, because of its lack of concreteness, does not lend itself well to quantitative measurement (Burkhart, 1989), which might be a reason for the limited amount of research in the area. Existential qualities of spirituality include but are not limited to joy, hope, peace, caring, courage, reverence, awe, and purpose in life. These concepts lend themselves more to qualitative measurement, in which subjectivity is valued in understanding the whole.

Caring Behaviors

Halldorsdottir and Hamrin (1997) conducted a phenomenologic study of cancer patients that explored both caring and uncaring nursing behaviors as perceived by the patient. These researchers identified three caring behaviors: a) a companion in the "cancer trajectory", b) a mutual trust and caring, and c) a sense of well-being, solidarity, empowerment and healing (p. 122). They also identified three uncaring behaviors: a) perceived barrier to healing and well-being, b) mistrust and disconnection, and c) unease and discouragement.

In an effort to determine if patient's perceived caring needs were addressed in a new patient classification instrument, Fagerstrom, Eriksson, and Engberg (1999) interviewed 75 patients from Finland using a phenomenological-hermeneutical method. Seventeen caring needs were identified as a result. Twenty-three of the respondents expressed needs that encompassed the dimensions of body, mind and spirit as identified by the authors, however, physiologic needs were predominant in the needs identified. Caring needs included: to be seen holistically, comforted, well-being and security addressed, hope supported, guidance provided, welcomed, treated with dignity and to have devotional needs supported. The most consistent theme that emerged was that the nurse helped the patient to recover. Interestingly, perceived spiritual caring needs were not addressed in the classification system, while physical and psychological needs were. The authors suggested that the classification system be supplemented by a "caring perspective".

Nine women recovering from hip repair surgery were interviewed in a phenomenological study by Kralik, Koch and Wotton (1997) aimed at understanding what patients perceived as important about nursing care. Two major themes emerged: engagement and detachment. Engagement was supported by the minor themes of nurses approaching the patient in such a manner that conveyed that nothing was too much trouble in their care, consulting with the patient, smiling and using humor, having the qualities of being kind and compassionate, knowing what was needed without having to be asked, being available, friendly, warm, and using a gentle touch. The theme of detachment was supported by such perceived behaviors as "treating the patient as a number" (depersonalization), being too efficient or busy, conveying that the patient should "try harder" or encouraging to the extreme, not sharing information with the patient, even when asked, having "rough hands", and approaching the job of nursing as "just a job" or "just doing what they are told". From the patient's perspective, engagement was directly related to perceived quality of care.

Clark and Wheeler (1992) investigated the meaning of caring based on the experience of six staff nurses and concluded that caring incorporated four major categories: a) being supportive, b) communicating, c) caring ability, and d) pressure (meaning that the nurses believed that pressure and stress either in the workplace or in their personal lives impeded their ability to care). Nurses also indicated that the quality of care they perceived they gave was hindered by patients who "shut them off" (p. 1289).

In a 1999 Finnish qualitative study, Fredriksson synthesized research in nursing and caring utilizing hermeneutic analysis. Citing Nelms (1996), presence was described as both 'being there', which indicates attention by the nurse and 'being with', or an act of mutual giving and receiving. The latter making both giver and receiver more vulnerable in trusting and sharing. Touch was also interpreted to be either necessary to carry out a task, a form of nonverbal communication, or a protective strategy on the part of the nurse to reduce exposure to emotional pain. Listening was described as an active and deliberate attention to another, essential in developing a relationship. These three concepts, presence, touch and listening, were viewed as central to developing a caring conversation between nurse and patient.

Tumblin and Simkin (2001) examined pregnant women's perceptions of their expectations of the nurse's role in general during labor and delivery in an informal survey of women who had never had children. The women were surveyed in their third trimester, during a childbirth class. The survey asked participants to write responses to the question: "What do you think your nurse's role will be during labor and delivery?" (p. 53). Themes included physical comfort, emotional support, information and instructions, advocacy, and technical skills.

Radwin (2000) described eight attributes of quality nursing care: professionalism, knowledge, continuity as reflected by continued encounters, attentiveness, coordination of activities, partnership, individualization of the patient, rapport and caring. These attributes were described by cancer patients in a grounded theory study conducted in a Boston area medical center. Attributes of non-quality care were addressed in part by Hewison (1995) in an earlier observational study conducted in England. He concluded that most nurse/patient interactions were superficial, routine and talk-oriented. It was suggested that nurses exert a 'power over' relationship as indicated by language used in communication with their patients. This power attribute was perceived as a barrier to any meaningful communication. Larrabee and Bolden (2001) identified five themes in their qualitative descriptive study of 199 hospitalized adults. The themes were: providing for patient needs, treating the patient pleasantly, caring, being competent, and providing prompt care.

Appleton (1993) conducted a phenomenological hermeneutic study with 17 participants to identify nursing process as art. In this study, both nurses and patients provided descriptions of the nursing experience as art. Participants described nurses as being present when they focused on the patient as a whole person with the encounter as a temporal moment in the entirety of the lifespan. Patients indicated they wanted the nurse to be considerate and kind. The art of nursing was described by patients as very special when time was taken to care and the perception was that the nurses were giving their very best. From the nursing perspective, providing opportunities for patients to realize their potential was identified as part of the art of nursing. Themes included ways of being, being with, creating opportunities for fullness of being, transcendent togetherness and the context of caring.

Understanding the transactional nature of the basic care needs of patients was illustrated by a Danish study. Adamsen and Tewes (2000) conducted focus group interviews of 120 patients and 22 nurses in a Danish hospital addressing basic nursing care. Fully one third of the patient-identified problems with care were neither noted on the chart, nor known by the nurse caring for them. From the patient's perspective, basic care needs (e.g., pain management and nutritional needs) were being overlooked. Clearly nurses cannot meet needs of which they are unaware.

Patient Expectations of Spiritual Care

Two studies were identified that addressed specifically the spiritual aspect of care. Conco (1995) conducted a phenomenological study with 10 participants who identified themselves as Christian to determine what constituted spiritual care from the perspective of the patient. She identified three themes: enabling transcendence of the situation for a higher meaning, enabling hope and establishing connectedness. Conco concluded that connectedness was simply caring. Sellers (2001) interviewed six key and 12 general informants residing in the Midwest regarding their perceptions of spiritual nursing care. She identified five spiritual themes in this ethnonursing study: 1) Spirituality is a motivator in the search for meaning through connectedness; 2) Spirituality involves a lifelong search for meaning; 3) Spirituality is expressed and practiced uniquely; 4) The environment influences spirituality; and 5) Nurses can enhance spirituality by establishing a caring presence with both the patient and their family. According to Sellers, spiritual nursing care can be achieved by listening attentively to others' stories, individualizing care, approaching the patient with sensitivity and respect, and maintaining a good sense of humor.

From the perspective of client as the community, Chase-Ziolck & Gruca, 2000) studied religious congregations as a nontraditional site for nursing practice, with an emphasis on health promotion and spiritual care. The authors used naturalistic inquiry as a framework for their descriptive exploratory study of patients' perceptions of interacting with nurses in their congregations. Participants described ways they felt cared for by the nurse, to include 'being there' and 'being with'. Because the setting was in the community, emphasis was on interpersonal caring actions rather than technical caring actions. Several participants described the setting (their church) as supporting the feeling of tranquility, peace and care and illustrated the connection between faith and health.

Caring is identified as a universal culturally dependent phenomenon. With that premise, patient expectations of care were examined by Cortis (2000) in an ethno-linguistic study. Twenty male and eighteen female participants from a Pakistani community in the United Kingdom participated. There was a link between caring, culture and spirituality as demonstrated by the importance of relationships to self and others. The importance of developing the nurse-patient relationship in order for caring to be perceived was evident. As a whole, the perception was that nurses had limited observation, empathy, and communication skills, and that the "assessments they experienced had been mechanistic and ritualistic rather than the framework for developing a therapeutic relationship with them" (p. 59). The author concluded that more effective cultural assessment was needed to foster a therapeutic relationship.

Summary

Quantitative studies regarding issues related to spiritual care and patient/family perceptions of care were limited mostly to Likert type questionnaire administration. Purpose in life studies revealed that commitment and psychological well-being were positively associated with purpose in life. Death anxiety, however was not. Quantitative studies of spirituality mainly measured elements of religiosity from the Judeo-Christian perspective. Findings revealed that spiritual dimensions were not limited to religiosity. Studies also support that terminally ill persons indicate a greater spiritual perspective. Touch was revealed to be important in care, however patients perceived instrumental touch (touching medications and machinery) more than personal touch (holding the hand). One study supported that self-esteem was a predictor of perception of nursing care and that pain was a predictor of perception of nursing care. Finally, studies support that the manner that care is delivered is more important to patients than the content of that care.

Qualitative studies examining the expectations of patients related to spiritual care were limited. For the most part, the literature addressed patient expectation themes of technical competence, caring, nursing as art, and quality of nursing. A meta-analysis gave more insight into care, but did not address specific spiritual themes. There was a significant amount of literature that addressed the ramifications of nursing care using the lens of the nursing shortage and managed care, all from the viewpoint of the nurse.

Caring behaviors were explored in several phenomenologic studies, identifying basic caring needs as: to be seen holistically, to be comforted, to have hope supported, to have guidance provided, to feel welcomed and to be treated with dignity. Additional caring behaviors identified included smiling, a gentle touch, for the nurse to be available, and to be treaded as a person, not a number. One study found nurses actual behaviors to be superficial and talk oriented. Only two studies addressed spiritual needs specifically. Themes that emerged included enabling hope, supporting connectedness to self, the nurse and to a higher power, and to facilitate search for meaning. Caring presence was seen as enhancing spiritual care.

Therefore, this literature review supports that spirituality is the essence of what it is to be human, and is central to health and the healing process. Nevertheless, it is difficult to define. Concepts associated with spirituality include hope, connection to self, others and a higher power, purpose or meaning in life, caring presence, religion, ritual, comfort, motivation, transcendence, well-being, values, beliefs, harmony, prayer or meditation, self-awareness, and even self-esteem. It is not evident whether or not these concepts are precursors of, or the result of spirituality.

Spirituality is often confused with, or a term used interchangeably with religion. Given that, spiritual needs are often referred by nurses to a chaplain or minister. No literature reviewed in this study addressed directly the spiritual needs of individuals who identify themselves as nonreligious or atheistic. Being a component of holism, spiritual care is within the purview of nursing. Indeed, it is an ethical responsibility of nursing.

A common thread in defining spirituality is that it involves a search for meaning or purpose in life, relationships with self, others and a higher being, and hope. The search for meaning or purpose in life can include any ideals or practices that contribute to a meaningful life. Meaning can only be ascribed by the individual. The role of the nurse in spiritual care is to understand the importance of spirituality to health and healing and to establish a trusting, caring relationship with the patient. It is not understood from the literature that patients would expect spiritual care from their nurse.

Methodology

Humanistic phenomenology is a framework for examining the lived experience of hospitalization and patients' expectations of care during that hospitalization. All participants were given an opportunity to reflect on their experience of hospitalization first by recounting their remembrances of their hospitalization by relating it in story form. Individual perceptions of hospitalization were very meaning-laden and as stories were elicited, the circumstances of hospitalization were expressed in words, gestures, tone and in a cadence unique to each participant.

Setting

The setting for this study was south-central United States. Two metropolitan statistical areas (MSA) located in bordering states were represented. Major economic influences for both MSAs included cattle, oil, and industries such as tire and tool manufacturing. Both MSAs serve a much wider rural population, and each are supported economically by separate military installations and small state universities. The larger MSA has a population of approximately 120,000 and the smaller, approximately 80,000.

Participants

Participants in this study were solicited via purposive sampling. Criterion sampling (soliciting interviews from any persons who meet the qualifications of the study and opportunistic sampling (following leads from participants and other informants) as described by Erlandson, Harris, Skipper, and Allen (1993) were used. The concepts of spirituality and perception of spiritual care are value laden and often used interchangeably with the concept of religion. Therefore, recruitment of participants evolved and, incorporating the strategy of maximum variation (Miles & Huberman, 1994), resulted in the solicitation of both self-identified religious and non-religious participants. Participants were interviewed until redundancy, which was indicated after nine interviews. In order to assure that no new substantive information would result from interview, two additional interviews were conducted. The quality of the content of the interviews indicated redundancy. Therefore, a total of 11 interviews were conducted. Data collection was conducted between May 2002 and January 2003.

Data Generation Strategies

All potential participants approached by the researcher consented to participate in the study. Participants were told that study participation would involve an interview lasting approximately one to two hours. All interviews were completed in about a one-hour time frame. The range of interview times was 30 minutes to 1 hours and 20 minutes. In order to elicit an unbiased sense of participants' expectations of nurses, the concept of spirituality was not mentioned as a focus of the study during participant recruitment with two exceptions. Some aspects of spirituality, such as building relationships, may not be recognized as such my the participants. It was important to get the flavor of the lived experience, which may have included aspects of spirituality, prior to introducing it as a topic and risking leading participants into telling the researcher what she wanted to hear. One participant was known to be atheistic. In order to assure that he was not "blindsided" by the interview questions regarding spirituality, he was told during recruitment that spirituality was an aspect of holistic nursing care and was a focus of the study. One participant knew through personal conversation, prior to recruitment, that the focus of the study was spirituality and requested to be included in the study. At the end of the interview, participants were told that one of the purposes of the research was to learn patients' expectations regarding spiritual care (as defined by holistic nursing standards of practice) from nurses. A written summary of the findings was available upon request to participants after compilation and analysis of the data. No participants indicated they wanted a summary of the findings.

Interviews were scheduled after either telephone or direct communication with potential participants. Informed consent was obtained at the time of the scheduled interview and a pseudonym of the participant's choosing was identified. Participants were asked, first to relate a story about a specific nurse or an experience with nursing care while they were hospitalized. Based on what the participant related, follow-up questions were asked in order to address the following basic questions:

1.   What did you expect from your nurse when you were hospitalized?
2.   How do you define or describe good nursing care?
3.   Did you expect spiritual care from a nurse?
4.   How do you define or describe spiritual nursing care?

Again, depending on the responses, nursing behaviors considered by nurses to embody the spiritual dimension of holistic practice would be offered, such as, "The spiritual component of care includes developing a trusting relationship with your nurse so that those things that give meaning to your life, such as art, music, meditation, relationships, or faith are acknowledged, supported and facilitated." I provided this definition if participants defined spiritual care only in terms of religious practice in order to elicit deeper description or discussion of the term "spiritual" or "spirituality". Therefore, I provided my definition in five of the eleven interviews.

Interviews were conducted at a time convenient to the participants, at a place of their choosing. Eight participants chose to be interviewed in my office. The office door was closed and distractions were minimal. Three participants were interviewed in their own business offices per their request. All interviews were audiotaped with permission. Audiotapes were used in this study to insure the accuracy of interview date as well as to record the exact words, tones, and emphasis conveyed by the participants. The reasons for this were twofold. First, meaning is conveyed by more than just words alone. Pauses, sighs, time for reflection, tone, choice of words, and voice modulation are also important in gleaning the full meaning of the words. Second, I could focus attention on being present with the participant and his/her interview rather than being distracted by constant note-taking. This attention during the interview would help to establish a trusting relationship. Audiotapes were only available to the participant and the principal investigator. While the proposed interview content had been piloted in interviews already conducted and found to elicit responses related to the topic, I remained flexible and use further clarifying questions as needed in each specific situation.

Two participants became tearfully emotional during the interview process. These two participants were given the option of terminating the interview or the audiotaping, and both elected to continue with the audiotaped interview process. All participants were told that they could contact me at any time after the interview for questions or additional comments. No participants contacted me for additional questions or comments. Participants did ask some questions during the course of the interview itself. In order to not interrupt the flow of the participant's stories, demographic data that were not made apparent during the course of the interview were collected at the end of the interview process. Demographic data included age, gender, race/ethnicity, marital status, religious preference, number and ages of children, diagnosis for which hospitalized, number of hospitalizations, level of education, occupation, and age at the time of hospitalization.

Interviews began with having each participant tell a story about being hospitalized. This strategy was appropriate. First, rich data were obtained. Second, participants seemed to become more at ease as they progressed in the telling of their story. Several participants were very concerned about the details such as dates, times, and names of their physician – the facts of their hospitalization – as they began their narratives. As they became immersed in the storytelling, I noticed that the event itself took on more importance. The narratives dictated follow-up questions.

Plan for Data Analysis

Audiotapes were made of each interview and transcribed verbatim. The analysis method described by Giorgi (1970) fit well with the data obtained and my own personal thought processes. Data were then analyzed using the phenomenologic method described by the psychologist Giorgi to identify patterns and themes. This method is based on reflection, an ordered, repetitive examination of the data to derive implications and meaning. Procedurally, the steps of the Giorgi method are:

1. Interview the participants.
2. Read the description (verbatim transcription) to get a sense of the whole.

3. Re-read and reflect on the description several times and identify individual units (patterns and themes).

4. Eliminate redundancies in the patterns and themes, clarifying each by relating them to each other and to the whole.

5. Continue to reflect on the patterns and themes, transforming meaning from concrete language into the language or concepts of the science (nursing literature).

6. Integrate and synthesize meaning into descriptive structure communicated to others.

I transcribed all interviews. After transcription, I read through each transcribed interview while listening to the audiotape until I was sure of accuracy of the transcription and had reflected on the meaning of the interview. Any additional nuances of tone, inflection and pause in narrative were noted in this process. An interview summary was written for each interview, to include exemplars of any themes or patterns noted.

Steps to Insure Methodological Rigor

Credibility was established by this investigator's 18 years of nursing experience and having prolonged engagement with the participants. Each interview lasted between 30 minutes and one hour 20 minutes. In addition, member checks were accomplished by requesting elaboration or clarifying concepts with each participant during the course of their interview. After reflecting on the interviews and rereading transcriptions, no questions arose that required follow-up interviews. No participant contacted me after the interview to add any comment or clarification. A nurse colleague, experienced in phenomenological methodology was asked to review the transcribed interviews (with participant aliases) and provide feedback regarding her impression of the interviews and to discuss emergent themes and patterns. This peer debriefing was ongoing throughout the data analysis process.

Transferability was addressed by eliciting rich description and providing thick description of the interviews. Any pertinent noises, sights, facial expressions, gestures and tones were included in field notes. Sampling was purposive to insure maximum variability of the phenomena of perceptions of nursing care during hospitalization.

Dependability and confirmability of the data were addressed by an audit trail to include audiotapes, transcriptions of the interviews, field notes of the investigator, notes of the peer debriefer, and interview summaries of each interview. I kept notes on the interview transcript and added to those notes each time I reread the transcripts as warranted. These notes addressed general impressions of the interviews, the settings, collaborative data, and historical data, which might impact the tone of the interview. For example, one participant consented to be interviewed and subsequently was diagnosed with a terminal illness. Concerned that the interview timing would not be in this person's best interest, I offered this participant the option of not being interviewed. She declined, stating that she really wanted to talk about her hospitalization. I believe the interview process was cathartic for this individual.

A methodological decision was made, for ethical reasons, to inform one prospective participant that spirituality and spiritual care would be discussed when soliciting his participation. Methodologically, this topic was not going to be addressed prior to the interview to attempt to avoid having participants "tell the researcher what she wants to hear". This participant was known to be atheistic, and I believed that he might feel entrapped without this information up front. He chose to participate and even brought Internet sites and literature to the interview to, as he stated, help me to understand his belief system.

Protection of Human Participants

None of the participants voiced any concern for loss of confidentiality, however, the principal investigator was the only individual with access to the identity of the participants. Pseudonyms (aliases) were self-assigned by the participants. Two participants became tearful during the course of their interviews, but both elected to continue the interviews. One participant referred to family members by name during the course of their interview and requested that the family member's name not be used. The family member's name was not used. No participant voiced any concern about being audiotaped.

Demographic Data

A total of seven women and four men participated in the study. The age range of participants was 36 to 59 years. All participants self-identified as Caucasian. All participants graduated from high school. Three participants had 2 to 3 years of college, five had baccalaureate degrees, one had a masters degree and two participants possessed doctoral degrees. Three participants self-identified as secretaries, one as a homemaker, one as a teacher, two as students, one as a broadcast engineer, two as university professors, and one as a retired police officer. Ten of the participants were married and one was in a committed relationship. Ten reported having 1 to 3 children while two reported having no children. The range of number of hospitalizations (requiring at least one overnight stay) of the participants was 1 to 13 times. Religious preference of the participants included Protestant (two Baptist, one Methodist, one Disciple of Christ, one Presbyterian, one Episcopalian, and one no-preference), Catholic (one), Agnostic (two), and Atheist (one).

Findings

The experience of hospitalization evoked strong feelings on the part of the participants, both positive and negative. The nature of the disease process and the number of times hospitalized varied with the participants, but it was clear that each experienced a sense of vulnerability, exacerbated by uncertainty that contributed to the event of their hospitalization being a very significant life event. Although each related experience was unique, there were some commonalities among participants in the experience of hospitalization and with the nurses who provided their care. Four major themes emerged in data analysis (Davis, 2005):

1. Definitions of "good" and "bad" nursing care
2. Expectations of surveillance and competence
3. Spiritual care expectations and definitions
4. Time and the nursing shortage

The focus of this paper will be spiritual care expectations and definitions. While all participants were able to define what they believed to be spiritual care and spirituality, nine of the 11 participants did not expect spiritual care from their nurses. In fact, one adamantly did not want it. Spiritual care was chiefly defined in terms of religious affiliation or religious practices or rituals such as prayer. Nurse referral to a chaplain or minister was, in general, thought to be the extent of nursing involvement in spiritual care. When provided with my definition of spiritual care, developing a trusting relationship with the nurse so that those things that give meaning to life such as art, music, meditation, relationships, or faith are acknowledged, supported and facilitated, participants generally agreed that spiritual care, thus defined, would be good for the nurse to do, but did not expect it. Shorter lengths of hospital stay, that preclude developing a relationship with the nurse, and workload of nurses were offered as rationales for not expecting spiritual nursing care.

Robbi had no expectations of spiritual care, but stated she would like to experience it, "I find it very comforting when I realize that the nurse and I have that connection." Lena also had no real expectations, but she articulated, "I usually think of it in terms as being requested by the patient. It sort of takes a request by the patient in a formal sense, someone to pray with or read literature with or whatever."

George defined spiritual care as something to be referred to the minister and would not expect spiritual interaction from nurses, citing lack of time on the part of the nurse. Even so, he gave the impression that nurses are not expected to attend to every wish of the patient, but to their needs, and spiritual care was not considered to be a need in the hospital setting.

> [Nurses are] extremely busy. I think most patients realize that. It's sort of like you're not expecting you know, a body servant or anything, or there as a personal kind of a counselor. You're mostly there as an individual patient that just has to wait their turn. You don't really look on it as the be all and end all. You don't see them really all that often. If you call on them they arrive, or something that has to be done procedurally they'll be there, but other than that, you hardly ever see them. They don't come in and say 'hi, how are you feeling' or generally chit chat for a little while… Well, I'm sure that if they had time, it would be nice.

Carol became tearful and was given the option of terminating the interview when spirituality was introduced as a topic. She was recently diagnosed with a terminal illness and had been in and out of the hospital for testing and pain management several times over the weeks preceding the interview. She began discussing the fact that she was not a deeply religious person. Although raised in a religious household, Carol began to question the religion she grew up with when she stated college and "reading more", to include reading about evolution. She went on to describe her feelings regarding religion and a higher being, stating that it just "didn't add up", referring to creation theory and the presence of a higher being. When asked to describe spiritual nursing care she described emotional comforting, a 'being with' on the part of the nurse. However, her conception of spirituality was mainly religion and religious practices, and the role of the nurse was limited to referral if indicated to a minister.

> I would think it would be a nurse coming in and telling me that 'you're going to get through this', possibly offering to get a minister in if I wanted one or something like that. I don't look on it as somebody taking my hand and saying a prayer with me. I don't look on it as that. I think if you want spiritual guidance or you want spiritual help that a nurse is going to know how to get it for you.

After hearing my definition of spiritual care, Carol was thoughtful, and agreed that all individuals have something that is important, that gives meaning, to them. She added that it is important to know someone, to develop a trusting relationship with the nurse, for some issues related spiritual care, such as things that give meaning to life, to be shared with another. When a more personal relationship develops with the nurse, she believed that this more personal information was shared because the patient feels more comfortable.

> Those things come out. Like you might say music relaxes me. You would you expect the nurse to pick up on that and offer to bring in a radio or something. That, to me would be providing spiritual care to you... Some people are annoyed by music. Every person has something that is extremely important, to me.

Diane did not expect spiritual care from her nurse, but when asked what it was, she could clearly describe it. Diane saw spiritual care as multidimentional. Elements of caring presence, 'being with', what she terms "people skills", such as being gentle, unhurried, developing a relationship, were included in her definition of spiritual care. She added that nurses should not detract from the healing environment of the hospital. Basically, if the nurse can't help, at least he/she should not be harmful, and this is included in the spiritual care of the patient.

> ...Like don't rush out of the room. Skills, actual people skills that could be taught that, and one is gentle tone of voice, touch gently. Maybe they don't give a hoot about you, but, you're not worse for their coming in the room. You know, you are not worse for connecting with them. They [nurses] say, 'do you want anything' and you are trying to answer and then before you know it... they're gone. [Laughs] Actually, now that you say it, connectedness is exactly what it takes. An actual concern, you know. I think you can draw pain away from people or do things for people. It's kind of a Christian based belief -that we can lift our burdens kind of thing. It's to form some kind of bond, [along] with that, empathy and sincerity. That you involve yourself enough to lift some of the burden off the patient. If someone can take you out of yourself for a moment. So, there you go.

Being recognized as an individual was considered to be part of spiritual care.

Carol also related that being made to "feel human" was important to spiritual care and was important to her. She indicated that she was comforted when the nurse wanted to help her, even if she was capable of caring for herself, because she saw that as acknowledging her, that she was seen as having worth as a human being.

> Just make you feel human. ...I appreciate that more than anything. You know, I'm not a problem patient. I'd just as soon do something myself than to ring a buzzer and have someone

do it for me. And, I like to be acknowledged that way, you know, like, 'Mrs. ____ why didn't you call me to do that'. Oh, I'm fine. I can do it. 'Well next time call me.' [laughs] You know … most of the nurses are like that.

Mary also found it helpful to be recognized as an individual. She recounted that nurses who cared for her when she was hospitalized for pneumonia treated her as a "whole person", which greatly enhanced the healing environment. This sense of acknowledgement as a human being was accomplished by nurses taking time to form a personal relationship with her. Mary's perception was that the nurses were fully present with her in their interactions.

> …and the nurses who took care of me here at [hospital] really made me feel like they cared about me as a whole person. There was a man nurse and a number of women nurses and, I really got the impression that they didn't think of me as the lungs in room 406, that they thought of me as this real person, who's sick and we're going to treat the whole person and try to get better. They would take the time to visit with me and I knew they had all the people they had to see and all the meds they had to get out and this enormous amount of work to deal with, and they would spend a few minutes to see how I was doing as a person in addition to dealing with the pneumonia. But they really made me feel like they cared about me as a whole person.

Mary further clarified that the sense of being treated as a whole person was enhanced by the fact that the nurses talked to her. In addition to the verbal communication, demeanor and body language contributed to the overall sense of being cared for by nursing staff.

> Some of it was the talking itself. Some of it was the nonverbal communication, the looks on their faces, the, probably open body language although I couldn't tell you that. So, I'm going to say probably it was the body language thing, facial features and open body language. But I really did feel like they cared about me more than just the lungs in 608.

David, self identified as atheistic, was told that spiritual care, as an element of holistic care would be included in the interview when he was recruited in an effort to ensure that David did not feel entrapped as the interview progressed. As a result, although he consented to the interview, David conducted the majority of his interview in a defensive mode, leaning forward in his chair with hand on his knees and he seemed to have prepared some comments prior to arriving at the interview. In fact, he brought an article printed from an Internet site, written by a physician, supportive of atheistic beliefs. As the interview progressed, he seemed to become more at ease, leaning back in his chair and pausing more between responses. At the conclusion of the interview, he continued to converse about atheism and spirituality. He strongly associated the word "spiritual" with religious beliefs, which he was ardently opposed to, and therefore was opposed to the word. He believed that the term "meaningful" was more helpful than "spiritual" for nurses to use in their definition of holistic care, and that there were things that gave meaning to life, such as music. He did not, however, expect the nurse to be concerned with what he found meaningful in life, including developing any personal kind of relationship with his nurse. He stated that providing comfort was appropriate but believed that nurses should operate under the axiom of "doing no harm", to include care that the patient might "need" as opposed to "want", the implication being that providing the patient with what they want might be doing harm. David also stated that he did not have the expectation that the nurse be able to intuit what the patient might want. If the patient wants something, according to David, he or she must ask for it.

> I think there are great limits to that [spiritual care] and great dangers that the nurse has to be aware of. You know.... should a nurse pray with a patient if the patient is praying for the strength not to get a blood transfusion and they don't get the blood transfusion? If they might die—should the nurse aid and abet that wish to make the patient feel more comfortable with that? How does that conflict with the Hippocratic oath? And I think her duty to medicine and her duty to science and her duty to patient care should always supercede what the patient wants if there is a potential conflict.

Although most participants identified religious aspects of spirituality such as prayer and developing a relationship to a higher being, definitions of spiritual care included referral to nature, connectedness to self and others, and music. Robbi stated that the nurse conveys the spiritual side of care by her actions. In addition, she stated that spirituality includes getting to know someone and the "little things like family or pets that you're interested in." She also mentioned nature as spiritual, and important to her. She implied that nature was one of those "little things" which could be shared in building a relationship with her nurse.

> ...don't you just love it when the trees leaf out? There are some questions that, on the surface, sound very unimportant, but I think they convey a lot about a person and how they connect with the earth and, you know, as a part of each of us.

Lena spoke of spirituality having a formal and an informal component. She described her early experience with what she termed a fundamentalist religion with very strict and judgmental practices. She had since rejected those fundamentalist beliefs. Her life choices were not congruent with the religious practices of her childhood and of her family. She was divorced and entered into a lesbian relationship. These life choices continued to create angst in that her family members condemned her lifestyle choices based on their religious beliefs. Clearly, Lena was a spiritual person, but maintained no religious affiliation. Lena reflected that spirituality had a formal or religious component as well as an informal component that included sympathy, empathy and reassurance.

> I think the way I define spiritual for myself personally is a much more informal thing. And its much more about that sensitivity and providing someone empathy or reassurance. Or in cases you can't really reassure as much, because you've lost something you're not going to get back, but ... just offer to listen, and sympathy are much more important than that formal spiritual advisor or leader. I think if I was hospitalized today, I would still be the same way, I wouldn't necessarily be looking for anyone to come and pray with me or read the Bible to me but I would feel better just having someone to talk to for a little bit. Or to listen to me, or to let me cry, you know... You know that informal [spirituality] I think is more important for me personally, because I think you spiritually minister to someone through those [listening and offering sympathy and reassurance]. And it's completely, its nondenominational, or not church affiliated in any way. And it wouldn't matter to me if the nurse were Christian, Jewish, Hindu, Islamic. I mean, that part would not be important to me. These are their own personal beliefs. But you know I come from a very conservative fundamentalist Christian background and in my life I have found that [pause] that whole viewpoint as - people from that kind of background tend to convert people, think that they can be saved, comfort people, aren't very comforting really at all and in fact are really offensive to me, you know. You know, all those

things I have heard growing up over and over again. And that would upset me if I had a nurse come in and say those kinds of things to me. I would have a real problem with that.

Mart offered more insight into differences in religious and spiritual beliefs and indicated that, if the nurse held a different belief, spiritual care may be detrimental to the patient. She brought up a very salient point. She reinforced the point that all religious practices are not the same, even within the same religious heritage. Mary self-identified as Episcopalian. She strongly believed that denominational religious beliefs are not necessarily the same. She also strongly believed in the power of prayer and was concerned when anyone offered to pray for her. Because of the differences in beliefs, it was possible that, however well-meaning, the proffered prayer may be in contradiction with her beliefs. She defined spirituality as "a connection between myself and a higher power", but was clear that there was no expectation of spiritual care from her nurse, in fact, it would not be welcome.

> ... and I don't expect my nurses to do anything related [to spirituality]. In fact...I'm Episcopalian. And, people of other denominations say they're praying for me, it often annoys me because their belief systems are so very different from mine, so no I really don't expect spiritual care from the nurse.

Because Mary valued being treated as a whole person, I attempted to further clarify if spirituality was included in her definition of holism. When asked about her definition of holism from an education standpoint, she responded.

> That we educate not just the mind, ah, intellectually, but we are concerned with what we call the whole child. We're concerned with social relationships that the kids, about how he deals with his family, we're concerned that his physical needs be met - his nutrition, is he well. So we're concerned, but we draw a very sharp line between spiritual and non-spiritual kinds of concerns because of, if we step on the line, and I know some horror stories of... one that comes to mind right now is a little first grader whose dog died, and was crying and one of his teachers- The child said, 'my dog died, will he go to heaven?' and she said no, honey, I'm sorry, but dogs don't go to heaven. And, ah, of course this kid was traumatized. So, we draw a real hard line that we don't involve ourselves in anything spiritual. Physical self is cared for and the social self is cared for and certainly the intellectual self is cared for.

Given her definition of holism, Mary was asked if she expected that from her nurse. She responded in the affirmative, "Yeah, I expect that from my nurse. I expect her to be concerned and to be sure: Do I have any family? Am I getting um, cards coming? And are people coming to visit me?"

Lee referred to relationships in his definition of spiritual nursing care. Important relationships for him included those of family. Also important to him was developing a relationship with his nurse. He identified caring as the key component of spiritual nursing care. He also viewed coaching, encouraging and exhibiting genuine concern as key to spiritual care.

> ...my family being there for some of my surgeries, you know, I really want them to know what's going on, Let em know 'he's doing fine'. [pause] As far as the music...that doesn't play a part so much. Bottom line is caring. To me that's spiritual. Caring for your patient, caring for your [the patient's] parents, or your family that are asking questions also...You

know, you're flat on your back and pretty helpless. Having somebody there who's going to take care of you. Every factor. Whether it's you know, a sponge bath, or taking you to the restroom, or you know, waiting for you to come out, you know, wheeling you here and there if you have to. Pushing. That's a big thing too. Pushing me to get up and get around… Coaching. Coaching me a little bit. And ah, wanting to see you get better, and wanting to see you leave. Not to get rid of you, but you know that you've made it through it and you're going to be fine… I think you have to have kind of a bond, a rapport. If you get off on a bad foot, you may not get someone. You know, pain in the butt, you're not going to get anything. It goes with personality also. You know, personality of the patient and the nurse.

He added that he did expect spiritual care, developing a bond and coaching, from his nurse, but stated, "I think that it makes the recovery time and the hospital stay a lot nicer."

Harold defined spirituality as "…kind of leans toward the religious aspect of things. But, I am not one who needs this." However, although he did not need or expect spiritual nursing care, he acknowledged that some patients do have religious needs when in the hospital and the nurse should have the skill to intuit such need.

This is a case of a nurse needs to learn, I think, to be able to read a person and read something along those lines…To kinda bring the obvious out in the open. Give you a light you've never seen before. Give you an idea…. where you can help yourself. They can help you bring this out… Of course if they know how. And it should be taught.

Debbie, a nursing educator, did not expect spiritual nursing care. She defined spirituality more in terms of her own religious beliefs, to include prayer. She agreed with my definition of spiritual nursing care, however, and went on to describe an incident in which she allowed family members to visit a patient outside of visiting hours because she knew it was important and a comfort to her Hispanic patient. She added that, with caring, you are "sensitive to what that patient needs for support. And then you do as much as you can to give that support."

Diane saw religion as different from spirituality. This distinction was revealed at the end of the interview when gathering demographic data. When asked if she had a religious preference, she replied that religion and spirituality were two different things. She defined religion as an "organized, group of same faithed believers who gather and share to express worship." She envisioned spirituality as,

Well spirituality to me is connectedness to the whole, with God. First with God, and then, through that, is connectedness with everything, and that has nothing to do with religion. Although, I can see where you get there through religion, or that's a good way to teach about, faith, or God or the Bible, Talmud, but spirituality to me is that communication with God, connectedness with God or with [something] larger than yourself. That there is, you know, life or being beyond your limits. Like we're all cells in an organism. The organism is God, maybe. When I hear, 'we are of God', I believe that. I feel a part of something, whether it's through my thoughts or deeds or actions, I feel like it affects everything around me almost. What we do matters. I mean, I don't go around, I'm not a peace nut or anything, and I have bad days, but I think it affects other people and I don't think its right to do those things. And the reason I think we're connected is because I don't have a way of not believing in God. I can't. We're all part of something bigger. We're all blades of grass. Mostly we're connected because of the world. We live on this planet together. If there are lots of possibilities there will be wars here or there or there are lots of possibilities there will be shooting, I just can't take the stress of the hostility and people are mean and the government doesn't care, and the first person they see on the subways spits on them. I understand that. I'm a part of that, so I have to care about it. Even evolution just blows my mind. Music is almost a direct line to spirituality. It's a healing sort of thing. That's another thing. Some people heal better through some visual or auditory stimuli, at least for me... That's another thing, taking a walk it the morning. And music, almost puts you in a meditative state. The way to concentrate is to get out of your normal way of thinking and it's very external. When you walk, your senses, all that input from nature can overwhelm. Just to breath. But music, you hear as well as play. Right away, playing music can put me in a better state- calm. And if I'm not in a place to play music, then listening, but playing is a different thing. Listening's fine, but it's not the same. Falling into it. Music and art, why would you do that if you didn't have hope or being compelled to make something beautiful almost, or to create. What's the point of that if [voice trails off]. There's something it does."

David, an atheist, objected to the term "spiritual" because of the religious connotations, but did see himself as a whole being, not distinguishing between mind, body and personality. He viewed spirituality as a label that had no meaning to him.

I don't know what spirit means and I don't believe in the duality of body and mind. My brain is my mind. There is no such thing as of mind and of body. Without the body there is no mind so I don't see the point in splitting the two... I'm a very analytical, laid back kind of person, and I think labels like that would probably best describe my personality most of the time. Everybody has down or off days in terms of characteristics, but I can display the other ones at times, but those [analytic and laid back personality] are probably my dominant ones.

When I related the definition of spirituality I had developed, he replied that the term "meaningful" as opposed to "spiritual" was a good label:

Well then I would term meaningful as a good label there, and philosophical probably a better label as well, because the word spiritual has way too much other baggage attached to it that I don't buy into. So,... if nurses are to provide fulfillment in patient's philosophical realm and help make their experience as being meaningful to them then, if that assertion is true then I think those are better labels to use. But if that is, if my definition is what you mean by spiritual then feel free to use it [the term spiritual] as linguistic shorthand [basically giving permission to use the term, spiritual] as long as we both understand what we are talking about."

Toward the end of the interview, when responding to demographic data, David identified religious preference as "atheist' and seemed to be watching me carefully to gauge my reaction to this. We both stood and moved toward the door. At this point, David seemed to be less guarded and asked, good-humoredly, if there was anything else he could "spout off" about. It was as if he could relax now that the formal part of the interview was over. He suggested that using the word "mood" instead of "spirit" would be more appropriate.

I still don't like the term spiritual, but I'm very uh, you know, who wouldn't be spiritual if it's defined the way you are defining it... How's your mood. That's a way of assessing spirit. Feeding the spirit—keeping the mood stable and healthy. If you're somebody who's questioning some very deeply held beliefs - that can be a very painful disturbing process. Does that mean its bad? Should a nurse try to alleviate that, or should she try to encourage you, or should she just stay out of it and stick to giving meds to make you feel better physically, and respect the boundaries of your personal conscious and thinking and decisions on matters like that?

Discussion

Humanistic nursing is predicated on the assumption that, while each person is unique, and each patient will respond uniquely to care, however, humans are more alike than different and value is also placed on that common humanness (Patterson & Zderad, 1985). While Benner (1985) and Rogers (1972) clearly indicate that nurses cannot understand health and illness by studying only the mind and body, but by studying the whole in context, it is believed that understanding the experience of the spiritual dimension of care will enhance the integrality of holistic care. Because of the existential nature of humanistic nursing, what nurses do should be perceived by patients in their care (Patterson & Zderad, 1985). Discussion will be organized around the research questions of this study.

1. Are the Explicit and Implicit Actions of Nurses to Address Body, Mind and Spirit Recognized by Their Patients?

Participants in this study were able to discern actions by nurses, both implicit and explicit, which addressed holistic care as well as implicit and explicit actions by nurses, which detracted from holistic care. Actions addressing physical care (the body) were readily discernable and described. Actions which addressed mind and spirit were also readily discernable and described, but not necessarily using the terminology of mind and spirit. In stories of hospitalization in general, and when asked to relate a story of good nursing care, patients were able to distinguish qualities of good nursing care and bad nursing care. Good nursing care included descriptions of experiences congruent with holistic nursing care, to include spirituality. Participants described being made to feel special or being treated as a human being, and good nurses as being kind, caring, and willing to share themselves. Of note, the stories of both good and bad nursing care were very vivid and detailed, even though some of the instances occurred over 30 years ago. Bad nursing care, as described by the participants, was the antithesis of good nursing care, and included behaviors suggesting lack of kindness and lack of caring, such as talking about a patient in a derogatory manner in the hall, not meeting basic care needs, addressing the patient with a lack of respect, and not seeing the patient as an individual. Good and bad nursing care seemed to have such an impact on the participants that incidents of good and bad nursing care were easily and vividly recalled. As Cathy, who recalled neither good nor bad nursing care from her hospitalization pointed out, " You know, you remember things like that, and I have no negative memories".

Good nursing care was described very clearly and articulately. Data were similar to those reported by Sellers (2001) in her study of Christian patients' perceptions of spiritual nursing care. Participants in that study were also able to describe effective and ineffective nursing care. Effective care reflected elements such as caring presence, compassion, active listening, respect, and a sense of humor. Sellers reported ineffective care as participants perceiving they were not being seen as a person; that nurses were insensitive or focused on procedures. Body, mind and spirit were addressed in the concept of presence as described by Benner (1985), to include both 'being there' and 'being with', and were described by patients in their narratives about good nursing care. Benner, in her description of expert nursing care found that the personhood and dignity of the patient were recognized by the expert nurse and the resultant actions of the nurse were perceived by the patient. Physical presence, 'being there', involves touching, assessing, doing, hearing and represents the routine level of physical nursing care, whereas psychological or therapeutic presence, 'being with', involves the therapeutic use of self, to include both verbal and nonverbal communication, with the intention of establishing a meaningful connection with the patient (Taylor, 2002; Watson, 1999).

Participants in this study had an expectation of competence of their nurses which was addressed in the physical presence, 'being there', of the nurse. These participants expressed an expectation of nursing knowledge and skill, correct, prompt attention to physical needs, administering medications in a timely manner, and assessing and attending to pain. Sourial (1997) proposed that physical care was perceived as more important to patients than psychosocial or existential care, and that nurses may take physical care for granted, in that physical care was seen as an imperative, whereas psychosocial or existential care was only provided if there was time. Eriksson (2001) likewise identified professional skill as important to perception of care. Latham (1996) reported that, overall, physical care was of more value to patients than spiritual care. This was certainly reflected in the stories and expectations verbalized by participants in this study. Physical care was a universal expectation and was universally valued by the participants in this study. Participants expected physical care more than they expected spiritual care. Spiritual care was greatly valued, but not expected.

Brush and Daly (2000) use the terms 'being here' and 'being there', and assert that presence is essential in spiritual caregiving. Although not specifically identified as elements of spirituality, study participants stressed that being seen as an individual, as a human being, was important. 'Being there' was a cardinal element in participants' descriptions of good nursing care and reflected 'being there' as described by Brush and Daly or the more common term in the literature, 'being with' (Benner, 1985; Burkhardt & Nagai-Jacobson, 2002; Chase-Ziolck et al, 2000; Nelms, 1996; Taylor, 2002; and Watson, 1999). Arthur Frank (1991), a trained sociologist, was profoundly affected by his own experience with illness and wrote of this experience with illness and hospitalization. He stressed that care only begins when differences (individualities) are recognized. Participants in the current study described good nursing care as being seen as individuals, as a human being. Caring was perceived as more than attending to physical needs in a technically competent manner only if the participants were seen as individuals. These data indicate that while the commonality of being human gives value, being seen as an individual allows persons/humans to feel valued; and the feeling of value is predicated by being cared for as an individual with a disease or health condition, not treated as a disease or health condition of a human. Most poignantly, "The common diagnostic categories into which medicine places its patients are relevant to disease, not to illness. They are useful for treatment, but they only get in the way of care (Frank, 1991, p. 45)".

Sharing of self by the nurse was a recurrent concept in the data. It was described as an integral part of being accepted as an individual by the nurse and of developing a trusting relationship. This humanistic holistic perspective, to include compassion, was also reflected as being considerate, kind and pleasant by participants. These characteristics were also described by Appleton (1993) as desires of patients. More than performing tasks, presence requires an openness on the part of the nurse to 'being with' a patient (Burkhardt & Nagai-Jacobson, 2002), and that openness reveals both the being of the nurse and the being of others, to include the patient (Nelms, 1996).

Appleton (1993) conceptualized the 'other' aspect of presence - that of patient presence, and the patient's way of being there as someone needing care and feeling vulnerable during hospitalization. The response of the nurse to the patient's presence would then result in comfort and reduced vulnerability. The participants' desires for touch, both touch needed for physical care, and comforting touch, are explicit in the concept of caring presence. Touch is identified in the theoretical literature as an element of presence (Burkhardt & Nagai-Jacobson, 2002; Swanson, 1999; Watson, 1999) and in research literature as indicative of caring (Fredriksson, 1999; Mulaik et al, 1991). Participants in the current study described being vulnerable and of being comforted in their descriptions of good nursing care. Data suggested a lack of comfort and a continued sense of vulnerability in stories of bad nursing care. I conclude that the hallmark of the conceptualization of good nursing care seemed to focus on existential spiritual care activities that the nurse performed that helped to reduce those feelings of vulnerability, specifically, not only seeing patients as human beings, but treating patients with kindness, gentleness and comforting touch. The mutuality of presence, both recognizing patients' presence as described by Appleton and offering nursing presence, is consistent with the existential nature of humanistic nursing and my assumption that nursing is holistic. Recognizing the presence of the patient and responding with caring presence, to include interventions of comforting touch, kindness, gentleness, and recognizing individuality are not expectations of patients when hospitalized, but are certainly recognized and appreciated as elements of good nursing care.

Adamsen and Tewes (2000) found a discrepancy in patient perception of the care they received and the care perceived as being giving by nursing staff. Perceptions of pain, sleep and rest, and problems that impact quality of life, although generally recognized by nursing staff, were underestimated by nursing staff according to patient perceptions. There was some evidence that this perception of care also occurred in the narratives provided by participants in this study. While pain management was not brought up as an issue, some participants reported such issues as noise in the hallways, nursing activities that interfered with sleep and having to wait an inordinate amount of time for assistance with nausea. The collective tone of the narratives was that nurses were very busy, not that there was a discrepancy in the perception of needs. If care was not perceived, participants were quick to defend the nurse by acknowledging the nurses were too busy. In addition, participants felt the need to be protective of nurses' time, almost a reverse-caregiver role. Patients were aware of problems that impacted quality of life while in the hospital such as waiting for a nurse to respond to a call light, or perceptions of noise in the hallway that interfere with rest. Patients were also protective of nurses' time, and quick to offer excuses (lack of time) for issues that affected the patients' quality of life while in the hospital, such as inordinate noise and not responding in a timely manner.

The phenomenological study by Kralik et al., (1997) considered what patients perceived as important about nursing care, and identified two major themes: engagement and detachment. Engagement was supported by the minor themes of nurses approaching the patient in such a manner that conveyed that nothing was too much trouble in their care, consulting with the patient, smiling and using humor, having the qualities of being kind and compassionate, knowing what was needed without having to be asked, being available, friendly, warm, and using a gentle touch. The theme of detachment was supported by such perceived behaviors as "treating the patient as a number" (depersonalization), being too efficient or busy, conveying that the patient should "try harder" or encouraging to the extreme, not sharing information with the patient, even when asked, having "rough hands", and approaching the job of nursing as "just a job" or "just doing what they are told". Similarly, Tumblin and Simkin (2001), Larrabee and Bolden (2001) and Radwin (2000) identified physical comfort, emotional support, providing instruction and information, attentiveness, coordination of activities, individualization and technical skills as expectations of the nurses' role by patients. Most of the behaviors identified by Kralik et al, Tumblin and Simkin, Larrabee and Bolden, and Radwin were also identified by the various participants in this study as elements of good nursing care. Individualization and "treating me as a human being", being seen as a unique individual, but also the commonality of being human, was repeatedly mentioned as exemplary of good nursing by participants in this study. However, participants did not identify all behaviors as having been exhibited by their nurses. Specifically, the concept that the nurse should convey that nothing is too much trouble in their care was not generally perceived. In fact, body language and demeanor of nurses toward the participants indicated that the nurses did not have time to be fully present. Participants believed they should be protective of the nurses' time because they did not want to trouble the nurses. Hewison (1995) described nurse/patient interaction as being superficial and routine, and suggested nurses had a 'power over' relationship with patients in their care. This superficiality is not conducive to communication or relationship building, and could explain in part the tendency of patients in the current study to believe they were infringing on nurses' time if they requested anything perceived to be outside the routine.

2. Are the Actions of Nurses to Address Spiritual Health Perceived by Patients as Fulfilling Their Expectations?

Although not couched in the same terminology, participants in this study perceived actions that address spiritual health and described these actions in their descriptions of good nursing care. Conversely, actions that did not offer caring presence were often defining characteristics of bad nursing care. In their own experience of spiritual nursing care, participants generally believed that spiritual nursing care involved attending to religious aspects of spirituality. Although actions to address caring presence, 'being with', were certainly appreciated, they were not an expectation. In addition, actions to address any religious aspects of spiritual care on the part of the nurse, were not only not expected, they were often unwelcome, as indicated by Mary, who, as a devout Christian, did not want to be prayed for because "they might be praying for the wrong thing".

Spiritual care begins with presence (Burkhardt & Nagai-Jacobson, 2002) and is the basic way that spirituality is integrated into nursing care (Davidhizar et al., 2000). In addition, the spiritual component of presence has two distinct aspects, the existential qualities and actions such as kindness, touch empathy, and connectedness, and spirituality as expressed by religiosity to include religious rituals and prayer. The North American Nursing Diagnosis Association (NANDA) now recognizes the distinction between existential spirituality and religious spirituality, and has revised nursing diagnoses to reflect spirituality and religiosity separately (Burkhart, 2001).

Of note, although elements of both 'being there' and 'being with' were described as good nursing care by the study participants, and were certainly perceived by the participants, only physical presence, 'being there' was expected. Participants described the expectation of competence and watchfulness over physical needs as being important and a characteristic of good nursing. However, spiritual and psychological care, described in the 'being with' aspects of presence, was not an expectation. Participants described aspects of existential spiritual care, 'being with', such as touch, empathy, relatedness, eye contact, and kindness, as welcome and helpful, but not expected from the nurse. The aspects of 'being with' associated with religiosity, such as prayer, were expressly not expected, and in some cases, potentially detrimental, according to study participants.

Expectations are commonly based on experience. Participants expressed that the nurses were too busy or did not have time to do more than attend to physical needs. Hewison (1995) observed that most nurse/patient interaction was superficial, routine and talk-oriented and suggested that nurses had a 'power over' relationship with patients, which was a barrier to any meaningful communication between nurse and patient. Data generated by Hewison's study reflected that 'power over' and being treated in a routine manner as opposed to as an individual was indicative of bad nursing care. Indeed, some participants identified such behavior as indicative of bad nursing care. Perhaps this could be an explanation for participants in this study having no expectation of existential spiritual care, and emphatically not being desirous of any religious aspects of spiritual care. Because patients in the hospital have a sense of vulnerability, it would neither be expected nor wanted for anyone seen as having 'power over' to delve into anything that in essence defines them as a human being.

3. What Actions by Nurses are Perceived as Spiritual Interventions by Patients?

Spiritual interventions perceived by participants in this study were centered around the religious patterns of spirituality such as prayer or referral to clergy, and knowing when to make such referral. Activities of presence such as touching, exhibiting care and concern, communicating to include listening and explaining medical care, making the participant feel less vulnerable, and sharing of self were also perceived, but not necessarily labeled or recognized as being spiritual by participants. However, such activities were recognized as elements of "good" nursing care. One participant identified the act of caring to be spiritual and described such attributes as coaching and exhibiting humor as evidence of spiritual care from his nurse. This was consistent with the humanistic framework. The existential nature of care includes an element of reciprocity, meaning that what is conveyed should be perceived as being conveyed (Appleton, 1993; Burkhardt & Nagai-Jacobson, 2000; Patterson & Zderad, 1988; Taylor, 2002).

Touch was identified as conveying caring, connectedness and a sense of 'being with' by two participants. Results of the study conducted by Mulaik et al (1991) also indicated that patients viewed touch as indicative of caring and that touch by the nurses was important in care. The study by Mulaik et al also indicated that 59% of respondents also reported that touch indicated control on the part of the nurse and should not be used often. Although, specific questions about touch were not included in the current study, participants did not mention perceiving touch as a means of control.

Two qualitative studies (Concho, 1995 and Sellers, 2001) that addressed patient's perceptions of spiritual care described spiritual interventions consistent with those described in this study. Participants in both Sellers' and Conco's studies were self-identified as being Christian, and described establishing a caring relationship, presence, listening and giving of self (sharing) as included in effective nursing care. In addition, they reported that people feel connected to others who share the same spiritual beliefs and examining meaning or purpose in life was described as spiritual caregiving by participants. This finding was not borne out in the current study, which, via sampling for maximum variation, recruited both religious and nonreligious participants. While one participant in the current study reported finding comfort if she and the nurse had common religious beliefs, other participants reported not having any expectation of spiritual care, other than to be referred to clergy. In addition, one participant in the current study, an atheist, expressly did not want the religious aspects of spiritual care and objected to the word "spiritual". Of note, another participant, self-identified as Episcopalian, reported being leery of nurses who offer to pray for her because they may not share her specific religious beliefs and may pray for the wrong thing, even if they are Christians.

4. How Do Individuals Define Spiritual Care?

Spiritual care was defined by participants in this study mainly in terms of religiosity – religious beliefs, prayer, needs provided by a minister, and connection to a higher power. Three individuals defined spiritual care as caring and went on to describe behaviors associated with nursing presence such as empathy, sympathy and "being there for you". Two participants specifically differentiated between religion and spirituality, identifying religion in terms of a belief pattern and spirituality in terms of nursing presence. These same concepts were identified by participants in the Sellers (2001) study, in which spiritual care was characterized as nurses understanding the unique human experience by establishing a caring relationship to include being present, listening, respecting and giving of self. Conco (1995) reported that spiritual care was given when caregivers shared their own beliefs in a supreme being with the patients. This idea of sharing of beliefs was identified by two participants in this study, who went on to indicate that spiritual care as described by Conco would have been welcomed. As was also found in the current study, both Conco and Sellers reported spiritual care as having strong religious connotations. I found that spiritual care was defined by patients mainly in terms of religiosity, and is neither expected, nor desired, from nurses in the hospital. To a lesser extent, spiritual care was described by behaviors consistent with nursing presence as described in the literature.

Religious aspects of spirituality are addressed in the literature by studies using various Likert type questionnaires to describe or measure components of spirituality such as purpose in life, life salience, ego strength, self image, perceived well-being, religious orientation, and existential wellbeing (Ellison, 1983; McCutcheon, 1998; O'Neill & Kenny, 1998; Shek, 1991). Religious aspects of spirituality dominate the content of these questionnaires. In defining spirituality, participants in the current study also discussed some of the same concepts measured in the various questionnaires including belief systems, religious orientation and practices such as prayer, and meaning or purpose in life. However, the majority of participants defined spirituality in terms of religious affiliation, belief in a higher being, and religious practices such as prayer. They acknowledged that that which gave meaning or purpose to life could be important, but primarily, spirituality was synonymous with religiosity. Of note, those participants who self-identified as agnostic and atheistic identified spirituality in terms of religion as strongly, or more strongly than participants who self-identified as Christian. Other consistent themes included in definitions of spirituality were appreciating nature, music, taking time to determine what is meaningful to the patient, active listening, being with, sharing self, demonstrating that the patient was valued and seen as a human being, and connection to others and to a higher power.

Reker, Peacock and Wong (1981) and Drolet (1990) utilized questionnaires designed to explore concepts associated with spiritual beliefs such as life purpose, death acceptance and symbolic immortality. Interestingly, these concepts were not mentioned as elements of spirituality by participants in this study. On the other hand, no participant specifically excluded these concepts from spiritual beliefs either.

The defining characteristics of spiritual care are also consistent with definitions of spiritual care in the theoretical literature. Quantitative studies of spirituality have been conducted largely with regard to religiosity (Giblin, 1997; Reed, 1987; Richards, 1991). Spiritual care is often confused with, or used interchangeably with religiosity. Given that, spiritual needs are often referred to a chaplain or minister. Burkhart (2001), in her report for the Spirituality and Religiousness Diagnosis Working Group, North American Nursing Diagnosis Association (NANDA) acknowledged that, in clinical nursing, spiritual nursing care has historically been defined in terms of religious preference or practice. Recognizing that this conceptualization does not address patients who do not have religious affiliations, this working group developed separate definitions for spirituality and religiosity. The new definition of spirituality encompasses the concepts of purpose in life, connection to self, others and a higher being, art, music, literature and nature.

In summary, consistent with the literature, participants in this study defined spirituality primarily in terms of religiosity or religious practices such as prayer. Other experiences used to define spirituality included appreciating nature, music, taking time to determine what is meaningful to the patient, active listening, being with, sharing self, demonstrating that the patient was valued and seen as a human being, and connection to others and to a higher power.

Although the data generating strategy for this study was to achieve maximum variation in respondents, the majority of the respondents self-identified as Christian, limiting responses, particularly in defining spirituality, to those reflecting Christian belief systems. Even those participants self-identified as agnostic or atheistic responded based on their own knowledge base or background, which was in all cases, Christian. The resulting data was rich, but the particular perspectives of Islam, Judaism and Eastern teachings and beliefs were not represented and could further enrich the understanding of spirituality and spiritual care.

In addition, all the respondents were Caucasian. Even within the same religious belief system, here Christianity, there are a wide variety of interpretations and practices among different ethnic and cultural groups. That variability was not reflected in this participant group. Because both religious and spiritual practices are largely influenced by cultural and ethnic traditions, the lack of variability related to culture and ethnicity is a limitation of the current study, particularly in understanding the phenomena of spirituality and spiritual care.

Questions in this study related specifically to caring practices of nurses in a hospital setting. One of my assumptions was that the participants would respond truthfully. I have no reason to believe that participants did not respond truthfully during their interviews. However, because I was known to the participants to be a nurse, it is possible that the participants told me what they thought I wanted to hear.

Many hospitals in the United States have religious sponsorship or affiliations while others are secular for profit and not for profit institutions. I did not ask, nor was it apparent in the collection of data for this study if participants were hospitalized in religious or non-religious affiliated hospitals. Examining responses to the study questions and narrative stories in light of whether or not participants were hospitalized in a religious-based institution could have added to a deeper understanding of the phenomenon of patient expectations of spiritual care by their nurses.

Recommendations for Future Studies

Further research is warranted to explore the concept of spiritual care as part of holistic nursing practice. Participants in this study were able to describe good and bad nursing care. Based on the responses of participants in this study, one of the most compelling conclusions I have reached with regard to spiritual care is that existential spiritual care is the hallmark of good nursing care. Conversely, lack of existential spiritual care was a definitive characteristic of bad nursing care. Clarifying and exploring the meaning of spiritual nursing care is therefore imperative in investigating quality nursing care practices and nursing education.

One of the potential limitations of this study, was that a nurse conducted the interviews, and participants responses were influenced by that fact. It is equally possible that participants were more considered in their responses because a nurse cared enough to ask questions about their hospitalizations. To address the potential for biased responses, either positive or negative, during the course of the interview, a non-nurse researcher could ask the interview questions. Comparisons could be drawn between responses elicited by a nurse, as in this study, and those elicited in a future study by a non-nurse. Hypothetically, responses elicited by the non-nurse researcher should be comparable to those elicited by the nurse researcher.

The lack of variability related to cultural and ethnic traditions is a possible limitation of the current study. Both religious and spiritual practices are largely influenced by cultural and ethnic traditions. Although one participant was atheistic and two were agnostic, the religious and cultural traditions of all participants in this study were Christian-based. It would be appropriate to address spiritual care perceptions through the lens of cultural and ethnic traditions. It would also be interesting to solicit respondents with more diverse religious backgrounds. It would also be exciting to explore perceptions of spiritual care among children of various developmental levels.

Spiritual care perceptions in this study were investigated from the perspective of the patient. Having a better understanding of the expectations regarding care in general and spiritual care specifically from the perspective of the patient, it seems logical to interview nurses regarding their perceptions of the care they provide, to include spiritual aspects of care. It would be interesting to present the findings of this study to a focus group of practicing nurses and discuss practice implications. Within the framework of humanistic nursing, there should be no difference in the perceptions of spiritual care between nurse respondents and patient respondents. In addition, nurses descriptions of exemplary nursing characteristics should parallel the characteristics of good nurses as described by the participants in the current study

Many scientific studies have been conducted that indicate there is a relationship between stress and the immune system. Does spiritual caregiving have a measurable effect on stress? Do religious beliefs or lack of a belief system have an effect on stress or perception of stress? Given that there is a measureable effect of stress on the immune system, if stress is ameliorated by spiritual care, the immune system would be enhanced. On the other hand, if stress is exacerbated by a lack of or inappropriate spiritual care, the immune system would be weakened. Religiosity of the patient may have a similar effect on stress perception and therefore the immune system. A future study could be conducted exploring the relationship between spirituality and religiosity, stress, and the immune system.

Conclusion

This study resulted in several interesting findings. First, nursing presence was seen by patients as important and elements of nursing presence were used to describe good nursing care. 'Being there', with elements of nursing competence (knowing what is going on and technical proficiency), as well as nursing surveillance (keeping track, notifying physicians as warranted, watching carefully), was a universal expectation of nurses. 'Being with', the existential spiritual element of presence (kindness, gentleness, caring touch) was the most defining characteristic of good nursing care as described by participants, but was not expected. Sharing of self, and element of existential spiritual care is generally discouraged in my experience as a nurse, both in nursing schools and in hospital settings, but was clearly appreciated from the patients' perspective. All participants were able to define spirituality, most frequently in terms of religiosity and religious practices such as prayer. Spiritual nursing care was most frequently described as recognizing the need to refer the patient to a minister. The religious element of spirituality was not expected or wanted, by some, adamantly.

Time was a strong recurrent theme. Perceptions of nursing not having time (scurrying in the hallways, not talking to the patient when in the room, not making eye contact) were mentioned by 9 of the 11 participants. Perceiving the nurses as too busy led to patients not requesting care. This perceived lack of time was then offered as a reason for not expecting existential spiritual care. Sourial (1997) concluded that nurses viewed physical care was an imperative, whereas psychosocial or existential care was only provided if there was time. This is consistent with study participant's perceptions.

The framework for investigating the concept of time with relation to patient care is provided in the theory of humanistic nursing (Pattrson & Zderad, 1988). Humanistic nursing recognizes that, in the transactional nature of nursing, there is an intersubjectivity between nurse and patient that results in a timing of behaviors aimed at developing the patient's human potential. In general, the findings of this study were congruent with the literature with the exception of patient expectations of spiritual interventions by their nurse. In addition, the theoretical framework of humanistic nursing was appropriate to describe the phenomenon of spiritual care and supports continued analysis and implementation of spiritual care.

The research questions of this study were addressed in the narratives of the participants. Findings of this study contribute to the understanding of the role of the nurse in providing spiritual care within a holistic nursing care framework. The opportunity to continue to research spiritual care, to include clarifying and reinforcing spiritual dimensions of care as it relates to individuals and to populations is illuminated.

References

[1]   Adamsen, L. & Tewes, M. (2000). Discrepancy between patients' perspectives, staff's documentation and reflections on basic nursing care. *Scandinavian Journal of Caring Science,* 14, 120-129.

[2]   Appleton, C. (1993). The art of nursing: The experience of patients and nurses. *Journal of Advanced Nursing, 18,* 892-899.

[3]   Benner, P. (1985). Quality of life: A phenomenological perspective on explanation, prediction, and understanding in nursing science. *Advances in Nursing Science, 8(1),* 1-14.

[4]   Bensley, R. (1991). Defining spiritual health: A review of the literature. *Journal of Health Education,* 22(5), 287-290.

[5]   Bohm, D. (Ed. Nichol, L.) (1996). On dialogue. New York: Routledge, Taylor & Francis Group.

[6]   Brush, B. & Daly, P. (2000). Assessing spirituality in primary care practice: Is there time? *Clinical Excellence for Nurse Practitioners,* 4(2), 67-71.

[7]   Burkhardt, M. (1989). Spirituality: An analysis of the concept. *Holistic Nursing Practice,* 3(3), 69-77.

[8]   Burkhardt, M. & Nagai-Jacobson, M. (2002). *Spirituality: Living our connectedness.* Albany, NY: Delmar.

[9]   Burkhart, L. (2001). Notes on NDEC: Report from the spirituality and religiousness diagnosis working group. *Nursing Diagnosis,* 12(2), 61062.

[10]   Carroll, B. (2001). A phenomenological exploration of the nature of spirituality and spiritual care. *Mortality,* 6(1), 81-99.

[11] Carson, V. (1989). *Spiritual dimensions of nursing practice.* Philadelphia: W.B. Saunders Co.

[12] Chase-Ziolck, M. & Gruca, J. (2000). Clients' perceptions of distinctive aspects in nursing care received within a congregational setting. *Journal of Community Health Nursing,* 17(3), 171-183.

[13] Clarke, J. & Wheeler, S. (1992). A view of the phenomenon of caring in nursing practice. *Journal of Advanced Nursing, 17,* 1283-1290.

[14] Concho, D. (1995). Christian patients' view of spiritual care. *Western Journal of Nursing Research, 17(3),*266-277.

[15] Cortis, J. (2000). Caring as experienced by minority ethnic patients. *International Nursing Review,* 47(1), 53-63.

[16] Cumbie, S. (2001). The integration of mind-body-soul and the practice of humanistic nursing. *Holistic Nursing Practice,* 15(3), 56-62.

[17] Davidhizar, R, Bechtel, G, & Cosey, E. (2000). The spiritual needs of hospitalized patients. *American Journal of Nursing,* 100(7), 24C-24D.

[18] Davis, L. (2005). A phenomenological study of patient expectations concerning nursing care. *Holistic Nursing Practice, 19(3),* 126-133.

[19] Dossey, B. (1998). Holistic modalities and healing moments. *American Journal of Nursing,* 98(6), 44-47.

[20] Dossey, B. and Dossey, L. (1998). Body-mind-spirit: Attending to holistic care. *American Journal of Nursing,* 98(8), 35-38.

[21] Drain, M. (2001). Quality improvement in primary care and the importance of patient perceptions. *Journal of Ambulatory Care Management,* 24(2), 30-46.

[22] Drolet, J. (1990). Transcending death during early adulthood: Symbolic immortality, death anxiety, and purpose in life. *Journal of Clinical Psychology,* 46(2), 148-160.

[23] Dyson, J., Cobb, M., & Forman, D. (1997). The meaning of spirituality: A literature review. *Journal of Advanced Nursing,* 26, 1183-1188.

[24] Ellison, C. (1983). Spiritual well-being: Conceptualization and measurement. *Journal of Psychology and Theology,* 11(4), 330-340.

[25] Eriksson, E. (2001). Caring for cancer patients: Relatives' assessments of received care. *European Journal of Cancer Care,* 10(1), 48-56.

[26] Erlandson, D., Harris, E., Skipper, B., & Allen, S. (1993). *Doing naturalistic inquiry: A guide to methods.* Newbury Park: SAGE Publications.

[27] Espland, K. (1999). Achieving spiritual wellness: Using reflective questions. *Journal of Psychosocial Nursing,* 37(7), 36-40.

[28] Fagerstrom, L., Eriksson, K., & Engberg, I. (1999). The patient's perceived caring needs: Measuring the unmeasurable. *International Journal of Nursing Practice,* 5, 199-208.

[29] Fontaine, K. (2000). *Healing practices: Alternative therapies for nursing.* Upper saddle River, NJ: Prentice Hall.

[30] Frank, A. (1991). *At the will of the body: Reflections on illness.* Boston: Houghton Mifflin Company.

[31] Frankl, V. (1984). *Man's search for meaning: An introduction to logotherapy.* New York: Simon & Schuster.

[32] Fredriksson, L. (1999). Modes of relating in a caring conversation: A research synthesis on presence, touch and listening. *Journal of Advanced Nursing*, 30(5), 1167-1176.

[33] Gilbin, P. (1997). Marital spirituality: A quantitative study. *Journal of Religion and Health*, 36(4), 321-332.

[34] Giorgi, A. (1970). *Psychology as a human science: A phenomenologically based approach.* New York: Harper & Row.

[35] Godkin, J. (2001). Healing presence. *Journal of Holistic Nursing.* 19(1), 5-21.

[36] Halldorsdottir, S. & Hamrin, E. (1997). Caring and uncaring encounters within nursing and health care from the cancer patient's perspective. *Cancer Nursing, 20(2),* 120-128.

[37] Hewison, A. (1995). Nurses' power in interactions with patients. *Journal of Advanced Nursing, 21,* 75-82.

[38] Howard, B. & Howard, J. (1997). Occupation as spiritual activity. *The American Journal of Occupational Therapy*, 51(3), 181-185.

[39] Kralik, D., Koch, T., & Wotton, K. (1997). Engagement and detachment: Understanding patients' experiences with nursing. *Journal of Advanced Nursing, 26,* 399-407.

[40] Larrabee, J. & Bolden, L. (2001). Defining patient-perceived quality of nursing care. *Journal of Nursing Care Quality,* 16(1), 34-57.

[41] Latham, C. (2001). Predictors of patient outcomes following interactions with nurses. *Western Journal of Nursing Research,* 18(5), 548-564.

[42] McCutcheon, L. (1998). Life role salience scales: Additional evidence for construct validation. *Psychological Reports*, 83, 1307-1314.

[43] McKinnon, N. (1991). Humanistic nursing: It can't stand up to scrutiny. *Nursing and Health Care*, 12(8), 414-416.

[44] McSherry, W, & Draper, P. (1998). The debates emerging from the literature surrounding the concept of spirituality as applied to nursing. *Journal of Advanced Nursing*, 27(4), 683-691.

[45] Meraviglia, M. (1999). Critical analysis of spirituality and its empirical indicators. *Journal of Holistic Nursing,* 17(1), 18-33.

[46] Miles, M. & Huberman, A. (1994). *An expanded sourcebook: Qualitative data analysis.* Thousand Oaks, CA: SAGE Publications.

[47] Mulaik, J., Megenity, J., Cannon, R., Chance, K., Cannella, K., Garland, L, & Gilead, M. (1991). Patients' perceptions of nurses' use of touch. *Western Journal of Nursing Research,* 13(3), 306-323.

[48] Mulholland, J. (1995). Nursing, humanism and transcultural theory: The 'bracketing out' of reality. *Journal of Advanced Nursing,* 22(3), 442-449.

[49] Nelms, T. (1996). Living a caring presence in nursing: A Heideggerian analysis. *Journal of Advanced Nursing,* 24(2), 368-374.

[50] Newman, M. (1989). The spirit of nursing. *Holistic Nursing Practice*, 3(3), 1-6.

[51] O'Neill, D, & Kenny, E. (1998). Spirituality and chronic illness. Image*: Journal of Nursing Scholarship*, 30(3), 275-280.

[52] Patterson, E. (1998). The philosophy and physics of holistic health care: spiritual healing as a workable interpretation. *Journal of Advanced Nursing,* 27(2), 287-293.

[53] Patterson, J. & Zderad, L. (1988). *Humanistic nursing.* New York: National League for Nursing.

[54] Polkinghorne, D. (1988). *Narrative knowing and the human sciences.* Albany: State University of New York Press.

[55] Quinn, J. (2000). The self as healer: Reflections from a nurse's journey. *AACN Clinical Issues: Advanced Practice in Acute Critical Care, 11(1),* 17-26.

[56] Radwin, L. (2000). Oncology patients' perceptions of quality nursing care, *Research in Nursing Health,* 23, 179-190.

[57] Reed, P. (1987). Spirituality and well-being in terminally ill hospitalized adults. *Research in Nursing and Health,* 10, 335-344.

[58] Reed, P. (1992). An emerging paradigm for the investigation of spirituality in nursing. *Research in Nursing & Health,* 15, 349-357.

[59] Reker, G., Peacock, E., & Wong, P. (1987). Meaning and purpose in life and well-being: A life-span perspective. *Journal of Gerontology,* 42(1), 44-49.

[60] Richards, P. (1991). Religious devoutness in college students: Relations with emotional adjustment and psychological separation from parents. *Journal of Counseling Psychology,* 38(2), 189-196.

[61] Ross, L. (1994). Spiritual aspects of nursing. *Journal of Advanced Nursing,* 19, 439-447.

[62] Rogers, M. (1972). Nursing: To be or not to be? *Nursing Outlook,* 20(1), 42-46.

[63] Sellers, S. (2001). The spiritual care meanings of adults residing in the Midwest. *Nursing Science Quarterly,* 14(3), 239-248.

[64] Shek, D. (1991). Meaning in life and psychological well-being: An empirical study using the Chinese version of the Purpose in Life Questionnaire. *The Journal of Genetic Psychology,* 153(2), 185-200.

[65] Sheldon, J. (2000). Spirituality as a part of nursing. *Journal of Hospice and Palliative Nursing,* 2(3), 101-108.

[66] Sourial, S. (1997). An analysis of caring. *Journal of Advanced Nursing,* 26, 1189-1192.

[67] Stranahan, S. (2001). Spiritual perception, attitudes about spiritual care, and spiritual care practice among nurse practitioners. *Western Journal of Nursing Research,* 23(1), 90-105.

[68] Streubert, H. & Carpenter, D. (1999). *Qualitative research in nursing: Advancing the humanistic imperative.* Philadelphia: Lippincott.

[69] Stuart, E., Deckro, J., & Mandle, C. (1989). Spirituality in health and healing: A clinical program. *Holistic Nursing Practice,* 3(3), 35-46.

[70] Swanson, K. (1999). What is known about caring in nursing science: A literary meta-analysis. In A.S. Hinshaw, S. Feetham, & J. Shaver (Eds.), *Handbook of clinical nursing research* (pp. 31- 60). Thousand Oaks, CA: SAGE Publications.

[71] Tanyi, R. (2002). Towards clarification of the meaning of spirituality. *Journal of Advanced Nursing, 39(5),* 500-509.

[72] Taylor, E. (2002). *Spiritual care: Nursing theory, research, and practice.* Upper Saddle river, NJ: Prentice Hall.

[73] Thomas, S. & Pollio, H. (2002). *Listening to patients: A phenomenological approach to nursing research and practice.* New York: Springer Publishing Company.

[74] Travelbee, J. (1969). *Intervention in psychiatric nursing: Process in the one-to-one relationship.* Philadelphia: FA Davis.

[75] Tumblin, A. & Simkin, P. (2001). Pregnant women's perceptions of their nurse's role during labor and delivery. *Perinatal Care,* 28(1), 52-56.

[76] Van der Zalm, J. & Bergum, V. (2000). Hermeneutic-phenomenology: providing living knowledge for nursing practice. *Journal of Advanced Nursing,* 31(1), 211-218.

[77] Van Manen, M. (1990). *Researching lived experiences.* London, Ontario: State University of New York Press.

[78] Watson, J. (1985). *Nursing: The philosophy and science of caring.* Niwot, CO: The University Press of Colorado.

[79] Watson, J. (1999). Postmodern nursing and beyond. New York: Churchill Livingstone.

[80] Watson, J. & Smith, M (2002). Caring science and the science of unitary human beings: A trans-theoretical discourse for nursing knowledge development. *Journal of Advanced Nursing, 37(5),* 452-461.

[81] Woolf, H (Ed.). (1975). *Webster's new collegiate dictionary* (6th ed.). Springfield MA: G&C Merriam Co.

[82] Wright, K. (1998). Professional, ethical and legal implications for spiritual care in nursing. *Image: Journal of Nursing Scholarship*, 30, 1, 82-83.

In: Trends in Nursing Research
Editors: Adam J. Ryan and Jack Doyle

ISBN 978-1-60456-642-0
© 2009 Nova Science Publishers, Inc.

Chapter 3

Factors Associated with Racially and Ethnically Diverse Children and Adolescent Immunization Rates in a Community Health Center

Richelle T. Magday Asselstine and *Victoria P. Niederhauser*
Shriners Hospital for Children – Honolulu,
1310 Punahou Street, Honolulu, HI 96826
University of Hawaii School of Nursing and Dental Hygiene,
2528 McCarthy Mall, Honolulu, HI 96822

Abstract

Background: Evidence of disparities in child and adolescent immunization rates are abundant in the literature (Niederhauser and Stark, 2005). These disparities occur in different ethnic groups, races, and socioeconomic classes. However, there is a lack of studies that examine factors associated with under-immunization rates in Asian and Pacific Islander (API) children and adolescents.

Community Health Centers (CHCs), who serve predominantly poor and minority populations, are in an ideal position to minimize gaps in child and adolescent immunization rates. The purpose of this study was to identify factors associated with under-immunization in racially and ethnically diverse children who seek health care services at a CHC in Hawaii. The setting for this study was at an urban CHC in downtown Honolulu that provides health care to a multi-ethnic population including many API immigrant families.

Methods: This was a cross-sectional descriptive design study. A sample of 400 children and adolescents, ages birth to 21 years, who received care at the CHC during a 12 month period of time, were randomly selected for participation in the study. Of the 400 who were selected, 369 medical records were available to review during the 1 month

* E-mail: rasselstine@shrinenet.org, Tel: 808-951-3670.

data collection period. The data collected from the medical records included age of child or adolescent (in months), gender, ethnicity, total household income, insurance status and type and date of childhood immunizations. For this study, a child was considered not up-to-date on their immunizations if they did not have the recommended immunization within one month of the due date. This study was approved by the Committee on Human Subjects, University of Hawaii at Manoa.

Results: The overall immunization rates for this sample was 41% up-to-date, 30% not up-to-date and 29% had no record of immunizations in their medical record. For the final analysis, the not-up-to-date and no record were merged into one category and considered not-up-to-date. There were 38% male and 62% female medical records reviewed. The total household income mean was $887 (range $0-$5153, SD $871). Sixty-three percent had insurance coverage, 35% had no insurance and 2% had no insurance information in the medical record. In the bi-variate analysis ethnicity (x^2 12.274, p= .015), insurance status (x^2 18.994, p= .000) and total household income (x^2 9.167, p= .010) were significantly associated with up-to-date status. In the logistic regression analysis, total family income and insurance status was associated with up-to-date status; when conducting the analysis with all three variables ethnicity was not significantly associated with immunization status.

Discussion: Overall the majority of children and adolescents in this study had sub-optimal immunization rates. The findings in this study are similar to findings in other studies of poor and ethnically diverse children and adolescents; immunization rates are significantly associated with having insurance, having a higher total family income and among the different ethnic groups. Interventions targeting increasing immunization rates in poor and ethnically diverse children are necessary to decrease disparities in this important public health intervention.

Introduction

Immunizations are among the greatest public health achievements and one of the most important public health tools of all time (Stern and Markel, 2005; US Department of Health and Human Services, 2000). Countries where routine immunizations are implemented have significantly better public health outcomes than countries not fortunate enough to benefit from immunizations (Eberwine-Villagrán, 2007). A recent study of childhood deaths in Northern India indicate that 61% of children who died of a vaccine-preventable disease were not immunized (Jha et al, 2006).

The United States Department of Health and Human Services' Office of Disease Prevention and Health Promotion (2000) created a national health initiative, Healthy People 2010 (HP 2010) with two goals; 1) increase quality and years of life and 2) eliminate health disparities. There are twenty-eight focus areas of HP 2010 with ten leading health indicators. As a leading health indicator, immunizations is a top ten focus for HP 2010 (CDC, 2007).

Background

Hawaii is an ethnically and racially diverse state with 75% of its population classified as a minority, including 42% Asian, 21% two or more races, and 9% Native Hawaiian or Pacific

Islander (U S Census Bureau, 2001). In the United States, Asian and Pacific Islanders (API) are projected to reach forty-one million, or a total of 11% of the population by the year 2050 (Barnes and Bennett, 2002; Reeves and Bennett, 2002; US Bureau of the Census, 2000 and 2001).

In the State of Hawaii, prior to 1999, childhood immunization rates were steadily above the national average and began to decline significantly thereafter (Altonn, 2002; Hawaii State Department of Health, 2002). In 2001, a time where the national average increased by one-percent to 77%, Hawaii's childhood immunization rates dropped from 82% in 1999 to nearly 73% in 2001 (Altonn, 2002). In response to the decrease in immunization rates, the Department of Health implemented strategies to improve the childhood immunization rates through a community action campaign that included spending more than $300,000 on radio ads in multiple languages. Three years later, the childhood immunization rates reached a record of 82.8% in the state, higher than the national rate of 80.9% (Dingeman, 2004). HP 2010's goal is to reach its target of 80% for the 4:3:1:3:3 (4 Diphtheria, Tetanus Toxoid and Pertussis vaccine (DTP), 3 poliovirus vaccine (Polio), 1 Measles containing vaccine (MCV), 3 Haemophillus Influenzae type B vaccine (HIB), and 3 Hepatitis B vaccine (HBV)) immunization series in children from 19 to 35 months by 2010; in 2006 Hawaii's rate was 78.8%, about 2% below the national goal (CDC, 2007; USDHHS, 2000).

In the literature, there is mounting evidence of the impact of socio-economic status (SES) on health outcomes and disparities in health indicators with racial and ethnic minorities (Javier, Huffman and Mendoza, 2007; Lee et al, 2007; Niederhauser and Markowitz, 2007; Niederhauser and Stark, 2005). Ethnic minority populations, including African Americans, Native Americans, Asian Americans and Pacific Islanders, are behind in achieving the goals of HP 2010 in "almost every health indicator, including health care coverage, access to care, and life expectancy" (Kagawa-Singer and Kassim-Lahka, 2003, p. 577). Due to numerous factors, both modifiable and non-modifiable, these populations have a greater mortality and morbidity rate than European Americans (Office of Minority Health and Bureau of Primary Health Care, n.d.).

There is a great disparity in childhood immunizations rates that extend across SES, racial, and ethnic backgrounds. The influence of various cultural beliefs, health care priorities, and parental values can impinge upon childhood immunizations, creating a larger disparity for these populations (Ghosh, 2003; Graberstein, 2001; Niederhauser and Stark, 2005; Niederhauser and Markowitz, 2007). The issues for families of low SES are multi-faceted and not only affected health, but are linked to education as well.

Previous studies in the literature report conflicting evidence on the association of ethnicity and childhood immunization rates. Several studies, some dating back to the 1970s, do not demonstrate an association with ethnicity and up-to-date (UTD) status and timelines of immunizations (Luman, Cauley, Stokley, Chi and Pickering; 2002; Marks, Halpin, Johnson and Keller 1979; Morrow et al., 1998). However other studies demonstrate that ethnicity and race are significant determinants of immunization status. Ehresmann et al., (1998) and Szilagyi et al., (2002) found a relationship between UTD status and ethnic minorities, specifically African Americans and Hispanics compared to Caucasians. Studies examining the relationship between UTD status and the API children are scarce. In a study looking at immunization rates in Chicago public schools, Dominguez and colleagues (2004) found that among the 13 month old ethnic minority children surveyed, Asians had the highest rates of UTD children. No study on Pacific Islander children and immunization rates were found in the literature.

Rosenthal et al., (2004) looked at four different medically underserved sites to conduct their study of immunization coverage in 19 to 35 month old children. Detroit, New York, Colorado and San Diego were the sites designated in the study and all yielded varying and conflicting results of UTD status ($p<0.0001$). However it is important to note that differences were not significant among the various ethnic groups. Factors associated significantly ($p<0.01$) with UTD status in this study were participation in the Vaccines for Children program, facility type (private, public, mixed or other), if the parent had the parent-held immunization card/record, and if the child was UTD at 3 months of age.

Some studies examining the relationship between insurance status and childhood immunization rates are found in the literature. Zhao, Mokdad and Barker (2004) conducted a study between 1993 and 1996 and found immunization status was significantly associated with insurance coverage. Children who were insured and those who were uninsured differed significantly as were the publicly insured and privately insured children. This study focused only on the 4:3:1:3 series, which includes "four or more doses of any diphtheria and tetanus toxoids and pertussis vaccine including diphtheria and tetanus toxoids, and any acellular pertussis vaccine (DTP4); three or more doses of any poliovirus vaccine (Polio); one or more dose of measles-containing vaccine (MCV); three or more doses of Haemophilus influenzae type b (Hib) vaccine and three or more doses of hepatitis B (HepB) vaccine" (p. 157). Coverage differences even varied between the different immunizations in this 4:3:1:3 series. Another study, looking specifically at publicly, privately, and underinsured children, validated the previous studies' findings concluding that there was an association between UTD status and insurance status (Santoli et al.,, 2004).

Kim et al., (2007) examined the effects of UTD status based on mother's income and educational status and found that mothers of lower SES with lower income levels had higher immunization rates. The researchers argued that one reason for these results was their study included educated mothers who based their decisions to immunize their children on controversial issues. The researchers concluded that income was not a reliable predictor to determine UTD status.

Purpose of the Study

The purpose of this study was to explore the relationship between health insurance coverage, ethnicity, and total family income on childhood immunization rates in an urban community health center (CHC) in Honolulu, Hawaii.

Research Questions

1. Is there an association between children/adolescents who are UTD with their immunizations and those who were not-up-to-date (NUTD) and their insurance coverage status?

2. Is there a difference among the total family income of children/adolescents who are UTD with immunizations and those who were NUTD with immunizations?

3. Is there an association between children/adolescents of different ethnic/racial groups and UTD status?

Methodology

Study design. This was a quantitative study, utilizing a cross-sectional descriptive design. A sample of 400 children and adolescents, ages birth to 21 years, who received care at the CHC during a 12 month period of time, were randomly selected for participation in the study. Of the 400 who were selected, 369 medical records were available to review during the 1 month data collection period. The data collected from the medical records included age of child or adolescent (in months), gender, ethnicity, total household income, insurance status and type and date of childhood immunizations. For this study, a child was considered NUTD on their immunizations if they did not have the recommended immunization within one month of the due date.

This study was part of a larger intervention study funded by the Hawaii Department of Health. In order to decrease barriers to immunizations, a free walk-in immunization clinic was established for children, adolescents, and young adults 6 months to 21 years of age during evening and weekend hours. The clinic was run by an Advanced Practice Nurse Practitioner, who conducted an initial health assessment, administered immunizations and provided information of follow-up care as necessary. The data collected for this study provided the baseline immunization rates for this intervention study (Niederhauser, Michaels and Ganeko, 2007).

Data analysis. The demographic variables used in this study included immunization status (UTD, NUTD, or no shot record available), total family income, ethnicity/race and health insurance status (insured or not insured). SPSS version 14.0 was used for the analysis. Statistical methods included cross-tabulation and Chi-Square analysis for nominal level data and independent sample t-test for interval/ratio data. Logistic regression was used to analyze the effects of the multiple independent variables (total family income, ethnicity/race, and health insurance status) on immunization status. A $p<.05$ value was considered as a significant value for this study.

Results

Demographic data. Three-hundred sixty-nine medical records were reviewed for this study. The mean age of the children was 10.95 years (range 6 months to 21 years of age, SD=6.61) and 62% were female. The average annual family income was $887.00 (SD=$871.00). Income was categorized into 4 groups, No income, $1-$999, $1000-$6000, and no record of family income in the medical record; the largest group (n=124) was in the $1-$999 (33.6%) total family income category, followed by 31% (n=115) in the $1000-$6000 group; nineteen percent (n=71) had no annual income. A summary of the demographic characteristics of the sample are found in Table 1.

Table 1. Demographic characteristics of the sample (N= 369)

SUBJECT	n	%
GENDER		
Male	141	38.4
Female	228	61.8
ETHNICITY		
Asian/Part Asian	71	19.2
Filipino	84	22.8
Hawaiian/Part Hawaiian	63	17.1
Pacific Islander	121	32.8
Other	18	4.9
Did not respond	12	3.3
INSURANCE		
Yes	233	63.1
No	128	34.7
Did not respond	8	2.2
IMMUNIZATION STATUS (3 categories)		
UTD	152	41.2
NUTD	112	30.4
No Shot Record	105	28.5
IMMUNIZATION STATUS (2 categories)		
UTD	152	41.2
NUTD	217	58.8
AGE CATEGORIES		
Birth to 18 mos.	35	9.5
19 mos. to 35 mos.	23	6.2
3 to 5 years	46	12.5
6 to 12 years	110	29.8
13 to 21 years	155	42.0
INCOME		
No income	71	19.2
$1 - $999	124	33.6
$1000-$6000	115	31.2
Did not respond	59	16.0

Insurance status and up-to-date with immunizations. There was a significant difference in the UTD status of children and health insurance status (x^2 18.994, p = .000). Further examination of the data revealed that for the 128 children who did not have health insurance, the majority were NUTD with their immunizations (73%, n=94); only 27% (n=34) of children who were not insured were UTD on their immunizations. For those children who had health insurance (n=223), one half (n=117, 50%) were UTD on their immunizations (Table 2).

Table 2. Bi-variate analysis of income, insurance, ethnicity/race and UTD status

	Up-to-Date		Not-Up-to-Date	
	n	%	n	%
Insurance*				
Yes	117	50	116	50
No	34	27	94	73
Total Annual Family Income**				
None	21	30	50	70
$1-$999	56	45	68	55
$1000-$6000	60	52	55	48
Ethnicity/Race***				
Asian/Part Asian	35	49	36	51
Filipino	24	29	60	71
Hawaiian/Part Hawaiian	25	40	38	60
Pacific Islander	60	50	61	50
Other	5	28	13	72

* p= 0.000, ** p=0.010, *** p= 0.015

Total family income and up-to-date with immunizations. The average total family income was $1021.50 for children who were UTD and $781.24 for those NUTD on their immunizations. The difference among the income mean of children who were UTD with immunizations and those who were NUTD with immunizations was significant ($t = 2.432$ and $p = .016$). For further analysis, the income was divided into 3 categories, no income, $1-999, and $1000-6000. No total family income over $6000 was identified in the medical records review. There was a significant difference in the income categories in this study (x^2 9.167, p =.010); the children with no family income had the lowest immunization rates (Table 2).

Ethnicity/Race and up-to-date with immunizations. The participants of this study were categorized into five ethnic/racial groups: 1) Asian/Part Asian (n=71), 2) Filipino (n=84), 3) Hawaiian/Part Hawaiian (n=63), 4) Pacific Islander (n=121), and 5) Other (n=18). The Pacific Islander and Asian/Part Asian children had the highest UTD immunization rates. The Other category, which included Caucasian, Hispanic and African American populations, and the Filipino population had lowest rates of UTD children (28%, 29% respectively). There was a significant difference between the ethnic/racial groups and UTD status ($x^2$12.274, p = 0.015). The Filipino, Pacific Islander and Other groups had the greatest disparities in childhood UTD and NUTD status (Table 2).

Ethnicity/Race, total family income, insurance status and up-to-date with immunizations. All of the variables of interest (total family income, insurance status, and ethnicity/race) were entered into a logistic regression model. This model demonstrated a non-significant Hosmer and Lemeshow test (p=.143), indicating the data fit the model (Munro, 2005). In addition, the model with the three predictors was statistically reliable in distinguishing between children who were and were not UTD (-2 Log likelihood 386.120; x^2 (7) 25.162, p = .001). This model was able to classify 67% of the children who were NUTD and almost one half (49%) of those children who were UTD; the overall model correctly classified 59% correctly. In the final analysis, only insurance status (p=.001) and the no income category (p=.048) were able to predict child immunization status. In other words, those children with no total family income were more likely to be NUTD; conversely, those children with insurance were less likely to be NUTD on their immunizations.

Table 3. Logistic regression model for total family income, insurance status and immunizations status

Variable	b	Wald Chi-Square	p	Odds Ratio	95% Confidence Interval for Odds Ratio	
					Lower	Upper
Ethnicity/Race						
Asian/Part Asian	-.823	1.821	.177	.439	.133	1.451
Filipino	-.148	.057	.811	.862	.256	2.908
Hawaiian/Part Hawaiian	-.374	.361	.548	.688	.203	2.331
Pacific Islanders	-.629	1.130	.288	.533	.167	1.700
Other		4.528	.339			
Total Annual Family Income						
None	.676	3.923	.048	1.966	1.007	3.838
$1-$999	.299	1.189	.275	1.349	.788	2.309
$1000-$6000		4.031	.133			
Children with Insurance	-.885	10.131	.001	.413	.239	.712
Constant	1.054	3.048	.081	2.871		

Note: All ethnicity/race categories were compared to the "Other" category, Total Family Income was compared to the "$1000-$6000" category.

Discussion

In the final analysis, this study revealed differences in immunization rates in children and adolescents based on insurance status and total family income. These findings are similar to other studies that examined factors associated with under-immunization in children (Bundt and Hu, 2004; Lee et al, 2007; Rosenthal et al, 2004; Santoli et al, 2004; Zhao et al, 2004). Other variables associated with UTD status include not only the child's health insurance status but also insurance type, education, and residence in a metropolitan area (Zhao et al, 2004).

In the logistic regression analysis, ethnicity/race was not significantly associated with UTD, however, three out of the five categories (Filipino, Pacific Islander and Other) were significant in the bi-variate analysis. In this study, the Asian/Part Asian children had one of the highest percentages of UTD status. Two other studies in the literature demonstrated high immunization rates in Asian children compared to other ethnic and racial groups (Chu, Barker and Smith 2004; Dominguez, Parrott, Lauderdale and Daum 2004). Chu, Barker and Smith (2004) found that the disparity between Caucasian children and Asian children narrowed approximately 0.8% each year from 1996 to 2001. Asian parents were less likely to believe that all children should receive the same immunizations (78%) when compared to Hispanics (97%), Caucasians (95%), and African-Americans (94%). Furthermore, the researchers demonstrated more Asian parents believed that their children were either likely or very likely to become ill after receiving immunizations as compared to 46% of African-American parents, 29% of Hispanic parents, and 10% of Caucasian parents. Santoli et al (2004) did not classify Asian, Filipino, Hawaiian and Pacific Islander separately, but did have an Other category. Through a bi-variate analysis, "child's race/ethnicity and insurance status; household income; maternal age, marital status, and educational level; location of usual source of well-child care; and WIC participation" (pg. 1961) were associated with UTD status, but through a multivariate logistic regression, only the location of the child's usual care and maternal educational level were significantly associated.

Most studies in the literature group Asians (including Filipinos) with Pacific Islanders (including Native Hawaiians); this study raises some questions about the validity of this approach. It is important to note that because of the large amount of Filipinos in the sample, they were placed in their own category instead of grouping them with the Asian/Part Asian group. In addition, because of the size and differences among these groups, Hawaiians/Part Hawaiians and Pacific Islanders were placed in different groups; however most studies combine these two groups into one category. The finding in the bi-variate analysis demonstrated differences in immunization status among the sub-ethnic and sub-racial groups, warranting further exploration. In addition, separating these groups makes it difficult to compare results accurately with other studies.

Another interesting finding was that even among the different income categories, there were differences in the UTD status of children. Those children coming from families with no annual income had the lowest immunization rates, with 70% NUTD. Although Kim et al (2007) disputes that low income is not an indicator of UTD status, Bundt and Hu (2004) would disagree. Bundt and colleagues found that family income, health insurance status, race/ethnicity, mother's education and age, and type of residence setting (military base or non-military base) were associated with UTD status.

Although this study identified factors associate with under immunization, all of the immunization rates in this study were sub-optimal. Even if all the children and adolescents that had no shot record in their medical records were UTD, there would only be a 59% UTD rate, well below the national HP2010 goal of 80%. These findings support that interventions need to be targeted across all ethnic, racial, income and insurance groups to improve immunization rates in children and adolescents.

This study was based on a medical record review; therefore all of the children included in the study had been seen at the CHC during a 12 month period of time. Despite this fact, many children and particularly adolescents and young adults did not have immunizations recorded in their medical records. These findings support the need to address immunization status at all health care provider visits and accurate and timely documentation of the rates in the medical record. In addition, implementing a policy to immunize children, adolescents, and young adults at every health care visit would improve immunization rates.

Limitations. There are a number of limitations in this study. First, this was a cross-sectional study; the results only represent a snapshot in time and may elicit different results if another time frame was chosen. Having a longitudinal study can eliminate some indirect variables such as vaccine availability and economic changes which can affect insurance status and family income.

The study also relied on data obtained from a medical records review. One hundred and five children/adolescents (28.5%) had no shot record in their medical record. These children were classified as NUTD when in fact it may not necessarily mean they were NUTD, merely that there was no documentation available at the time data was collected. Follow-up surveys and discussion with parents regarding their child's immunization status, especially in the case of missing shot records, could have provided more accurate results of UTD versus truly NUTD.

This study was limited to one urban CHC and therefore cannot be generalized to other CHCs or populations. Including data from additional CHCs or underserved areas would further validate the findings from the study. However, the study was strengthened by using a random sample of all children seen at the clinic during a certain time period, thus the results can generalize back to that particular population.

This study was a retrospective chart review. Studies such as Luman and colleagues (2002) determined if immunizations were completed in a timely manner versus status at the time of the study. This study did not consider an immunization as UTD if it was not within a month of its due date. The child may have been UTD at that time of medical record review, but if an immunization was "late," was considered NUTD.

Conclusion. Insurance status and total family income are major factors in whether or not children are UTD with their immunizations (Dominguez, Parrott, Lauderdale and Daum, 2004; Rosenthal et al, 2004). Targeting poor and un- and under- insured children, adolescents, and young adults with interventions that increase access, availability and cost-effective immunizations can improve the overall immunization rates and decrease disparities in this important public health intervention.

References

Altonn, H. (2002, October 23). Health officials unsure why rate of childhood immunizations has been declining. *The Star Bulletin.* Retrieved on March 1, 2006 from *http://starbulletin.com/2002/10/23/news/story7.html.*

Barnes, J.S., and Bennett, C.S. (2002). *The Asian population: 2000. Census 2002 brief.* Washington, DC: US Department of Commerce.

Bundt, T.S. and Hu, H. (2004). National examination of compliance predictors and the immunization status of children: Precursor to a developmental model for health systems. *Military Medicine, 169: 795-803.*

Centers for Disease Control (2007). National, state, and local area vaccination coverage among children aged 19-35 months – United States 2006. *MMWR Weekly, 56*(34); 880-885.

Chu, S.Y., Barker, L.E., and Smith, P.J. (2004). Racial/Ethnic disparities in preschool immunizations: United States, 1996-2001. *American Journal of Public Health, 94*(6): 973-977.

Dingeman, R. (2004). Childhood vaccination rate hits records 82.8% in state. The Star-Bulletin. Retrieved on December 1, 2007 from *http://the.honoluluadvertiser.com/article/2004/Aug/06/ln/ln27a.html.*

Dominguez, S.R., Parrott, J.S., Lauderdale, D.S., and Daum, R.S. (2004). On-time immunization rates among children who enter Chicago public schools. *Pediatrics, 114*(6): 741-747.

Eberwine-Villagrán, D. (2007). Best buys for public health. *Perspectives in health, 11*(1). Retrieved on December 14, 2007 from *http://www.paho.org/English/DD/PIN/Number23_article1.htm.*

Ehresmann, K.R., White, K., Hedberg, C., Anderson, E., Korlath, J.A., Moore, K.A., and Osterholm, M.T. (1998). A statewide survey of immunization rates in Minnesota school age children: implications for targeted assessment and prevention strategies. Pediatr Infect Dis J.;17:711–716.

Ghosh, C. (2003). Healthy people 2010 and Asian American/Pacific Islanders: Defining a baseline of information. *American Journal of Public Health, 93*(12), 2093-2098.

Grabenstein, J. (2001). Overcoming immunization disparities based on ethnicity. *Pharmacy Practice Management Quarterly, 20*(3); 23-30.

Hawaii State Department of Health (2002). DOH officials meet with top health care providers to discuss strategies for infant immunization. Retrieved on April 15, 2006 from *http://www.hawaii.gov/health/about/pr/2002/02-66imm.html.*

Javier, J.R., Huffman, L.C. and Mendoza, F.S. (2007). Filipino child health in the United States: do health and health care disparities exist? *Preventing Chronic Disease: Public Health research, Practice and Policy, 4*(2): 1-20. Retrieved on December 11, 2007 from *http://www.cdc.gov/pcd/issues/2007/apr/pdf/06_0069.pdf.*

Jha, P., Gajalakshmi, V., Gupta, P.C., Kumar, R., Mony, P., Dhingra, H., and Peto, R. (2006). Prospective study of one million deaths in India: rationale, design, and validation results. *PLoS Medicine, 3*(2); 191-200.

Kagawa-Singer, M., and Kassim-Lahka, S. (2003) A strategy to reduce cross-cultural miscommunication and increase the likelihood of improving health outcomes. *Academic Medicine, 78*(6):577-587.

Kim, S.S., Frimpong, J.A., Rivers, P.A., and Kronenfeld, J.J. (2007) Effects of maternal and provider characteristics on up-to-date immunization status of children aged 19 to 35 months. *Am. J. Public Health* 97(2).

Lee, G.M., Santoli, J.M., Hanna, C., Messonnier, M.L., Sabin, J.E., Rusinak, D., Gay, C., Lett., S.M., and Lieu, T.A. (2007). Gaps in vaccine financing for underinsured children in the United States. *Journal of the American Medical Association, 298(6)*:638-643.

Luman, E.T., Cauley, M.M., Stokley, S., Chi, S.Y., and Pickering, L.K. (2002). Timeliness of childhood immunizations. *Pediatrics 111:* 935-939.

Marks, J.S. Halpin, T.J., Johnson, D.A. and Keller, J.R. (1979). Risk factors associated with failure to receive vaccinations. *Pediatrics, 64*:304-309.

Morrow, A. L., Rosenthal, J., Lakkis, H.D., Bowers, J.C., Butterfoss, F.D., Crews, R.C., and Sirotkin, B. (1998). A population-based study of access to immunization among urban Virginia children served by public, private, and military health care systems. *Pediatrics, 101* (2):1-10.

Munro, B.H. (2005). *Statistical Methods for Health Care Research*, 5th ed. Lippencott Williams and Wilkens, Philadelphia.

Niederhauser, V.P. and Markowitz, M. (2007). Barriers to immunizations: Multiethnic parents of under- and unimmunized children speak. *Journal of the American Academy of Nurse Practitioners 19*: 15-23.

Niederhauser, V., Michael, M., and Ganeko, R. (2007). Simple solutions to complex issues: Minimizing disparities in childhood immunization rates by providing walk-in shot clinic access. *Fam. Community Health*, 30, (2S), pp s80-s91.

Niederhauser, V.P. and Stark, M. (2005). Narrowing the gap in childhood immunization disparities. *Pediatric Nursing, 31*(5). Retrieved on November 15, 2007 at *http://www.pediatricnursing.net/ce/2007/article10380388.pdf.*

Office of Minority Health and Bureau of Primary Health Care. (n.d.). *Reducing health disparities in Asian American and Pacific Islander populations: A provider's guide to quality and culture seminar.* Retrieved November 12, 2007 from *http://erc.msh.org/provider/informatic/AAPI_Disparities_HealthStatus.pdf.*

Reeves, T. and Bennett, C.S. (2002). *The Asian and Pacific Islander population in the United States: March 2002.* Washington, DC: US Department of Commerce.

Rosenthal, J., Rodewald, L., McCauley, M., Berman, S., Irogoyen, M., Sawyer, M., Yusuf, H., Davis, R., and Kalton, G. (2004). Immunization coverage levels among 19- to 35-month-old children in 4 diverse, medically underserved areas of the United States. *Pediatrics, 113*(4): 296-302.

Santoli, J.M., Huet, N.J., Smith, P.J., Barker, L.E., Rodewald, L.E., Inkelas, M., Olson, L.M., Halfon, N. (2004). Insurance status and vaccination coverage among US preschool children. *Pediatrics, 113:* 1959-1964.

Stern, A. M. and Markel, H. (2005). The history of immunizations and immunizations: Familiar patterns, new challenges. *Health Affairs, 24*(3): 611-621.

Szilagyi, P.G., Schaffer, S., Shone, L., Barth, R., Humiston, S.G., Sandler, M., and Rodewald, L.E.. (2002). Reducing geographic, racial, and ethnic disparities in childhood immunization rates by using reminder/recall interventions in urban primary care practices. *Pediatrics*,110(5): 1-8.

U.S. Bureau of the Census. (2000). *Projections of the resident population: Middle series projection, 2050 to 2070, by race, Hispanic origin, and nativity.* Washington, DC: US Department of Commerce.

U.S. Bureau of the Census. (2001). *Profiles of general demographic characteristics 2000: 2000 census population and housing.* Washington, DC: US Department of Commerce.

U.S. Department of Health and Human Services (2000). Healthy People 2010. Washington, DC: U.S. GPO. Retrieved on December 15, 2007 from *http://www.healthypeople.gov/.*

Zhao, Z., Mokdad, A.H., Barker, L. (2004). Impact of health insurance status on vaccination coverage in children 19-35 moths old, United States, 1993-1996. *Public Health Reports, 119,* 156-162.

In: Trends in Nursing Research
Editors: Adam J. Ryan and Jack Doyle

ISBN 978-1-60456-642-0
© 2009 Nova Science Publishers, Inc.

Chapter 4

Quality of Life and Coronary Artery Bypass Surgery: A Longitudinal Study

Geraldine A. Lee
Division Of Nursing and Midwifery,
La Trobe University, Melbourne, Australia
Preventive Cardiology, Baker Heart Research Institute,
Melbourne, Australia

Abstract

INTRODUCTION: Cardiovascular disease (CVD) remains a significant worldwide health problem leading to premature death and chronic illness with Coronary heart disease (CHD) accounts for 52% of CVD cases with 16 million cases of CHD in the US. One of the treatment options for those with CHD is Coronary Artery Bypass Surgery (CABG). The aim of the surgery is to alleviate symptoms such as angina and breathlessness, prevent further Myocardial Infarctions (MIs) and reduce the progression of CHD.

METHOD and AIM OF STUDY: A study was undertaken in the United Kingdom five years after CABG. Patients from a previous study agreed to participate in a follow-up study five years after cardiac surgery. Participants were asked to complete a quality of life questionnaire, the Short-Form 36 (SF-36) and questionnaires on their psychological well-being (anxiety and depression symptoms). Neuropsychological assessment was also performed at the follow-up. The assessments of psychological well-being and neuropsychological tests were previously completed prior to surgery.

RESULTS: One hundred and nine patients were interviewed face-to-face. The SF-36 component summaries of the patients indicated that their physical (PCS) and mental (MCS) health was relatively good (45.8 and 53.6, respectively, with 0 = worst health and 100 = best health and 50 being the mean score). Lower PCS scores were associated with comorbid illness. Psychological well-being (anxiety and depression) was found to correlate with the SF-36 physical and mental component summaries ($p < .001$) at the time of follow-up.

Deficits in neuropsychological scores five years post CABG were found in 28% of the patients with no correlation between the SF-36 component summaries and the neuropsychological assessment five years after CABG suggesting that these deficits do not interfere with patient perceived HRQoL.

DISCUSSION: The significance of psychological well-being were highlighted in the hierarchical regression analysis with pre-operative angina scores and the following data five years post CABG; comorbid illness, anxiety and depressive symptoms and physical activity, accounting for 37% of the variance in PCS. Pre-operative anxiety, interim myocardial infarction and the following data five years post CABG: age, diet scores, anxiety and depression symptoms, accounted for 60% of the variance in MCS.

CONCLUSION: The findings demonstrate that patient perceived HRQoL five years after CABG is generally good. However, it is negatively affected the presence of anxiety or depression symptoms at follow-up. The findings have implications for healthcare professionals and highlight the importance of anxiety and depression after surgical revascularisation.

Introduction

Cardiovascular disease (CVD) remains a significant worldwide health problem leading to premature death and chronic illness with 17.5 million deaths reported worldwide in 2005 [World Health Organisation (WHO) 2008]. The main forms of the disease are Coronary Heart Disease (CHD) and cerebrovascular disease (stroke). In 2005, CHD accounted for 7.6 million deaths and stroke accounted for 5.7 million deaths [WHO, 2008]. It is the leading cause of death worldwide with a projected increase in incidence in both the high income and low to middle income countries by 2015 with 20 million deaths from CVD predicted [WHO, 2008].

Recent statistics from the American Heart Association (AHA) reported that an estimated 80.7 million Americans (1 in 3) are living with some form of CVD [AHA, 2008]. What is important to note is that CVD stills accounts for more deaths than any other single cause or group of causes of death in the United States since 1900 (with the exception of 1918) [National Institute of Health, 2001]. In 2004 in the US, there were 869,000 deaths from CVD. Of these, CHD accounted for 52% of deaths (451,000) [AHA, 2008]. The main manifestations of CHD are angina pectoris and acute myocardial infarctions (AMIs). From the 2005 figures, the prevalence of AMI was 8.1 million and 9.1 million angina cases. Although the mortality rates from CHD have steadily declined over time, a substantial increase in those living with some form of CHD is evident. As well as over 17 million suffering AMIs or having angina, a further 5.3 million have heart failure.

To add to this, projected figures for 2008 estimate that 770,000 individuals will have a new coronary event and a further 430,000 will have a recurrent attack. An additional 190,000 silent first AMIs are predicted with 600,000 new AMIs and 320,000 recurrent AMIs [unpublished data from Atherosclerosis Risk in Communities Study]. The estimated direct and indirect cost of CVD in the United States for 2008 is $448.5 billion [AHA, 2008]. What becomes apparent from these statistics is that CHD continues to be a major health problem, both for the individual and the healthcare budget in terms of healthcare professionals' time and resources.

Various inter-relationships exist between background, behavioural and physiological factors relative to the development of CHD and MI. Background factors include reduced height, low birthweight, sex, social class, race and geographical location. Behavioural factors include reduced physical activity, a poor diet (increased saturated fats, saturated fatty acids, decrease in antioxidants and excessive alcohol intake), smoking and stress. The physiological factors associated with CHD include hypertension, increased plasma insulin and increased plasma cholesterol, decrease in antioxidants and increased plasma fibrinogen. This demonstrates that CHD is multifactorial and arises from an interaction of these risk factors, leading to atherosclerosis and thrombogenesis.

The prevalence of risk factors within the US population has been reported by AHA. With hypertension, the estimated 2005 prevalence was 73 million. With hypercholestraemia, 48% (106 million) of the US population have raised levels of total cholesterol (NHANES 2001-04). This was for levels above 200 mg/dL with a further 17% of the population (37 million) having levels above 240 mg/dL [National Cholesterol Education Program Expert Panel, 2002]. Given these significant figures, it would be expected that these individuals would be on appropriate medication but less than half are on any kind of lipid-modifying treatment and less than half of even the highest-risk persons (with symptomatic CHD) are medication [AHA, 2008]

Another growing problem (literally) is obesity with an estimated 142 million adults overweight (66% of the population) and of these 67 million adults classified as obese [AHA, 2008].Diabetes is another risk factor associated with CHD and the 2005 prevalence among adults was 15 million (7.3% of the adult population) [National Diabetes Statistics website]. The Framingham Heart Study have reported a doubling in the incidence of diabetes over thepast 30 years, with the most significant increase during the 1990s.

A key question is why does CHD remain so prevalent? The answer lies in the incidence and continued increasing prevalence of modifiable risk factors associated with CHD. The nine risk factors include cigarette smoking, abnormal blood lipid levels, hypertension, diabetes, abdominal obesity, a lack of physical activity, low daily fruit and vegetable consumption, alcohol overconsumption and psychosocial index [INTERHEART Study investigators, 2004]. These nine risk factors were identified in the INTERHEART study which carried out a case-control study of 52 countries and found these nine risk factors accounted for over 90% of the risk associated with initial AMI. The important aspect of these nine risk factors is that they are *all modifiable*. The researchers also noted that the effects did not change according to gender, ethnicity or geographical location which makes these results applicable to any population group worldwide.

Previous studies have highlighted the high exposure of those with CHD to at least one risk factor for CHD. The researchers identified three major risk factors: (i) high total blood cholesterol levels, or current medication with cholesterol-lowering drugs; (ii) hypertension, or current medication with blood pressure-lowering drugs; current cigarette use; and (iii) clinical report of diabetes [Greenland et al., 2003]. Another study estimated that more than 90% of CHD events will occur in individuals with at least one elevated risk factor and approximately 8 percent will occur in people with only borderline levels of multiple risk factors [Vasan et al., 2005]. When examining the three main risk factors (hypertension, current smoking and raised serum cholesterol), it becomes evident that those with the three major risk factors have a significant increased risk of fatal CHD. The NHANES II Mortality Follow-Up Study report the risk for fatal CHD was 51% lower for men and 71% lower for women with none of three major risk factors compared to those with one or more risk factors [Mensah et al., 2005].

The importance of risk factor management and lifestyle modification interventions highlight the success of reducing global cardiovascular risk and this is approach is gaining momentum but only in those who have experienced cardiovascular events such as MI as opposed to those *with* associated risk factors [Lear et al., 2006]. Formal clinical guidelines now exist in the USA for the treatment of CHD and the treatment of risk factors developed by the National Lipid Association [National Lipid Association website] and the American Heart Association in conjunction with the American College of Cardiology [Grundy et al., 1999]. In the UK guidelines have been published by the National Institute for Health and Clinical Excellence (NICE). These guidelines endorse the same risk factors and agree on their management, for example, reducing high blood pressure and elevated serum cholesterol, promoting physical activity and maintaining ideal body weight [INTERHEART Study investigators, 2004; Aldana et al., 2003; The Multiple Risk Factor Intervention Trial Research Group, 1996].

Although great advancements have been made in terms of medical interventions, pharmacology and genetics, the prevalence of these risk factors highlights quite strongly the reason why CHD continues to be such a significant health problem. Not only does CHD impact on the individual in terms of symptoms, but also on their family, employment and their role in society. If a person has a chronic condition with symptoms, this can mean an inability to perform activity of daily living (ADLs) and impact on physical and psychological well-being.

There are three main coronary arteries; the right coronary artery, the left main stem branches into the circumflex and the left anterior descending. Coronary arteries have a very small diameter and atherosclerosis is a pathological process resulting in the narrowing of these main arteries leading to CHD. It involves a localised inflammatory response to endothelial injury and subsequent platelet aggregation and fibrin mesh formation. This condition results in the formation of thrombi, leading to further narrowing causing angina. A complete occlusion of the coronary artery occurs with rupture of the plaque causing an AMI. With theories that various biological mediators are involved in atherosclerosis, the hypothesis on the aetiology of CHD is constantly evolving. The inflammatory response hypothesis is gaining favour, with inflammatory markers reportedly increased in people with CHD [Danesh et al., 2004: Pai et al., 2004]. While treatment of the inflammatory process is recommended, there is no consensus on interventions [Paoletti et al., 2004].

Symptoms and Treatment of Coronary Heart Disease

The two major symptoms associated with CHD are angina and breathlessness. Angina requires medical investigation to determine if the pain is related to CHD and to establish the degree of coronary artery narrowing. Many terms are used to describe the chest pain associated with angina: for example, crushing, stabbing and heaviness. The pain sometimes radiates down the right arm or through the jaw. Angina is usually precipitated by an increased myocardial workload with an increased oxygen demand in the presence of such arterial narrowing within coronary arteries. Not all patients with CHD experience chest pain, so other clinical tests are necessary to determine if their chest pain is cardiac in origin. Another recognised symptom of CHD is breathlessness, especially if it is associated with minimal exertion. Pathologically, breathlessness may be due to other conditions such as respiratory diseases and, therefore, the cause of the breathlessness must also be established.

Clinical objective tools are used to quantify the level of symptoms with the most popular classifications used are the New York Heart Association (NYHA) [The Criteria Committee of the New York Heart Association, 1974] and the Canadian Cardiovascular Society (CCS) scales [Campeau, 1976]. These tools classify symptoms from mild/asymptomatic (Class I) to severe (Class IV). Although the NYHA classification is used widely for cardiac patients, there has been very little research on its reliability and validity over the last 25 years. Some research has suggested concerns with using the NYHA [Bennett et al., 2002; Goldman et al., 1982]. However, others report excellent inter-rater and intra-rater reliability rates of 90% [Kubo et al., 2004]. In general, many studies continue to use the NYHA classification for cardiac patients. These clinical tools should be used in conjunction with asking the patient to describe their symptoms (in their own words) and how these symptoms affect their daily activities (for example; can they climb stairs, walk up an incline, etc). Usually severity of symptoms can be correlated with physical health and the corresponding improvement of symptoms is reflected in improved functional status which extends to very old patients [Huber et al., 2007].

Other clinical tools used to detect signs of CHD include electrocardiographic exercise testing and angiography. These tests are used to determine the extent of the atherosclerosis. Coronary angiography is usually carried out to identify the location and severity of the stenosis (the angiogram can detect blockages in coronary arteries from a minimal to total occlusion). The severity of angina and breathless symptoms together with the angiography results and the patient history will determine treatment required [American College of Cardiology/American Heart Association Task Force on Assessment of Diagnostic and Therapeutic Cardiovascular Procedures, 1999].

Based on the diagnosis, the most common types of treatment for CHD are behavioural risk modification, medical pharmacological therapies and interventional procedures (both medical and surgical). The most common treatments are Percutaneous Coronary Intervention (PCI) involving ballooning of the artery (angioplasty) and stent insertion. The commonly performed surgical procedure is CABG. These procedures are conducted to alleviate angina and breathlessness symptoms, increase exercise tolerance which will hopefully lead to better functional capacity and physical activity levels, and allow individuals to perform daily activities independently and without symptoms.

CABG is customarily performed through a median sternotomy with the patient placed on a cardio-pulmonary bypass machine (CPB). Radial arteries and saphenous veins are used as grafts along with the internal mammary artery (IMA) from the left subclavian artery [Malinowski et al., 2006]. Arerties are advantageous over saphenous grafts as arteries show greater long-term graft patency. Radial arteries are also commonly used conduits and also show good long-term patency [Desai et al., 2004; Possati et al., 2003].

A percentage of patients are now undergoing bypass surgery on the beating heart (that is, off the cardio-pulmonary bypass machine). It is a technique which permits surgery on multiple coronary vessels without the use of the CPB. Off-pump Coronary Artery Bypass Graft Surgery (OPCAB) is an alternative to conventional on-pump surgery. The operation can be minimally invasive or involve a midline sternotomy. A more recent technique is totally endoscopic robotically assisted coronary artery bypass surgery (TECAB).

CABG remains the main surgical method of coronary revascularisation in multi-vessel CHD since it was first used in 1970. In 2005, 461,000 CABG were performed in the US [AHA, 2008], while in 2003 29,000 CABG were performed in the United Kingdom [Allender et al., 2007]. The cost of CABG is substantial and estimated at $85,653 per case while the cost of PCI is PCI $44,110 [AHA, 2008].

Although the numbers of individuals undergoing CABG is relatively steady, the most recent figures highlight an increase from 2004 to 2005 from 427,000 procedures in 2004 to 461,000 in 2005. The reasons for the significant numbers undergoing CABG are an ageing population and higher incidence of diabetic and higher risk patients undergoing the operation.

Two important questions in relation to CABG are: What is the mortality risk from the operation (both short-term and long-term) and what are the morbidity risks with this surgery?

A consistent theme in studies carried out since the first CABG is the evaluation of the surgery in terms of mortality. A distinction is made in the literature between 'operative mortality' which refers to mortality within 30 days of surgery, and 'long-term mortality' which refers to survival rates at various time points post-operatively. The most frequently reported time points are one to five years and 10 to 15 years after surgery. The current mortality rate is 2.1% [AHA, 2008] with the peri-operative risks are cerebrovascular accidents (1% to 2%), peri-operative MI (5%), with the overall death risk of 1% to 2% in most UK cardiothoracic centres [Society of Cardiothoracic Surgeons of Great Britain and Ireland, 2001]. Bridgewater et al., [2003] reported a 30 day mortality of 1.7%. The studies acknowledge that over time, as the operation was carried out more frequently, the mortality rate decreased.

Mortality figures from the operation and in the post-operative period are one of the indicators of its success [Huber et al., 2007; Bridgewater et al., 2003] Researchers have identified a number of variables associated with mortality and morbidity including the number of grafts, left ventricular function, the use of IMAs, bypass and ischaemic times and the age of the patient [Michalopoulos et al., 1999; Pocock et al., 1995].

The introduction of OPCPB has shown significantly lower mortality rates compared to those on CPB (p<0.001) [Nathoe et al., 2003; Cleveland et al., 2001; Plomondon et al., 2001]. Nearly 10% of procedures in one site were carried out off-pump [Cleveland *et al.,*

2001]. The operative mortality was 2.9% in the cardio-pulmonary bypass group and 2.3% off-pump (p< 0.001). Although OPCPB shows lower in-hospital mortality and complications rates three years after the operation, there were lower revascularisation rates in CPB patients [Hannan et al., 2007].

Specifically relating to survival five years after CABG, the rates reported range from 94.6% [Stahle et al. 1994] to 90% [Yusuf et al. 1994, Kirklin et al. 1989] and 79% [Herlitz et al., 1999]. Other researchers report survival rates of 80% to 85% [Fitzgibbon et al.,1996; Doliszney et al., 1994; Rowe et al., 1989]. The most recent five year mortality figures from the American College of Cardiology/American Heart Association Taskforce on Practice Guidelines for Coronary Artery Bypass Graft Surgery [1999] recorded a survival rate of 89.8%. Huber et al. [2007] reported a 70% survival in 61 octogenarians who underwent CABG while one large study reported survival of 83% [Koch et al., 2007]. The rate reported varies and this may be partly explained by changes to CABG procedure over time and also in the type of patients undergoing surgery (including older, sicker and with more comorbidities at the time of operation).

Within the literature there is no formal or structured approach in relation to morbidity and CABG. Some authors include survival mortality only after surgery, while others include factors such as non-fatal MIs and being pain-free in the context of CABG. In this paper, all non-fatal consequences are included in the morbidity category.

Many of the factors implicated in operative mortality also contribute to post CABG morbidity for example, older age, graft occlusion and incidence of post-operative MI and being painfree after CABG. Older patients, those over the age of 70 years, are predominantly featured as being at higher risk of problems post CABG, including operative mortality and morbidity [Zaidi et al., 1999; Ivanov et al., 1998]. Increasing age and cardiac surgery are paradoxical in that older patients who undergo CABG are statistically at the greatest risk of complications but also derive the greatest benefits if they survive [Deiwick et al., 2001; Fruitman et al., 1999]. An important issue, which has been documented, is the possibility of post-operative problems being under-reported. It is suggested that in-hospital morbidity from CABG may be underestimated due to the transfer of patients to other wards and referring hospitals [Pande et al., 2003; Lazar et al., 2001].

One of the problems with bypass grafts is that over time they may partially or completely occlude. Graft patency can decrease over time due to early thrombosis, subintimal fibrosis and late atherosclerosis. Aspirin has been clinically proven to improve graft patency post CABG and thus reduce graft occlusion [Possati et al., 2003; Gavaghan et al., 1991].

MIs have been reported after CABG and research has identified the small but consistent benefits in survival of MI post CABG if beta-blockers are commenced before bypass surgery [Ferguson et al., 2002]. Painfree in this context is defined as free from angina, that is, with no symptoms of any chest pains which could be attributable to angina and this is an important outcome after CABG. The reported range of painfree patients five years after CABG is from 63% to 80% [Rogers et al., 1990, Kirklin *et al.* 1989; The European Coronary Surgery Study Group 1979].

One of the biggest problems that can occur peri-operatively is neurological complications which can result in permanent neurological impairment (such as cerebrovascular accident-stroke) and transient neurological complications such as delayed awakening and post-operative delirium, confusion and impaired memory. If neurological complications occur, they can have a negative impact on physical and functional health in those affected and thus, they are an important aspect of CABG. One of the major complications is stroke with the current incidence now approximately 1% to 3% [Loponen et al., 2003]. Previous rates of stroke were recorded at 5% [Breuer et al., 1983], and although serious neurological complications are decreasing, neuropsychological morbidity is persisting [Al-Ruzzeh et al., 2006].

So how do we measure these neuropsychological deficits (that is poor memory, attention and concentration)? Neuropsychological assessment is a recognised technique in assessing for minor disturbances and the aim of the tests is to observe changes in performance between the tests. Neuropsychological tests can be performed to assess the short- and long-term impact of cardiac surgery on the brain using an established battery of tests examining memory, attention, concentration, reaction time, perceptuomotor skills and visuo-constructive skills [Newman and Stygall, 1997]. Declines in all these tests have been reported after cardiac surgery [Abildstrom et al., 2000; Mahanna et al., 1996; Stump, 1995]. These declines manifest as problems with their memory and concentration and the speed of their motor responses [Van Dijk et al., 2000; Newman and Stygall, 1997; Vingerhoets et al., 1997; Mahanna et al., 1996]. A range of post-operative test intervals are in the literature, usually these are eight days, six weeks, one year and five years [Pugsley et al., 1990; Newman et al., 1987; Savageau et al., 1982].

The majority of studies demonstrate a decline in cognitive functioning at discharge from hospital and an improvement from the time of surgery to six and eight weeks [Sellman et al., 1992]. Studies in which tests were completed at six months post-surgery have concluded that impairment in memory, concentration and hand-eye co-ordination have a negative effect on patients and on their ability to carry out daily activities (that is affects physical abilities) [Khatri et al., 1999]. It would seem pertinent to examine if deficits are present five years after CABG and whether they affect physical health.

Causes of Neuropsychological Deficits

An important point to consider are the causes of neuropsychological deficits and this area remains controversial. Cerebral micro-emboli can be detected during cardiac surgery via Doppler monitoring of the middle cerebral artery [Pugsley, 1989]. These micro-emboli have been implicated in the aetiology of cognitive dysfunction associated with cardiac surgery. The causes of neuropsychological deficits have been a contentious issue. Some studies have demonstrated that cognitive outcomes for patients worsen with a greater number of emboli [Barbut et al., 1997; Stump et al., 1997]. Some of the factors implicated in neuropsychological deficits are cerebral micro-emboli, the CPB, genetic predisposition and ageing [Abildstrom et al., 2000; Borowicz et al., 1996; Newman et al., 1994]. One genetic marker being investigated is apolipoprotein E status but currently there is no consensus on the role of ApoE and cognitive dysfunction. A few intervention studies using agents believed to be neuroprotective and as yet none has proven to have great efficacy in neuroprotection [Arrowsmith et al., 1998].

Although much of the literature highlights the short-term incidence of neuropsychological deficits, the longer-term incidence such as five years after revascularisation is not as clear. There is evidence to support the decline in patients' neuropsychological functioning five years post CABG [Stygall et al., 2003; Selnes et al., 2001] with one study recording deficits in 46% of patients five years after surgery [Newman et al., 2001b]. Given these results, it appears that neuropsychological functioning after CABG is an area that requires further investigation and in particular does the presence of neuropsychological deficits after CABG affect functional health of individuals? Although we could easily examine cognitive functioning in relation to CABG and report any neuropsychological deficits related to revascularisation, it is important to examine patient perceived health-related quality of life (HRQoL) in relation to cognitive functioning after CABG especially in the longer-term such as five years after the operation. Before examining cognitive functioning five years after CABG, we will first define quality of life (QoL) and in particular HRQoL.

Quality of Life

Although clinical data has a role in contributing to overall knowledge, QoL studies can also provide information for future patients. The application of QoL can be for health needs assessments, clinical care, resource allocation and clinical trials for example. The goal of medical healthcare and interventions is to improve patients' QoL in relation to the disease [Jenkins 1992; Stewart et al., 1992; Spilker 1990] and establishing if a particular treatment is beneficial [Sandoe and Kappel in Nordenfelt, 1994].

Many authors have commented on the lack of a consensus on a definition for QoL [Smith et al., 1999; Bowling 1995; Shumaker and Naughton 1995; Wenger et al., 1984]. What becomes apparent from the literature is that certain concepts are relevant when focusing on measurements of health outcomes or interventions. These concepts include health, functional ability and well-being (both physical and psychological).

The goal of bypass surgery for cardiac patients is not to 'cure' them but to eliminate or reduce symptoms and reduce the risk of future MIs. This intention is an important consideration in assessing HRQoL in patients who have undergone CABG [Wenger et al., 1984]. It would seem that the risks and complications from interventions, along with the patient's perception of their QoL, would generate clinical and subjective reports of meaning for those caring for patients (in particular cardiologists and nurses). The majority of studies are observational but it is possible to identify important costs and benefits to patients having a particular treatment.

HRQoL refers to patients' functional disabilities in relation to a particular disease or disability such as cardiovascular disease. Given that this paper is concerned with evaluating QoL, the QoL examined will *specifically* be health-related QoL (HRQoL). A review of some of the literature highlights the lack of consensus on what concepts should be included [Stewart and King 1994; Walter 1992; Mayou 1990, Van Dam, 1986; Fava and Magnani, 1988]. Lukkarinen [2005] performed methodological triangulation in those with CHD (n=19) and suggested that as well as HRQoL questionnaires, researchers should undertake qualitative approach (namely interviews) to capture psychosocial aspects. Although this approach is valid, the application of psychological well-being and social support questionnaires could address this concern adequately.

There has been some specific work on QoL conceptualisation in those with CVD. Wenger et al. [1984] have written extensively on the topic and stated that QoL should encompass the measurement of several aspects of the patient: their ability to function carrying out daily activities, productivity, and performance of social roles, intellectual capability, emotional stability and well-being. The authors maintained that three major factors reflect HRQoL: functional capacity (including physical, intellectual, social and emotional functioning), perceptions (levels of well-being and satisfaction with life) and effects of the symptoms of disease. Bowling [1995] reviewed the literature on the indicators used for measuring QoL in people with heart disease and reported the frequently reported criteria from the studies as mortality, morbidity, graft patency, symptoms (angina and breathlessness) and pain. The least reported criteria were: activity levels, social activities, and financial and psychological status amongst others. She goes on to quote Wenger and what should be included in HRQoL in cardiovascular studies: physical capabilities, emotional status, social interactions, intellectual functioning, economic status, and self-perceived health status. Similar lists are reported by other authors [Fletcher et al., 1992; Williams et al., 1985]. The physical symptoms and their associated psychological problems (depression and anxiety) have been studied in CABG [Lindsay et al., 2000; Rumsfield et al., 1999]. One paper showed that poor HRQoL after cardiac surgery identified patients at risk of reduced long-term survival [Koch et al., 2007]. These studies validate the proposed examination of HRQoL after CABG in this paper.

In light of this literature in relation to those with CHD, for the purpose of this paper, relevant HRQoL concepts have been identified as:

- physical health (which incorporates physical functioning and being able to carry out daily activities)
- severity of symptoms (angina and breathlessness)
- emotional well-being / mood (namely anxiety and depression)
- social support (that is the ability to socialise if, and when, the individual desires to do so, with no limitations from physical or emotional health)

By inclusion of severity of symptoms along with physical and emotional well-being and social support; these tools can measure patients' functional status after CABG. Hofer et al. [2006] have suggested that treatment *should* relieve symptoms *and* improve functional status as well as prolonging life. This view was also reiterated by Hawkes et al. [2006] who identified the importance of investigating physical, psychological and social variables after CABG.

There are many HRQoL tools available and one that is widely used in the cardiac population is the Short Form-36 Health Survey (SF-36)[Ware et al., 1994]. It is easy to administer and has good psychometric qualities. The questionnaire examines HRQoL relative to physical health (physical functioning, physical role limitations, bodily pain, energy and general health perceptions) and emotional health (mental health, social functioning and emotional role limitations). The role limitations allow both physical and mental health problems to be evaluated.

Five year follow-up studies after CABG have been undertaken [Herlitz et al., 2000a; 2000b; Caine et al., 1999; Herlitz et al., 1999; Treat-Jacobsen, 1998]. Caine et al., [1999] re-examined the 100 male patients and 84 participated, while only 50% responded using a postal method (n=876) in Herlitz et al., [2000a]. Both these studies chose the Nottingham Health Profile (NHP) to determine HRQoL five years after CABG. A strong association was reported by Caine et al [1999] between presence of symptoms and restrictions in activities both socially and at home (p<0.01) while Herlitz et al., [2000a] also noted a significant association between breathless symptoms and physical activities such as walking, dressing and at rest (p<0.0001). Herlitz et al., [2000a] found improvements in physical activity, chest pain and dyspnoea symptoms regardless of the patient's age. They also observed an inverse association between age and physical activity limitations prior to five years but not at the five year follow-up. This association with decline in physical activity and ageing is not an unusual finding. The older patients identified tiredness as the reason for restricting their physical activity; those with dyspnoea also reported limitations at the five year follow-up.

Examining symptoms demonstrated a correlation between the severity of symptoms and HRQoL. With respect to chest pain and angina, a total of 34 (40%) out of 84 patients had symptoms five years after their operation [Caine et al., 1999]. In the same cohort, dyspnoea was a problem for 50 patients (60%) and symptoms of angina and breathlessness were significant in prevalence when compared to one year post CABG (p<0.001). Of 32 patients who had no dyspnoea pre-operatively, 17 patients continued to be asymptomatic five years after surgery [Caine et al., 1999]. In a second group with no dyspnoea pre-operatively (n=29), three had breathless symptoms five years after surgery. The researchers concluded that absence of breathlessness prior to surgery had the ability to differentiate outcomes five years after surgery and indicated that operative dyspnoea is associated with poor left ventricular function and thus predictive of functional ability.

Both studies attempted to predict HRQoL five years after CABG from their data and concluded that a decline in physical functioning is compatible with the expected decline in graft patency. However no association was found between the pre-operative ejection fraction and symptoms at five years post CABG by Herlitz et al., [2000b], a finding which opposes the five year follow-up by Caine et al., [1999]. Herlitz reported that poor pre-operative QoL was a strong predictor of a reduction in HRQoL five years after surgery with the three independent predictors were being female, a history of diabetes mellitus and a history of respiratory dysfunction, namely chronic obstructive pulmonary disease.

Another follow-up study by Treat-Jacobsen [1998] examined HRQoL five to six after bypass surgery in a cohort of 184 patients. Data were gathered by telephone interview and a functional status questionnaire. Areas addressed were physical, social and mental functioning, exercise behaviour and symptoms. The functional status questionnaire data demonstrated that 76% of patients had no reduction in their activities of daily living. This result is very positive, showing a high functional status in the cohort. The overall HRQoL rating was 6.7 out of a total of 10 (with the higher scores reflecting better health). The researcher acknowledged certain limitations in the design of the study. Patients were from an elective surgery group, of limited ethnic diversity (hence minimal cross-cultural comparisons could be made), the recording of pre-operative symptoms was retrospective and follow-up was at one point in time [Treat-Jacobsen, 1998].

The predictive value of QoL questionnaires, especially for mortality has been reported [Rumsfeld et al., 1999; Inouye et al., 1998; Inouye et al., 1993]. In the first known published paper using the SF-36 related to CABG surgery, researchers report on finding the PCS to be an independent risk factor for six month post-operative mortality. The Veterans study group [Rumsfeld et al., 1999] used a pre-operative SF-36 PCS score to predict mortality following CABG surgery (n=2,480 patients). They found the PCS to be a statistically significant risk factor for six month mortality after adjustment of known clinical risk factors. There was a 39% increase in the risk of six month mortality post CABG. The MCS was not a significant predictor in multivariate analyses. The researchers concluded that pre-operative SF-36 may be useful for pre-operative risk stratification in CABG. In a subsequent 8 year follow-up paper using the Duke Activity Status Index (DASI), the authors were able to identify poor long term survival after CABG when examining DASI after recovery from CABG [Koch et al., 2007]. Those with poorly perceived DASI had poor HRQoL which predicted survival in the longer term. The risk adjusted long-term survival hazard ratio of 0.98 per unit increase was reported (95% confidence limits, 0.97 to 0.98, p<0.0001). Both these studies highlight the importance of HRQoL and its role in long-term survival after CABG.

Psychological Well-Being: Depression and Anxiety

Many of the HRQoL questionnaires contain questions on the emotional status of the person and their mental health. As well as physical health, another important aspect of HRQoL is emotional well-being and this is particularly relevant in those with CHD (especially depression and to some extent anxiety).

Depression is a widely misused term. The DSM-IV manual offers definitions of the signs and symptoms of depression [American Psychiatric Association, 1994]. At least five of the following symptoms must be present in the same two weeks, occurring nearly every day; they must be noted by the patient or by others, and constitute a definite change from usual functioning [American Psychiatric Association website [n.d.]]:

- depressed mood
- decreased interest or pleasure
- significant weight loss or weight gain (when not dieting or when appetite is markedly decreased or increased)
- insomnia or hypersomnia (excessive sleep)
- psychomotor agitation or retardation
- fatigue or loss of energy
- suicidal thoughts

Clinical depression is a prevalent condition in the population with WHO reporting 5% to 10% of the population in Western Europe affected by major depression [WHO website, n.d.:

Health Evidence Network]. Clinical depression is a diagnosed condition requiring treatment and it should not be confused with depressive affect or depressive symptoms. Several questionnaires are used to measure depressive symptoms including the Beck Depression Inventory (BDI) which was developed to measure depression in psychiatric patients in the USA [Beck et al., 1961]. It is now commonly used in clinical research to detect depressive symptoms. The BDI focuses on the patient's attitudes towards him/herself; it questions their mood, attitudes, behaviours and symptoms. It explores their feelings of disappointment, guilt and failure in themselves and whether they feel suicidal.

The questionnaire employs a specific scale and it provides a measure of the severity of symptoms [Beck et al., 1961]. It consists of a 21-item inventory which allows self-rating on the severity of symptoms. Each statement has four response choices which are ranked according to severity, from neutral to maximum. The BDI score is divided into the following ranges: 0-9 (normal range), 10-15 (mild depression), 16-19 (mild to moderate depression), 20-29 (moderate to severe depression) and 30-63 (severe depression). It has good reliability and validity as reported in its use with both psychiatric and non-psychiatric respondents [Beck et al., 1988; Gallagher et al., 1982; Beck et al., 1961].

One study claims that up to a fifth of patients with CVD have major depression with the relative risk ranging from 1.5 to 4.5 [Sheps and Shepard, 2001]. Other studies estimate the rates of depression in those with CVD as between 20 to 35% [Lett *et al.*, 2004; Rozanski *et al.*, 1999]. The incidence of clinical depression in those with CHD is reported as being from 10% to 40% [Ruo et al., 2003; Sheps and Shepard, 2001]. In recent years, the relationship between clinical depression and mortality has been debated extensively [Baker et al., 2001; Ford et al., 1998; Glassman and Shapiro, 1998; Musselman et al., 1998; Barefoot et al., 1996]. One often reported finding is that those who had clinical depression also had CVD had a higher mortality risk [Ford et al. 1998; Schulz et al. 2000].

Physiological changes have been reported in CHD patients such as abnormal platelet function, increased sympathetic nervous system activity leading to arrhythmias and elevated inflammatory markers such as C-reactive protein for example [Lesperance et al., 2004; Ford et al., 1998; Glassman and Shapiro, 1998; Musselman et al., 1998; Laghrissi-Thode et al., 1997].

Researchers have examined depression and depressive symptoms and their impact on the physical health of patients with diagnosed CHD, post MI survival and those in recovery after cardiac surgery [Ruo et al., 2003; Irvine et al., 1999; Frasure-Smith et al., 1999; Musselman et al., 1998]. In the majority of studies, a relationship is reported between the presence of symptoms, a reduction in physical health and high rates of depression [Stafford et al., 2007; Cosette et al., 2001; Mayou et al., 2000; Irvine et al., 1999]. It is not surprising that the presence of depression has a negative effect on physical health. Physiological changes occur with depression and increased risk profiles associated with CHD was evident in these individuals.

Studies have examined patients' clinical depression at different time points after CABG from 3 to 6 months [Duits et al., 1998; Timberlake et al., 1997; Channer et al., 1988] to one year [McKhann et al., 1997; Gundle 1980] and two years after their operation [Strauss et al., 1991]. The studies found that those with depression pre-operatively were more likely to report problems post-operatively. Research reported that those with depression post-operatively were significantly associated with previous psychiatric complaints (mainly anxiety and depression) (p<0.005). From these studies, it would appear that there is a group of patients who have depression pre-operatively and also post-operatively. It would seem that other factors are involved although being symptom-free from CHD post CABG can result in patients no longer showing signs of depression.

Specifically five years after CABG, only mild depression has been reported in a few patients [Lindal et al., 1996]. The BDI was used and revealed that the previously high levels of depression were not evident, confirming the view of depression being strongly associated with functional disability in those with symptomatic heart disease. A 2003 study by Burg et al. examined depression post CABG using the BDI and reported scores of ten or more in 25 patients of the total number of patients examined (n=89). They found that those with the higher BDI scores had higher rates of hospitalisation (p<.04), continued pain six months post CABG (p<.01) and had failed to return to their previous activity level six months after surgery (p<.0001). The researchers concluded that depression was an independent predictor of medical and psychosocial morbidity. They also reported that those with pre-operative depression were more likely to have post-operative depression six months post CABG, a finding in line with previous studies.

Goyal et al., [2005] demonstrated that those with high levels of pre-operative depressive symptoms predicted a poorer physical functioning using multiple regression analysis. An increase in depressive symptoms two months post cardiac surgery also predicted poorer physical and psychosocial functioning six months after their operations. The researchers concluded that an association exists between depressive symptoms and HRQoL six months post surgery. Mallick et al. [2005] examined 963 patients who underwent CABG and found that pre-operatively a quarter had significant depressive symptoms. Of those assessed one year post CABG, patients who were younger, less educated, unmarried and a low level of social support had higher depressive symptom scores. A graded inverse relationship was reported between the pre-operative depressive symptoms and their physical functional status one year after their operation measured using the SF-36. Those with moderate to severe depressive symptoms were less likely to gain an improvement in physical functioning post-operatively, even following adjustment for more than 20 clinical variables. The predictive value of depressive symptoms was even stronger in women. This was the first study to examine HRQoL and depressive symptoms post CABG and demonstrated a lack of functional improvement in patients six months following CABG. These studies support the view that depressive symptoms affect physical HRQoL and are also reported by others (Hofer et al., 2006) where depression accounted for 6% of the change in SF-36 scores from pre-operative to post-operative HRQoL.

Rumsfeld and Ho [2005] acknowledge the evidence of both behavioural and physiological mechanisms in relation to CHD and ask some pertinent questions regarding the issue of depression and CHD:

> "Is depression a causal risk factor, directly related to cardiovascular disease and outcome? Or is depression a risk marker, indirectly related to cardiovascular disease through behavioural variables? Or is depression a secondary event, elicited by major medical events such as cardiac surgery?" [Rumsfeld and Ho, 2005: p. 250].

As can be seen, there are still many unanswered questions regarding the role of depression.

One common recommendation from the literature is the need for better psychological evaluation in patients undergoing cardiac surgery and better management of those with depressive symptoms with an aim of improving their HRQoL after surgery [Goyal et al., 2005; Ruo et al., 2003]. Other studies have demonstrated the benefits of anti-depressants in cardiac patients and report a reduction in cardiovascular mortality and morbidity in those treated with Sertaline [Berkman et al., 2003; Swenson et al., 2003; Glassman et al., 2002]. However the effects of anti-depressant medication post CABG has yet to be investigated.

Anxiety is another emotion investigated in CHD and CABG patients. Anxiety can be ·defined as a multi-system response to a perceived threat or danger causing biochemical changes in the body [Dr. J. E. Smith, Medical Library website, n.d.]. It can be brought on by various stimuli; for example, anticipating a negative event such as visiting the dentist or having an operation. In addition to physiological changes (such as increased heart rate and profuse sweating), anxiety entails subjective experience which potentially results is psychological changes. While anxiety is a normal response to stimuli, there are many categories of anxiety disorders, such as panic disorders, generalised anxiety disorder and post-traumatic stress disorder. The role of anxiety in relation to the development of CHD is not a well researched area. However there is some evidence to support the role of anxiety and the stress response with atherothrombogenesis (leading to atherosclerosis and CHD) [Todaro et al., 2007; INTERHEART study investigators, 2004].

The prevalence of anxiety in those with CHD has been reported at 36% with a lifetime report of anxiety disorder of 45% [Todaro et al., 2007]. Women had higher current and lifetime rates of anxiety disorder compared to men ($p<.001$). The authors recommended that greater efforts are needed to identify and treat anxiety in cardiology patients. Some studies have reported an association between anxiety and the development and recurrence of CHD [Shen et al., 2008; Todaro et al., 2007; Lavie and Milani, 2004]. A high prevalence of generalised anxiety and moderate to severe anxiety symptoms was reported in CHD patients [Lavie and Milani, 2004]. Similar to those with depression, younger patients had higher rates of anxiety than older patients and also reported abnormal risk profiles in anxious patients (such as abnormal platelet function and fibrinogen levels). This study also highlights the association between anxiety and physiological variables leading to atherothrombogenesis. A 12 year longitudinal study confirmed the importance of anxiety in relation to MI [Chen et al., 2008]. In the Normative Ageing Study, anxiety was found to be a predictor of MI in men over 60 years. The relative risk was 1.43 (95% confidence interval 1.17-1.75) after adjustment for health behaviours and medications and other psychological variables. Although there are many confounding variables that must be considered whilst examining the role of anxiety in CHD and subsequent CHD-related events, there is currently some evidence to support anxiety as an independent risk factor for CHD.

In relation to CABG; anxiety has been examined in the immediate pre and post-operative period (usually three-months post CABG) [Rymaszewska et al., 2003; Koivula et al., 2002; McCrone et al., 2001]. Studies have shown that anxiety is prevalent pre-operatively but declines in the short-term post-operative period, suggesting that it is related to the operation itself although others have found contrary findings. A study by Andrew et al. [2000], examining pre-operative or post-operative anxiety, depression and stress symptomology found that anxiety was significantly increased in the post-operative period after cardiac surgery. However, they urged caution and stated that somatic anxiety symptoms may not be a suitable measure in cardiac surgery patients. Other findings demonstrate that in the immediate post-operative period, anxiety rates remain high but decreases in the months after surgery. Patients who have an existing psychiatric disorder or anxiety disorder are more likely to have anxiety symptoms than those with no previous history. Patients' perceptions pre-operatively demonstrated that CABG was a major life event for most, with dependency on others and a threat of a sudden cardiac event of most concern Lindsay et al. [2000]. Anxiety at the time of a major operation such as cardiac surgery is an expected response but the clinical relevance of anxiety in the immediate post-operative period is unknown. Also what is uncertain is if post-operative anxiety has a role in predicting further CHD events in the longer-term or whether anxiety as a personality trait is more relevant.

Although anxiety is prevalent pre-operatively and post-operatively, an important issue is whether the presence of anxiety affects HRQoL. There is little in the literature about anxiety and HRQoL in CABG patients. One paper by Phillips Bute et al., [2003] examined HRQoL using the SF-36 one year post CABG in 280 patients and demonstrated that female patients reported a poorer HRQoL one year post CABG with higher levels of anxiety (p=0.03) and had limitations in their work activity (p=0.02) compared to males. Their conclusion was that women do not show the same long term benefits as men from CABG. Clearly, there is very limited literature on anxiety in relation to longer-term outcomes of CABG such as physical and emotional well-being.

The Spielberger State Trait Anxiety Inventory (STAI) was developed to detect levels of anxiety measuring an index of personality-trait based anxiety levels [Spielberger et al., 1983]. Two aspects of anxiety can be measured: state (transitory feelings of fear or worry) and trait (the stable tendency to respond anxiously to stressful scenarios) [Bowling, 1995]. The STAI consists of 20 items measuring state anxiety and 20 items measuring trait anxiety [Bowling, 1995]. This questionnaire remains one of the most widely used in clinical research. The rationale for examining anxiety after CABG is that the process of atherothrombogenesis may well continue after surgery if the person remains anxious leading to further CHD symptoms and potentially MIs.

Social Support

Within the last twenty years there has been much interest on the role of social support and its role in health. Social support can often be misinterpreted as formal help from local organisations but within the current context, it refers to support from family, friends, spouse or partner (as appropriate). Social support is commonly measured in studies examining the effect of diseases on individuals. Some studies have highlighted a direct association between social support and depression, anxiety, physical symptoms and self-reported use of health services [Holohan et al., 1996; Sarason et al., 1985]. Those with a high level of social support from family and friends had less symptoms of anxiety and depression and the severity of physical and psychological symptoms were less than those with little or no social support

[Sarason et al., 1985].Given these findings, social support would seem to be an important consideration in those with CHD while its role in the long term after CABG is unknown.

Research has shown that social support is influenced by many factors including age, change in circumstances (unemployment, retirement and death of a spouse for example). The other issue is the availability of social support through local resources. In areas of extreme poverty or geographical remoteness, there may be a lack of community services leading to poor social integration. The factors and issues surrounding social support are enormous and although marital status, gender, age, stress and mental health have been implicated as important, the overall inter-relationships are not so straightforward. Issues that affect social support are multifactorial and the importance of confounding variables such as alcohol consumption, smoking and pre-morbid psychopathology need to be taken into consideration when predicting the effect of social support on mortality. Thus, to what extent social support actually affects overall mortality is unclear although it would appear to play an important role.

Of importance is the fact that social support levels will differ between people and therefore subjective opinions need to be examined. An individual can have many social contacts but it is the frequency and type of contact that is relevant. However from objective measures that examine the number of social contacts per week or per month, this may give an accurate picture of actual or perceived social support. Health surveys in the UK reported that 25% of women between 65 and 74 years and 30% of women over the age of 45 were socially active in their communities [Cooper et al., 1999].The authors concluded that social support is beneficial to health and this is confirmed by others with low levels of social support associated with increased mortality [Vaillant et al., 1998; Berkman et al., 1993]. In men who were classified as "socially isolated" and having high levels of life stressors, they were found to have a four times greater risk of dying as compared to those with low measures in both. One hypothesis is that lack of social support when stress is present can lead to poor health-related behaviour such as increased smoking and alcohol consumption [Vaillant et al., 1998].

In relation to CHD; various studies have demonstrated a relationship between the individual's risks of dying from CHD increasing as the size of their social network diminished [Brummett et al., 2001] while the lack of social support was identified as a risk factor for CHD in a Swedish study [Orth-Gomer et al., 1993]. Alcohol and smoking may be mediators between social support and mortality making studies difficult to interpret [Valliant et al., 1998].

In relation to survival post acute MI, researchers showed a significant difference in fatality post MI related to married and unmarried patients. Married males had a reduced mortality compared to unmarried men [Chandra et al., 1983]. Ten year survival was also significant for married AMI patients. Although having a spouse is important, others believe that in those over 60 years, close friends and/or relatives are of greater importance than spouses [Seeman et al., 1987]. Indeed, two factors implicated in affecting recovery post MI are depression and lack of social support [Irvine et al., 1999; Berkman et al., 1992] which highlights the importance of social support in AMI patients.

In relation to CABG, the role of social support has been investigated [Yates 1995; Kulik and Mahler 1989; Radley and Green, 1987]. Social support from a spouse has a crucial role in the immediate post-operative period following bypass surgery [Radley and Green, 1987].

At a one-year follow-up, he found that those who "returned to normal" had the least change in their relationships and those who complained of pain had marked decline in their social contacts. The couples that were most prepared for surgery actually increased their social contacts and their own relationship was better. However he did find some patients who kept things to themselves and didn't wish to discuss issues with their families in order to get back to normal as quickly by avoiding discussion. Unfortunately no anxiety and depression measurements were performed. Social support in the immediate post-operative period also reduced hospital length of stay. Kulik and Mahler [1989] found that men who had many visits from their wives in hospital and perceived a high level of social support made a speedy recovery and were discharged 1.26 days earlier than those with lower levels of social support. Yates [1995] reported beneficial psychological recovery post MI from spousal support and health care providers. This highlights that the social support does not necessarily have to come from the spouse to aid recovery in cardiac illness. No studies examining social support five years after CABG have been found in the literature.

Methodology

Based on the reviewed literature, there is a need to examine subjective and objective data five years after CABG. The purpose of the study was to assess patients' HRQoL five years after CABG in terms of (i) physical health including symptoms of angina and breathlessness, (ii) psychological well-being incorporating anxiety and depression and (iii) social support which informs social functioning level. Several assessments were made on HRQoL using the SF-36, psychological well-being (namely depression and anxiety), dietary habits, physical activity, social support and their cognitive performance five years after CABG.

The questionnaires selected were the SF-36 [Ware et al., 1988], the Allied Dunbar National Fitness Survey diet sheet [Allied Dunbar, 1992] and a physical activity/exercise sheet [Wang et al., 1992]. Patients' perceived mood state was assessed using the STAI [Spielberger et al., 1983] and the BDI [Beck et al., 1961] and the Multidimensional Scale of Perceived Social Support (MSPSS) was used to measure social support [Zimet et al., 1988].

The data recorded prior to patients' bypass operation from the original study were examined. In the original study, a physician examined patients and elicited a full medical history. Routine blood tests, a chest X-ray and an ECG were carried out. Symptoms such as angina and breathlessness were scored and comorbid health problems (such as rheumatoid arthritis and asthma) documented. Prior to surgery and eight weeks post-operatively, a psychologist administered neuropsychological and mood assessment tests.

SF-36

The Short Form-36 (SF-36) is short, easy to administer and has good psychometric qualities [Ware et al., 1993].The SF-36 UK version 2 was used [Jenkinson et al., 1996].

The SF-36 covers eight domains measuring:

- Physical functioning with limitations in physical activities
- Role physical (usual role activity limitations)

- Bodily pain and its impact
- General health perceptions
- Vitality/Energy
- Social functioning (and the effect of physical and emotional problems on socialising)
- Mental health (psychological well-being).
- Change in health status

The eight profile scores can be aggregated into two psychometrically-based summary scores measuring physical and mental health; the PCS and the MCS respectively. The scores are from 0 to 100 with zero representing the worst possible state measured by the questionnaire and 100 denoting the best possible health state.

Angina and Breathless Symptoms

Two classifications are commonly used by physicians to score symptoms; the Canadian Cardiovascular Society Functional Classification (CCS) [Campeau, 1976] and NYHA [The Criteria Committee of the New York Heart Association, 1974]. Both classifications were used; symptoms in this study pre-operatively and at the five year follow-up. The questionnaires were completed by the researcher at the five year follow-up visit based on the information received from the patient concerning current symptoms relating to everyday activities.

Anxiety

The STAI [Spielberger et al., 1983] was used to determine levels of anxiety symptoms. This questionnaire consists of 40 statements (with the choice of answers ranging from "not at all", "somewhat", "moderately so" to "very much so"). The answers relate to how the patient is feeling at that particular moment. The STAI encompasses state and trait anxiety. The trait anxiety provides an index of personality-based anxiety levels whereas state anxiety levels provide an immediate measure of anxiety in the current situation (relevant to the follow-up visits of this study). The STAI consists of 20 items for measuring trait anxiety and 20 items for measuring state anxiety [Spielberger et al., 1983]. The trait was performed pre-operatively.

Depression

The BDI has been used mainly with patients and in research [Gallagher et al., 1982]. The BDI is a standardised, 21 item, self-report inventory for the measurement of depressed mood. The questions are aimed at identifying how subjects have been feeling in the previous week. The BDI scores are separated into the somatic (that is, physical) and cognitive related questions [Beck et al., 1961]. The somatic questions related to ability to work, tiredness, loss of appetite, loss of weight and concern about health. The remaining questions were concerned with mood. Each question offers a choice of four response statements.

Neuropsychological Testing

Trained psychologists administered the battery of neuropsychological tests. This battery consisted of the Rey Auditory Learning Test, Non-verbal Recognition Memory, Trailmaking A and Trailmaking B, WAIS Block Design Test, Tapping Test, letter cancellation, symbol digit replacement, choice reaction time and displaced reaction time. The tests were used because of their reported sensitivity to change [Pugsley et al., 1994] and their endorsement in the literature [Murkin et al., 1995]. Where available, parallel forms of the tests were administered to limit the effects of learning between each testing time.

Perceived Social Support

The Multidimensional Scale of Perceived Social Support (MSPSS) was used [Zimet et al., 1988]. There are three subscales each addressing a different source of support- family, friends and "significant other"(their spouse for example). It consists of a twelve-question scale, which asks about how the patient feels about the amount of social support they receive from family, friends and a significant other. The scale is a seven-point scale ranging from "very strongly disagree" to "very strongly agree". A total of twelve questions were asked with four each on family, friends and special person. The maximum score from each aspect is 28 and a minimum of four. The total score from all three sources is a maximum of 84 and a minimum of 12.

Dietary Questionnaire

The Allied Dunbar questionnaire was chosen to measure current diet. This questionnaire consists of eleven questions on eating habits [Allied Dunbar, 1994]. Each question has a choice of three answers and each answer is scored as one, two or three, depending on whether the diet is classified as "healthy" or "unhealthy". Scoring one means a healthy diet, whereas three is the least healthy option. A total score is calculated.

Physical Activity Questionnaire

The questionnaire was taken from Wang et al., [1992], adapted from Simons-Morton et al. [1988]. The questionnaire was composed of seven levels of activity from level one "sedentary" to level seven "competitive". An activity description was given for each level in terms of the minutes per day the activity is carried out, times per week and the effect on heart rate and perceived physical exertion. Patients were asked to nominate the level which related to their activity level over the previous month in an attempt to measure their actual physical activity level rather than elicit their view of their maximal ability. Activity examples were given to enable individuals to determine their current level, even if they were unaware of maximal heart rate and exertion rate.

Interim Data

Interim data refers to events that took place between CABG and the time of the follow-up visit. These data included patients' reported start or return of angina after CABG, MI incidence, the need for cardiac procedures (such as angiography) and hospitalisation.

Follow-up data

Patients were also asked for a list of their medications, to list any current illnesses and any other issues regarding their health in relation to their CABG operation.

Physical Component Summary and Mental Component Summary of the SF-36 were chosen as the dependent variables as these variables summed up the physical and mental health aspects (that is the eight domains) of HRQoL. Component summary scores have been used in previous studies [Pearson et al., 1999; Rumsfeld et al., 1999; Jenkinson et al., 1997; Ware et al., 1994]. They were also chosen as the summary scores of the patients' physical and emotional health can be used without substantial loss of information from the eight domains [Jenkinson et al., 1997]. A key question addressed here is whether the PCS and MCS are independent. Many researchers maintain that there is an inter-relationship between physical and psychological functioning. It would be difficult for questionnaire data to separate the two domains. The relationship is difficult to quantify and is probably bi-directional in nature [Cohen and Roderiguez 1995; Hyland 1992]. Thus, the decision to exclude these variables from the two hierarchical models was justified.

For the hierarchial regression, analysis was carried out on continuous and categorical data at various time-points (pre-operatively, peri-operatively and five years post CABG). The pre-operative data examined were gender, full scale IQ, anxiety using STAI and depression using BDI and symptoms (angina and breathlessness pre-operatively). Interim measures were hospitalisation, illness and angiogram. The peri-operative data were restricted to the numbers of grafts. The post-operative data examined at five years were symptoms (angina and breathlessness), SF-36 eight domains, diet score, physical activity level, neuropsychological change and psychological well-being (STAI and BDI measures of anxiety and depression symptoms respectively). These variables were examined to establish whether they correlated significantly with the SF-36 physical and mental component summaries. It was expected that those which inter-correlated highly would negatively affect the hierarchical regression analysis significance and would make it difficult to interpret the data.

Participants

All participants had been admitted to the Middlesex Hospital, London for their elective bypass surgery and had been subjects in a randomised control trial of the efficacy of a neuroprotective drug [Arrowsmith et al., 1998]. One hundred and sixty-two patients were recruited for the original study invited to return 4.5 to 5.5 years after bypass surgery to examine quality of life five years after CABG.

Study Population

All participants were admitted for elective bypass surgery. The inclusion criteria were patients undergoing elective CABGS aged between 18 and 75 years. Those who had a history of neurological or psychiatric conditions, previous drug or alcohol abuse and those undergoing emergency CABGS were excluded from the study. The hospital's Ethics Review Committee gave approval for the follow-up study.

Procedure

The follow-up study was carried out five years after surgery and all 162 patients were invited by letter to return to the hospital. The information sheet outlined the confidentiality and anonymity of the patient information and its use. Those who declined the invitation were not contacted again. Patients who attended the hospital visit completed questionnaires in a quiet room. The researcher was present to clarify any problems experienced in responding to the questions but not to aid the participants in their choice of answer. The data obtained in the study were stored and analysed confidentially in a password protected computer. Only the researchers had access to the data.

Statistical Analysis

The SPSS 10.0® statistical package was used for data entry and analysis within the managed PC system. Continuous data were analysed using independent t-tests and chi-squared analysis for categorical data.

Results

One hundred and sixty-two patients were recruited at the time of surgery originally, with 156 traced five years after CABG (96%). One hundred and twenty-eight (that is, 79% of the original sample) participated in the five year follow-up study with eighteen (11%) failing to attend appointments, four patients (3%) declining to participate in the five year follow-up and six patients (4%) had died from the time of surgery to the time of follow-up. One hundred and nine patients attended hospital for follow-up and completed questionnaires and were seen by the researcher and by the psychologists who performed the neuropsychological tests. Another nineteen patients completed some postal questionnaires but this data will not be discussed here.

A total of 109 patients completed the questionnaires at a face-to-face visit. Two patients who were assessed were excluded from the analyses as one had undergone a second CABG and the second was inebriated when he attended for the appointment. The follow-up time ranged from four years and 11 months to five years and six months after CABG. The sample consisted of 93 males (87%) and 14 females (13%) whose average age at follow-up was 66 years. The characteristics of the study sample at follow-up closely matched those of the original cohort and statistically, the patients were representative of the original cohort in terms of number of vessels grafted (t=.638, p= .625) and pre-operative MI incidence (χ^2= .286, df=1, p=.593). The majority of patients had three coronary grafts (n= 76, 71%) with two undergoing four grafts (2%) and a quarter of patients having two grafts (n=27).

Interim data from CABG to five year follow-up were collected. The angina-free interval varied. A total of 81 patients (64%) remained free of angina as reported at the follow-up assessment five years after CABG. In the time from bypass surgery to follow-up, four patients (4%) had an MI with 94% (n=101) reporting no interim MI. Data were missing on two patients (2%). All these patients had pre-operative MI and had severe angina pre-operatively (CCS Class IV pre-operatively). At follow-up, all had severe angina (CCS Class III) and two had breathlessness classed as NYHA Class III.Coronary angiograms were carried out on 10 patients (9%) after CABG. Hospitalisation was defined as spending one night or more in hospital as an in-patient for any illness from the time of discharge after CABG to the time of follow-up. A total of 16 patients (15%) had been hospitalised since their cardiac surgery up to the time of their follow-up assessment (χ^2= 39.35, df=1, p< .001).

The main classification groups in the International Classification of Diseases (ICD) were used to classify the presence of other illnesses, disorders and diseases as reported by the patient at the time of assessment. For example if a patient stated that they had asthma, it was classified as a respiratory system illness. Forty-nine percent of the patients had no illnesses at the time of the five year follow-up assessment (n=52) with the remaining 55 patients having a current illness (51%). The majority (28%) of those with reported comorbid illness suffered endocrine (n=14) (diabetes mellitus and thyroid dysfunction) or metabolic disorders and blood disorders (n=16) (anaemia in particular). A further 10 patients (10%) had musculoskeletal disease (the primary diagnosis being osteo-arthritis). Patients with illness had significantly higher rates of interim hospitalisation. The majority of patients remained on aspirin post CABG (Table 1). Over a third of patients were prescribed lipid-lowering drugs (n= 41) and a further 13 patients were taking anti-hypertensive drugs.

Table 1. Type of medication prescribed to assessed patients (n=107) at time of follow-up

Medication type	Yes =n (%)	No =n (%)	Missing=n (%)
Aspirin	105 (95%)	2 (2%)	0
Statins	41 (38%)	63 (59%)	3 (3%)
Diuretic	18 (17%)	86 (80%)	3 (3%)
Anti-hypertensive	13 (12%)	91 (85%)	3 (3%)
ACE inhibitors	14 (13%)	90 (84%)	3 (3%)
B blockers	19 (18%)	85 (79%)	3 (3%)
Anti-anginals	14 (13%)	90 (84%)	3 (3%)
Diabetes	7 (7%)	100 (93%)	0

Table 2. Comparison of classification of angina and breathless symptoms pre-operatively and at five years post CABG (n=107)

Symptoms	n (%) Pre-operative	n (%) Five years follow-up
CCS Class I	0 (0%)	68 (63.5%)
CCS Class II	9 (8.4%)	28 (27.0%)
CCS Class III	88 (82.3%)	10 (10.3%)
CCS Class IV	10 (9.3%)	1 (0.9%)
NYHA Class I	49 (45.8%)	72 (67.3%)
NYHA Class II	54 (50.5%)	24 (22.4%)
NYHA Class III	4 (3.7%)	11 (10.3%)
NYHA Class IV	0 (0%)	0 (0%)

Angina and breathless symptoms were measured pre-operatively and five years after CABG and a comparison of pre-operative and five year post-operative symptoms was made (Table 2). At five years post CABG the majority of patients had no, or minimal angina compared with pre-operative moderate ratings of moderate to severe angina. Ninety-six patients (90%) had CCS classification of I or II at five years follow-up. By combining and identifying the Class I and II as "asymptomatic" and identifying Class III as "symptomatic" no significant differences were observed between the symptomatic and asymptomatic groups (χ^2= 138.29, df=1, p<0.01).

Using the New York Heart Association classification a comparison was made between breathless symptoms pre-operatively and five years post CABG in the patients. By combining and identifying the Class I and II as "asymptomatic" and identifying Class III as "symptomatic" no significant differences were observed between the symptomatic and asymptomatic groups (χ^2=2.58, df=1, p= .347). A higher percentage of patients had no breathlessness compared to their pre-operative classification (NYHA Class I: 67.3% v. 45.8%, 72 v. 49, respectively) and no patients had deteriorated to NYHA Class IV on assessment five years post CABG.

The SF-36 results are presented in Table 3 with the mean scores along with standard deviations and the PCS and MCS. The scores are normative based scores, with a mean of 50 and standard deviation of 10. The scores are rated from zero to 100. One hundred represents optimal health with no physical or emotional health limitations and zero represents poor physical and mental health. Three domains scores are above the mean of 50 in the patients: "physical role", "emotional role", "mental health", "energy/vitality" and MCS.

Table 3. Mean SF-36 scores in eight domains, PCS and MCS of patients (n=107)

Variable	Patient score mean (SD)
Physical functioning	45.9 (11.8)
Physical role	50.4 (9.6)
Emotional role	51.8 (9.1)
Mental health	54.6 (9.9)
Social functioning	45.8 (9.1)
Energy/vitality	51.9 (10.1)
Bodily pain	47.5 (10.8)
General health Perceptions	49.8 (11.4)
PCS	45.8 (10.6)
MCS	53.6 (8.6)

Anxiety and depression was measured pre-operatively and five years post CABG. Table 4 compares the mean BDI and STAI scores pre-operatively and at five years post CABG. Using a paired t test, the results show a significant difference between the pre-operative and post-operative scores in the total somatic and total BDI scores (p<.05) and STAI anxiety score (p<.001) with lower scores at follow-up compared to pre-operatively.

Correlations were performed between the depression and anxiety scores five years after CABG and the component summary scores of the SF-36 (Table 5). Both PCS and MCS correlated significantly with the BDI and STAI scores from the five-year visit.

Table 4. Anxiety and depression mean scores and standard deviations pre-operatively and at five year follow-up (n=107)

Psychological well-being	Pre-operative Mean (SD)	Five years post CABG Mean (SD)	t value	p value (2 tailed significance)
Depression (BDI total score)	6.9 (4.3)	5.5 (4.5)	2.6	.011
Depression (BDI Somatic score)	2.8 (1.7)	1.8 (1.8)	4.4	<.001
Depression (BDI Cognitive score)	4.2 (3.3)	3.8 (3.8)	0.7	.470
Anxiety (STAI score)	37.2 (9.5)	32.2 (10.3)	4.8	<.001

Table 5. Pearson correlation coefficient between HRQoL and mood (depression) five years after CABG (using SF-36: PCS and MCS) and the BDI (n=107)

SF-36 component summary	BDI Correlation R=	p value (2 tailed)
PCS	-.478	<.001
MCS	-.711	<.001
	STAI correlation R=	p value (2 tailed)
PCS	-.246	<.05
MCS	-.577	<.001

All the domains and the component summary scores correlated highly with the BDI (p<.001). The STAI measure of anxiety correlated highly with all the SF-36 domains and component summaries (not shown). Dividing the BDI into somatic (that is, physical) and cognitive (that is, emotional) aspects, all eight domains of the SF-36 correlated with the somatic and cognitive BDI measures (all at p <.01).

With respect to neuropsychological deficits, a total of 28% had deficits five years after CABG. The pre-operative baseline scores were reduced in two or more tests when measured five years post CABG. Certain tests took longer to complete at five years compared to pre-operatively when examined as mean score differences between the two tests: block design, tapping test and trails A. A correlation was carried out between the SF-36 components summary scores and the change scores from the neuropsychological tests. The change score was calculated for each subject on each test by subtracting their post-operative performance from their preoperative performance. No correlations were found between the SF-36 component summaries and the neuropsychological changes scores five years after CABG.

The Multidimensional Perceived Social Support (MSPSS) [Zimet et al 1988] measured perceived social support. The total score was a maximum of 84 and a minimum of 43. The majority of patients perceived adequate social support from significant other, family and friends. The question over whether HRQoL was related to perceived social support was examined looking at the eight domains of the SF-36 and the composite scores (PCS and MCS). None of the SF-36 domains correlated with the MSPSS. A correlation was carried out between the social support questionnaire and psychological well-being (measuring anxiety and depression) at five years post CABG. In all the social support aspects and the anxiety and depression scores, no correlation was found. Similar results were found when the somatic and cognitive aspects of the BDI were examined.

Prior to performing hierarchical regression analysis, it was necessary to establish the correlations between variables at the various time-points. Correlations were found between pre-operative anxiety and depression symptoms ($p < .01$). Pre-operative change scores correlated with age ($p<.01$). Correlations were found between the interim MI and hospitalisation ($r = -.033$, $p<.001$). Correlations were also evident between PCS and interim hospitalisation ($r=.30$, $p<.05$) and interim illness and PCS ($r = -.23$, $p<.05$). A correlation was also found between MCS and interim MI ($r= -.24$, $p<.05$). Negative correlations were found between PCS and angina, breathlessness, physical activity levels, anxiety and depression five years post CABG. The MCS correlated negatively with angina, diet score, anxiety and depression at the five year follow-up (all $p<.001$).

Hierarchical Regression Analysis

Multiple hierarchical linear regression analyses were performed to examine which variables determined physical and mental QoL five years after CABG. Prediction could not be performed as the measures were concurrent (that is, some were from five years post CABG) and so prediction of HRQoL was not possible.

Entry into the model was used within blocks. For the purpose of entry into the regression, all variables with a correlation with a significance level $p< 0.05$ were used (with the exception of the component summary scores due to its collinearity and the inter-relationship between physical and psychological functioning [Cohen and Roderiguez, 1995].

Hierarchical Regression and the SF-36 Physical Component Summary

Six variables correlated with the PCS: pre-operative angina score (CCS), interim comorbid Illness, and the following five years after CABG -anxiety score (STAI), depression score (BDI) and physical activity. All were significant at $p<.01$. The MCS variable was omitted from the analysis as it is strongly correlated with the other variables and also correlated with the dependent variable, PCS ($r=0.26$, $p<.05$).

Variables were entered in five blocks as follows: pre-operative angina score, comorbid illness at the time of follow-up, anxiety and depression scores five years post CABG, and physical activity five years post CABG. With regard to the pre-operative data, the first variable used for regression was the pre-operative angina score using the Canadian Cardiovascular Society score (CCS) (Table 6). In the second block, comorbid illness at the time of follow-up was added to the equation and this, along with pre-operative angina, accounted for 5.5% of the variability (adjusted $R^2=.055$). In the third block where anxiety scores five years post CABG were added, these variables accounted for over 10% of the variability (adjusted R^2=.109). When depression scores five years post CABG were added to the analysis, these combined variables accounted for nearly 26% of the variability (adjusted R^2=.257). In the final equation physical activity level five years post CABG was included. The inclusion of this variable accounted for a further 11% of variability (adjusted R^2=.365).

These variables showed that pre-operative angina symptoms, comorbid illness, physical activity at five years, depression and anxiety scores at five years, and physical activity at five years accounted for a significant amount (36%) of the PCS variance when measured five years post CABG.

Table 6. Multiple regressions to determine SF-36 Physical Component Summary five years post CABG

		PCS	
Cum			Cum
	β	R2	Adjusted R2
Block 1			
Pre-operative angina Score (CCS)	-.072	.025	.016
Block 2			
Comorbid illness	-.171*	.073	.055
Block 3			
Anxiety scores five years post CABG (STAI)	.009	.134	.109
Block 4			
Depression scores five years post CABG (BDI)	-.339**	.285	.257
Block 5			
Physical activity 5 years post CABG	.359**	.395	.365

**p<.001, *p<.05

Hierarchical Regression and SF-36 Mental Component Summary

Seven variables that significantly correlated with the MCS (p<.01): Anxiety scores pre-operatively (STAI), interim MI, age and the following five years after CABG: diet scores and anxiety and depression scores.

In the first block, 4% of the variability was explained by anxiety (as measured by the STAI) pre-operatively. At the second block when post CABG MI was included, over 8% of the variability was accounted for (adjusted R^2=.084). When age was added to the block, these variables accounted for 16% of the variability (adjusted R^2=.167). In the fourth block, the addition of current diet scores accounted for 20% of the MCS variability (adjusted R^2=.202).

In the penultimate equation, the inclusion of anxiety scores five years post CABG accounted for a further 26% of variability (adjusted R^2=.462). In the final model, the addition of the depression scores at the time of follow-up accounted for 60% of the MCS (adjusted R^2=.606) five years after CABG (Table 7).

Table 7. Multiple regressions to determine SF-36 Mental Component Summary five years post CABG

MCS			
Cum	Cum		
	β	R2	Adjusted R
Block 1			
Pre-operative anxiety scores (STAI)	-.019	.052	.042
Block 2			
Interim MI	.074	.103	.084
Block 3			
Age at five years	.236**	.194	.167
Block 4			
Diet scores five years post CABG	-.020	.244	.202
Block 5			
Anxiety scores five years post CABG (STAI)	-.303**	.496	.462
Block 6			
Depression scores five years post CABG (BDI)	-.518**	.634	.606

**$p<.001, *p<.05

Discussion

The study aimed to examine quality of life five years post CABG. The SF-36 questionnaire revealed that the majority of patients rated themselves as having a good HRQoL and that physical illness can cause physical functioning limitations, it does not lead to emotional problems as seen by MCS. The majority of patients had minimal angina and breathless symptoms and a small number had concomitant illness at follow-up. Significant differences were observed from pre-operative depression and anxiety scores to five years after CABG. When correlations between component summary scores from the SF-36 and anxiety and depression scores five years after CABG were performed, all correlated significantly suggesting that psychological well-being negatively affects both physical and mental HRQoL five years after surgery. Neuropsychological deficits were evident in 28% of patients at the five year follow-up but no correlations were found between the deficits and SF-36 or psychological well-being. These results suggest no effect on patients' cognitive functioning at the time of follow-up. Examining patients perceived social support showed the majority felt well supported.

Use of a hierarchical regression model established that pre-operative angina scores, comorbid illness, depression and anxiety scores at follow-up and physical activity level were predictors of the PCS of the SF-36 (36.5% of the variance). Pre-operative anxiety, post-operative MI, current diet score, anxiety and depression at follow-up accounted for 60% of the variability of the MCS.

In relation to the relevant literature, the study showed a very high trace rate (96%)and this rate compares favourably with reports in the literature on other five year follow-up studies in patients who have undergone CABG [Herlitz et al., 1999] [Caine et al., 1999]. It proved possible to collect data from a high percentage of those traced (n=128, 79%).

Patients' non-attendance at the follow-up appointments accounted for 18 patients in the study (11%). Possible reasons for not returning may relate to the comparative younger age of this "group", making it likely that these individuals were working or had other time constraints. The total time commitment for the majority of patients of four hours, including travel time to the hospital, may have been a disincentive. Six patients had died since their bypass operation. This mortality rate (3.7%) is lower than the rates cited in three five year follow-up studies; which is between 5.4% and 10% [Stahle et al., 1994; Kirklin et al., 1989; Parisi et al., 1989]. The implication of this comparatively low death rate is that the cohort in this study came from the "better end" of the prognostic spectrum with better treatment and less severe CHD and it is a later study than others - assuming no major differences in surgical technique.

The clinical data examined in this study included symptoms, such as angina and breathlessness, of patients who had had CABG and those who required a second bypass operation, hospitalisation post CABG and medication at the time of follow-up. Angina and breathless symptoms were measured five years post CABG and the majority of patients were free from angina symptoms at five years (64.3%) with the remainder reporting some anginal symptoms. A similar UK five year follow-up study reported 60% painfree (that is, free from angina), with a lower mean age at surgery of 51 years compared to this study's mean age of 60 years at the time of surgery [Caine et al., 1999]. This figure of 60% replicates findings cited in other five year studies of between 63% and 80% painfree [Rogers et al., 1990; Kirklin et al., 1989; European Coronary Surgery Study 1979].

A small and statistically non-significant increase in breathless symptoms five years post CABG was found in patients who had no breathless symptoms pre-operatively. Those with dyspnoea NYHA Class III rose from 3.7% pre-operatively to 10.3% five years after CABG. Researchers have claimed that breathlessness is an important predictor of HRQoL [Caine et al. 1999; Herlitz et al.1999] and identified dyspnoea as a good indicator of severely impaired left ventricular function. However, as they did not report the breathlessness classifications at five years, the levels of dyspnoea using the NYHA classification are unknown and this makes interpretation of the findings difficult.

Five years post CABG, patients were asked which medication they were currently taking at the follow-up visit and the vast majority of patients continued on aspirin (over ninety percent). The modifiable associated risk factors of CHD have been well documented [INTERHEART study investigators, 2004; Greenland et al., 2003]. Over a third of patients were receiving statins for raised cholesterol and just over ten percent were taking ACE inhibitors, raising the possibility that their medical regimen was sub-optimal. The guidelines from the National Lipid Association in the US [National Lipid Association website] and NICE in the UK [NICE website] clearly advocate the use of statins in reducing elevated serum cholesterol [Grundy et al., 1999]. It is difficult to come to any definitive conclusions regarding their medication regimen from this study however suboptimal treatment of B-blockers and ACE inhibitors as secondary prevention medications after CABG has been reported [Goyal et al., 2007]. The researchers reported significantly higher 2-year death rates and MI rates in these patients suggesting better clinical outcomes could be achieved with optimal medication management.

The incidence of hospitalisation over the five year period was examined in these patients. Interim hospitalisation was taken as an indicator of ill-health from CHD or other conditions. The other five year follow-up studies offered no data on hospitalisation post CABG. The literature on hospitalisation rates and medication was too sparse to determine whether the present group was "typical" in these respects.

Given that some patients were hospitalised suggests the presence of comorbid illness. The incidence of comorbid illness post CABG was examined, the rationale being that reports of illness increase as people with known CHD get older [Chocran et al., 1996; Sjoland et al., 1996]. The main illnesses reported in the follow-up study were endocrine and metabolic (that is, diabetes mellitus and thyroid dysfunction), blood diseases (for example, anaemia) and musculoskeletal disorders (for example, osteoarthritis). Diabetes is a recognised cardiovascular risk factor and has been shown to lead to a greater risk of mortality in those with CHD [Vasan et al., 2005]. Overall, self-reported illness is sparsely reported and no conclusion can be drawn on the incidence of comorbid illness in this study.

Too few patients had angiograms post-operatively to determine long term graft patency. Caine et al. [1999] reported a re-operation rate of 3% within five years of the first operation. Re-intervention (that is, angioplasty or surgery) was cited at 3% in one study [Kirklin et al., 1989]. No five year follow-up comparative studies between CABG and PCI have been identified while a three year comparative follow-up demonstrated a higher number of coronary interventions in PCI patients than in the CABG cohort (that is, the PCI patients required further coronary interventions following their first procedure) [Hannan et al., 2005]. Further comparative studies of these two interventions are needed.

The SF-36 was chosen because of its wide use in cardiac studies and its ability to examine functional ability in cardiac patients [Deiwick et al., 2001; Fruitman et al., 1999]. The physical and mental health-related QoL in cardiac and CABG patients have been reported using the SF-36 although few studies have been conducted on CABG follow-up patients [Lindsay et al., 2000; Rumsfeld et al., 1999]. The fact that most reported a good HRQoL and had very few symptoms five years after CABG validates the inclusion of the SF-36 and measuring clinical symptoms and replicates other studies which have used a combination of questionnaires and measuring symptoms [Huber et al., 2007].

In this study five years post CABG, the patients interviewed in person scored between 45 and 55, indicative of a good HRQoL. A comparison to an age-matched population sample could not be carried out as the UK population normative data has only included a sample up to 64 years. This study's samples mean age at follow-up was 66 years. These findings are in line with previous studies in older cardiac patients with better SF-36 scores than the general population [Deiwick et al., 2001; Fruitman et al., 1999]. Scores greater than 50 were recorded in four domains of patients demonstrating above average results compared to normative population scores.

Correlations were found between mental QoL (using the SF-36) and psychological well-being (anxiety and depression symptoms using the STAI and BDI, respectively) five years after CABG. Both depressive and anxiety symptoms correlated with the domains on the SF-36. It would appear that depressive symptoms and functional ability are linked with symptomatic heart disease. These findings replicate previous studies [Sullivan et al., 1997] but other researchers have found no evidence of this relationship five years post CABG [Herlitz et al., 2000a; Lindal et al., 1996]. Other studies reporting HRQoL five years post CABG such as Caine et al. [1999] did not examine psychological well-being as part of the follow-up. Similarly, Herlitz et al. [2000a] report on symptom relief and briefly refer to an improved psychological well-being five years post CABG. Only a few studies so far has identified the effects of depressive symptoms on QoL after bypass surgery [Stafford et al., 2007; Mallick et al., 2005] but Mallick et al.'s study was only at one year post CABG. However the importance of depression and depressive symptoms has led to studies examining the efficacy of anti-depressants in those with CHD [Berkman et al., 2003; Swenson et al., 2003; Glassman et al., 2002]. Given the evidence supporting the abnormal physiological markers in those with depression and anxiety, these results need further investigation.

The incidence of raised physiological markers (such as C-reactive protein and platelets for instance) in patients with CHD and depression is currently topical [Lesperance et al., 2004]. The relationship between poor physical health in CABG patients with clinical depression has been reported [Doering et al., 2005]. The findings imply a complex relationship of physiological, behavioural and psychological factors and many questions remain unanswered about these mechanisms and their role in CHD [Rumsfeld and Ho, 2005]. Recent research on anxiety highlights its role in CHD and as an independent predictor of MI [Shen et al., 2008; Todaro et al., 2007]. These physiological markers were not examined five years post CABG. Future research should focus on investigating physiological markers with anxiety and depression symptoms in those with no known CHD, known CHD, post MI and after CABG. Examining these four distinct groups may answer some of the questions about physiological markers and psychological well-being.

Although a relationship was found between HRQoL five years post CABG and anxiety symptoms in this study; the relevant literature has focused on its prevalence pre-operatively and in the immediate post-operative period [Rymaszewska et al., 2003; Koivula et al., 2002; McCrone et al., 2001; Duits et al., 1998]. These researchers reported a decline in anxiety symptoms post CABG compared to the levels recorded pre-operatively. However, others have reported contrary findings with higher levels recorded post-operatively [Andrew et al., 2000]. Two studies have examined anxiety symptoms one year after CABG [Rothenhausler et al., 2005; Phillips Bute et al., 2003]. Although the evidence highlighting the presence of anxiety symptoms in patients pre and post CABG is available, further studies are required to determine its importance in psychological well-being in CABG patients at various follow-up times such as one, two and five years post CABG for example.

However an important fact was that patients generally regard themselves as healthy five years post CABG. One question is whether patients have changed their perceptions and beliefs since their operation. Psychological adaptation is one plausible explanation for their perceived HRQoL. Change in perceptions over time were not examined within this study but is an issue which warrants further investigation.

The hypothesis that neuropsychological performance would have declined over five years was supported. A deficit in the performance on the cognitive test battery was detectable in 28% of the five year follow-up patients. Newman et al. [2001b] also described deficits in 42% of patients five years after CABG; this finding was also predicted by cognitive function at discharge after CABG.

It was possible, of course, that these five year changes were due to cerebrovascular disease that also explained the vulnerability of these patients to the circulatory disturbance during CABG and to early post-operative cerebral complications. Many factors have been implicated in cognitive decline such as Apolipoprotein E and surgical technique of CABG but no consensus has been reached [Steed et al., 2001; Abildstrom et al., 2000]. Ageing has been strongly implicated by various studies but none of these researchers examined decline five years after CABG [Borowicz et al., 1996; Newman et al. 1994].

The data were also explored for evidence of any relationship between neuropsychological performance and perceived HRQoL. It was hypothesised that a decline in neuropsychological performance would correlate with poor mental HRQoL but no correlation was found. There is little literature on this subject. Although Newman et al. [2001b] reported a connection, the data were preliminary. The researchers concluded that from a patient's perception on their general health, a direct correlation existed with their cognitive function. No baseline HRQoL data was recorded warranting further research to examine this finding. In the only other five year study [Selnes et al., 2001], HRQoL was not measured and the only variables examined related to the pre-operative demographic data and interim medical incidents such as MI and PTCA.

The likely explanation for this negative finding is that the cognitive changes are, in general, minor. An alternative explanation is that neuropsychological changes are contaminated by the effects of anxiety. An important point here is that the patients report no cognitive problems and perceive a good HRQoL. However, the lack of a correlation between HRQoL and neuropsychological deficits suggests that patients regard themselves as "healthy" five years post CABG. The findings reflected in this study need to be replicated by other studies in order to support or refute the findings.

Perceived social support from spouse, family and friends was generally good in patients. No correlations were found with anxiety and depression scores and the SF-36. A very small group of patients reported very little perceived social support. A difference between actual and perceived support has been observed [The HEA health and lifestyle survey 1992]. The HEA survey found a diminished actual amount of social contact (with friends) in those older than fifty-five years but no difference was found in actual contact with relatives.

Further investigations dividing the total social support scale (an arbitrary division), showed no significance between those with lower perceived support and PCS or MCS scores. It was anticipated that mood would affect social support as those who were depressed would be less likely to socialise and interact with others and may perceive lower levels of social support from family and friends. Depression and anxiety symptoms did not affect perceived social support five years post CABG. This finding is contrary to others [Holohan et al 1999]. Having a spouse did not change perceived social support compared to those without a spouse (i.e. unmarried, widowed or divorced). It may be that friends and relatives play just as vital a role in social support as the spouse does as previously reported [Seeman et al 1997, Chandra et al 1983].

If social support is so fundamental then why is there no relationship between quality of life and mood or concomitant illness? One explanation is that the questionnaire may not be sensitive enough to detect social isolation or it may be that the patients perceived HRQoL with limited symptoms is a true reflection and has no impact on their social functioning ability.

Which Variables Can Determine Quality of Life Five Years after CABG?

The search for determinants of HRQoL five years post CABGS yielded a series of variables using the physical and mental component summaries of the SF-36 as dependent variables. Examining the determinants of PCS, pre-operative angina, comorbid illness and concurrent variables of anxiety and depression scores with physical activity accounted for 36% of the variance. Anxiety (pre-operatively and five years post CABGS) and depression symptoms also accounted for a considerable amount of variance with the MCS along with age, interim MI and diet scores accounted for 60% of PCS variance.

Examining the variables which accounted for some of the multiple regression anlayses; angina and comorbid illness accounted for some variance with the majority of patients limited in their physical functioning by the presence of angina. Age has also been identified as a predictor of long term survival [Koch et al., 2007]. Sjoland and colleagues have used exercise capacity to measure their physical functioning and thus HRQoL [Sjoland et al., 1996]. The variables of angina symptoms and comorbid illness in determining some of the PCS variability is not surprising. The presence of comorbid illness undoubtedly affects HRQoL and its presence can be used as a simple marker of physical health problems. Greater decrements in functioning and well-being were revealed in those with comorbid illnesses and supported by others [Koch et al., 2007; Brazier et al., 1992]. The decline in physical activity has previously been reported and in usually associated with a decline in graft patency, however to confirm this, repeat angiography and other clinical tests would need to be performed [Caine et al., 1999].

The value of using the component summary scores of the SF-36 as predictors of various aspects of health has been demonstrated [Pearson et al., 1999; Rumsfeld et al., 1999]. One important aspect of the SF-36 component summary scores is that the PCS and MCS are not independent and the inter-relationship between has previously been reported [Cohen and Rodriguez, 1995]. No studies demonstrating the predictive value of MCS have been published and thus further studies are required to examine if MCS has any predictive value in CABGS patients.

It would appear that all markers of physical well-being (symptoms like angina, physical activity level, anxiety and depressive symptoms at follow-up and comorbid illness) impact on reported HRQoL in the physical measures. Anxiety and depressive symptoms dominated reported mental HRQoL.

Twenty-nine percent of the variance of PCS and 40% of the MCS variability were explained by the anxiety and depression scores at the time of follow-up. Anxiety and depressive symptoms have been identified as predictors of outcome post MI [Mayou et al., 2000]. This is in accordance with HRQoL and depressive symptoms one year post CABGS and was the first to report the relationship between HRQoL and depressive symptoms [Mallick et al., 2005]. This was the first study to examine HRQoL using the SF-36 and depressive symptoms post CABGS and demonstrated a lack of functional improvement in patients six months following surgery.

The role of depression and depressive symptoms in CAD and CABGS has been reported. Sullivan and colleagues found depression in patients with CAD five years after diagnosis was significantly associated with angina, personality type and the level of spouses' emotional support [Sullivan et al., 1997]. In one three-month follow-up study, anxiety and depression accounted for 4% and 6% of the change in SF-36 scores from pre-operative to three month follow-up [Hofer et al., 2006]. In a review of the literature on predictors of QoL post CABGS, researchers reported that pre-operative depression is a predictor of post-operative psychological maladjustment [Duits et al., 1997]. Burg and colleagues reported depression as an independent predictor of medical and psychosocial morbidity in 89 patients post CABGS six months after surgery with higher rates of hospitalisation and continued pain [Burg et al., 2003]. Undoubtedly anxiety and depression affect physical QoL and further studies are needed in larger populations to determine their exact role in determining HRQoL.

This study has shown that both anxiety and depressive symptoms are strongly implicated in determining both PCS and MCS and their importance in patients' HRQoL post CABGS cannot be underestimated. The implications for healthcare professionals would be to increase screening of anxiety and depressive symptoms after cardiac surgery. Further research is needed to examine if cognitive interventions and/or anti-depressants could benefit patients and improve their physical and mental HRQoL. It appears that psychological well-being is as important as relieving symptoms.

Limitations of the Study

During, and on completion of, the study several issues were identified which were problematic. These were suggestive of limitations of the study or of unresolved questions which point the way for future studies. Although the trace-rate was high (96%), the follow-up participation rate was only 79%. Similar figures are reported by others five years post CABG [Caine et al., 1999; Herlitz et al., 1999]. It would be interesting to explore alternative ways of assessing those who failed to show up for appointments. The group accounted for 11% of the sample and valuable data would not have been collected if the postal data had not been included. An important area is whether there is some way of ascertaining the reason for patients' non-attendance. Individual circumstances or some aspect of the follow-up visit may have been behind their non-participation. Also, it is unknown whether any patients participated in rehabilitation programmes.

Recommendations for Future Research

Several recommendations are made in relation to future research in this area including the collection the collection of subjective and objective clinical data, neuropsychological assessment to detect neurocognitive decline and implementation of nurse led clinics in the community (where subjective data could be collected and patients advised and educated about their cardiac risk factors for example).

Subjective Health-Related Quality of Life Data and Objective Clinical Data

Of importance is the finding that the presence of comorbid illness does not negatively affect mental health. It suggests that psychological adjustment occurs in the face of physical limitations. The study thus indicates the value of patients' self-reported information, not as a substitute for clinical treatment and risk factor measurement but to assist the physician to establish the patient's functional capability and related physical limitations in relation to chronic illness. Indeed, one study has shown that subjective information from patients is as important as clinical data and reports an association between symptom status and health related HRQoL [Sousa and Williamson, 2003]. It is clear that clinicians' care of their post CABG patients would be enhanced by their awareness of patients' perceived HRQoL and of issues relevant to specific patients.

Neuropsychological Assessment

It would appear that there is a risk from CABG surgery of cognitive decline (even five years after CABG). Further research is required in a larger population to demonstrate whether there is late, neurocognitive decline post CABG. Alternatively, or as well, a sub-group of patients may be particularly vulnerable to cerebral injury and neurological degenerative disorders.

Cognitive dysfunction post CABG is probably a multi-factorial problem and now with the use of OPCAB surgery, further comparative neuropsychological testing can be carried out. The cardiopulmonary bypass has been singled out as a contributory factor to cognitive decline; therefore, less cognitive deficits could be expected in patients who have OPCAB surgery. A comparative study would help establish or eliminate the role of cardiopulmonary bypass in cognitive dysfunction. In conjunction with this proposed study, further studies need to be carried out on long-term cognition in older noncardiac surgery patients to obtain comparative data. Currently, there are limited data on this area.

The findings of this study raise the question of whether there are currently adequate resources and facilities in place for patients five years after CABG to monitor their HRQoL and to prevent further atherosclerotic progression. The study suggests that there is a need to maximise the benefits of surgery for the patient, with attention being paid to any comorbid illness, in both the hospital and community setting with immediate and long-term care. One study has suggested the implementation of a lifestyle intervention and risk factor modification should be considered after cardiac rehabilitation programmes to further reduce the global risk of cardiovascular events [Lear et al., 2006].

An area of future clinical interest might be establishment of nurse-led clinics (especially in relation to the administration of HRQoL questionnaires, the provision of health education, diet and exercise prescriptives). Although a few papers have been published on nurse-led clinics [Fitzsimons et al., 2000], there is no wide implementation of such clinics. Undoubtedly, cardiac rehabilitation has an important role to play in patient recovery. The nurse's role in increasing attendance and compliance cannot be underestimated.

Clinical Implications of This Study

Given that atherosclerosis is a progressive condition, it is important to examine HRQoL longitudinally (especially after interventions such as CABG). This body of knowledge can reveal problems in physical and emotional health. The completion of HRQoL questionnaires is not time consuming or expensive and questionnaires can be administered and allow further regular or intermittent clinical assessment if health problems are detected. The study revealed that some patients have physical health problems which were reflected in their poor reported HRQoL. Patients may require further interventions to manage conditions (such as chronic respiratory disorders and diabetes). The identified need for patient generated data suggests that researchers should devise, and test, appropriate clinical data gathering strategies.

The influence of mood on HRQoL cannot be ignored either and must be taken into account when HRQoL is assessed. This study has shown that both anxiety and depressive symptoms are implicated and anxiety symptoms correlated with neuropsychological performance five years after CABG. Deficits are present five years after CABG but the implications of this finding are currently not apparent. Interval neuropsychological testing on patients may elucidate whether these changes persist over time or whether the deficits can be attributed to increasing age or the presence of comorbid illness. However, with the known practice effect experienced with neuropsychological assessment, the interval between tests would have to be chosen carefully.

Conclusion

This study found that the majority of patients perceive themselves to have good HRQoL five years after CABG but highlight that anxiety and depressive symptoms have a negative effect on HRQoL. The innovative aspect of this study related to its use of both objective and subjective data. Examination of HRQoL from the patient's perspective has been shown to allow health professionals to combine their clinical objective findings with the patient's personal subjective experience. In doing so, the possibility of improving patient care is enhanced. This study has demonstrated clearly the value of this approach for patients undergoing CABG. The nurse can play an important role in this work. As such, the nurse will offer holistic care which has important implications for the patient and for other members of the healthcare team.

References

Abildstrom H, Rasmussen LS, Rentowl P, Hanning CD, Rasmussen H, Kristensen PA, Moller JT. (2000) Cognitive dysfunction 1-2 years after non-cardiac surgery in the elderly. ISPOCD group. International Study of Post-Operative Cognitive Dysfunction. *Acta Anaesthesiology Scandinavia, 44 (10),*1246-51.

Aldana, S.G., Whitmer, W.R., Greenlaw, R., Avins, A., Salberg, A., Barnhurst, M., Fellingham, G., Lipsenthal, L. (2003) Cardiovascular risk reductions associated with aggressive lifestyle modification and cardiac rehabilitation. *Heart Lung, 32,* 374-382.

Allender S, Peto V, Scarborough P, Boxer A, Rayner M (2007) *Coronary heart disease statistics.* British Heart Foundation: London.

Allied Dunbar (1994) *National Fitness Survey- Technical Report.* London: Allied Dunbar.

Al-Ruzzeh, S., George, S., Bustami, M., Wray, J., Ilsley, C., Athanasiou, T., Amrani, M. (2006) Effect of off-pump Coronary Artery Bypass Graft Surgery on clinical, angiographic, neurocognitive, and quality of life outcomes: randomised controlled trial. *British Medical Journal*; doi:10.1136/bmj.38852.479907.7C.

American College of Cardiology \American Heart Association Guidelines for Coronary Artery Bypass Graft Surgery: Executive Summary and Recommendations. (1999) A Report of the American College of Cardiology/American Heart Association Task Force on Practice Guidelines (Committee to Revise the 1991 Guidelines for Coronary Artery Bypass Graft Surgery) [online]. 1999. Available from: URL: *http://circ.ahajournals.org.cgi/content/full/100/13/1464/T3.*

American Heart Association (2008). Heart Disease and Stroke Statistics — 2008 Update. Dallas, Texas: American Heart Association.

American Psychiatric Association [n.d.] Depression Available from: URL: *http://www.psych.org/public_info/depression.cfm.*

American Psychiatric Association (1994) *DSM IV: Diagnostic and Statistical Manual of Mental Disorders (Diagnostic and Statistical Manual of Mental Disorders.* New York: American Psychiatric Association.

Andrew, M.J., Baker, R.A., Kneebone, A.C., Knight, J.L. (2000) Mood state as a predictor of neuropsychological deficits following cardiac surgery. *Journal of Psychosomatic Research, 48 (6), 537-546.*

Arrowsmith, J.E., Harrison, M.J.G., Newman, S.P., Stygall, J, Timberlake, N., Pugsley, W.B. (1998) Neuroprotection of the brain during cardiopulmonary bypass. *Stroke, 29,* 2357-2362.

Atherosclerosis Risk in Communities Study (ARIC). Unpublished data.

Baker, R.A., Andrew, M.J., Schrader, G., Knight, J.L. (2001) Preoperative depression and mortality in Coronary Artery Bypass Graft Surgery: preliminary findings. *Australia and New Zealand Journal of Surgery 71 (3),* 139-142.

Barbut, D., Lo, Y., Gold, J.P., Trifiletti, R.R., Yao, F.S.F., Hager, D.N., Hinton, R.B., Isom, O.W. (1997) Impact of embolization during coronary artery bypass grafting on outcome and length of stay. *Annals of Thoracic Surgery, 63,* 998-1002.

Barefoot, J.C., Helms, M.J., Mark, D.B., Blumenthal, J.A., Califf, R.M., Haney, T.L., O'Connor, C.M., Siegler, I.C., Williams, R.B. (1996) Depression and long-term mortality risk patients with coronary artery disease. *American Journal of Cardiology, 78,* 613-617.

Beck, A.T., Ward, C., Mendelson, M. (1961). An inventory for measuring depression. *Archives of General Psychiatry, 4,* 561-71.

Beck, A.T., Steer, R.A., Gartin, M.G. (1988). Psychometric properties of the Beck Depression Inventory: twenty five years of evaluation. *Clinical Psychology Review,* 8, 77-100.

Bennett, J.A., Riegel, B., Bittner, V., Nichols, J. (2002) Validity and reliability of the NYHA classes for measuring research outcomes in patients with cardiac disease. *Heart Lung, 31 (4),* 262-270.

Berkman, L.F, Blumenthal, J., Burg, M., Carney, R.M., Catellier, D., Cowan, M.J., Czajkowski, S.M., DeBusk, R. Hosking, J., Jaffe, A., Kaufman, P.G., Mitchell, P., Norman, J., Powell, L.H., Raczynski, J.M., Schneiderman, N.; Enhancing Recovery in Coronary heart Disease Patients Investigators (ENRICHD) (2003). Effects of treating depression and low perceived social support on clinical events after myocardial infarction: the Enhancing Recovery in Coronary Heart Disease Patients (ENRICHD) Randomised Trial. *Journal of American Medical Association, 289,* 3106-3116.

Berkman, L.F., Syme, S.L. (1979) Social networks, host resistance and mortality: a nine-year follow-up study of Alameda County residents. *American Journal of Epidemiology, 109,* 186-204.

Berkman, L.F., Vaccarino, V., Seeman, T. (1993) Gender differences in cardiovascular morbidity and mortality: thye contribution of social networks and support. *Annals of Behavioural Medicine, 15,* 112-118.

Borowicz, L.M., Goldsborough, M.A., Selnes, O.A., McKhann, G.M. (1996) Neuropsychologic changes after cardiac surgery: a critical review. *Journal of Cardiothoracic and Vascular Anaesthesia, 10,* 105-112.

Bowling, A. (1995) *Measuring Disease: a review of disease-specific quality of life measurement scales.* Buckingham: Open University Press.

Brazier, J.E., Harper, R., Jones, N.M.B., O'Cathain, A., Thomas, K.J., Usherwood, T., Westlake, L. (1992) Validating the SF-36 health survey questionnaire: New outcome measure in primary care. *British Medical Journal, 305,*160-164.

Breuer, A.C., Furlan, A.J., Hanson, M.R. (1983) Central nervous system complications of coronary artery bypass graft surgery: Prospective analysis of 421 patients. *Stroke, 14 (5),* 682-687.

Bridgewater, B., Grayson, A.D., Jackson, M., Brooks, N., Grotte, G.J., Keenan, D.J.M., Millner, R., Fabri, B.M., and Jones, M. on behalf of the North West Quality Improvement Programme in Cardiac Interventions (2003) Surgeon specific mortality in adult cardiac surgery: comparison between crude and risk stratified data. *British Medical Journal, 327,* 13-17.

Brummett, B.H., Barefoot, J.C., Siegler, I.C., Clapp-Channing, N.E., Lytle, B.L., Bosworth, H.B., Williams, R.B. Jr., Mark, D.B. (2001) Characteristics of socially isolated patients with coronary artery disease who are at elevated risk for mortality. *Psychosomatic Medicine, 63 (2),* 273-274.

Burg, M.M., Benedetto, M. C., Rosenberg, R., Soufer, R. (2003) Presurgical depression predicts medical morbidity 6 months after coronary artery bypass graft surgery. *Psychosomatic Medicine, 65,* 111-118.

Caine, N., Sharples, L.D., Wallwork, J. (1999) Prospective study of quality of life before and after coronary artery bypass grafting: outcome at five years. *Heart, 81,* 347-351.

Campeau, L. (1976) Grading of angina pectoris. *Circulation, 54,* 522- 523.

Chandra, R., Sikka, K.K., Kumar, S., Srivastava, D.K. (1983) A study of serum cholesterol and low-density lipoproteins in cerebrovascular disease. *Journal of Association of Physicians of India, 31 (11),* 697-700.

Channer, K.S., O'Connor, S., Britton, S., Wallbridge, D., Russell Rees, J. (1988) Psychological factors influencing the success of coronary artery surgery. *Journal of the Royal Society of Medicine, 81,* 629-632.

Chocron, S., Etievent, J.P., Viel, J.F., Dussaucy, A., Clement, F., Alwan, K., Neidhardt, M., Schipman, N. (1996) Prospective study of quality of life before and after open heart operations. Annals of Thoracic Surgery; 61 (1): 153-157.

Cleveland, J.C., Shroyer, A.L., Chen, A.Y., Peterson, E., Grover, F.L. (2001) Off-pump coronary artery bypass graftin decreases risk-adjusted mortality and morbidity. Annals of Thoracic Surgery; 72 (4): 1282-1288.

Cohen, S., Rodriguez, M.S. (1995) Pathways linking affective disorders and physical disorders. *Health Psychology, 14(5),* 374-380.

Cooper, A., Lloyd, G., Weinman, J., Jackson. G. (1999) Why patients do not attend cardiac rehabilitation: role of intentions and illness belief. *Heart, 82,* 234-236.

Cosette, S., Frasure-Smith, N., Lesperance, F. (2001) Clinical implications of a reduction in psychological distress in patients participating in a psychosocial intervention programme. *Psychosomatic Medicine, 63,* 257-266.

Danesh, J., Wheeler, J.G., Hirschfield, G.M., Eda, S., Eiriksdottir, G., Rumley, A., Lowe, G.D.O., Pepys, M.B., Gudnason, V. (2004) C-Reative Protein and other circulating markers of inflammation in the prediction of coronary heart disease. *New England Journal of Medicine, 350,* 1387-1397.

Deiwick, M., Roschner, C., Rothenburger, M., Schmid, C., Scheld, H.H. (2001) Feasibility and risks of heart surgery in very elderly: Analysis of 200 consecutive patients of 80 years and above. *Archives of Gerontology and Geriatrics, 32 (3),* 295-304.

Desai, N.D., Cohen, E.A., Naylor, C.D., Fremes, S.E. (2004) A randomised comparison of radial-artery and saphenous-vein coronary bypass graft. *New England Journal of Medicine, 351,* 2302-2309.

Dr. Joseph E. Smith medical library [n.d.] Anxiety. Available from URL: *http://www.chclibrary.org/micromed/00038160.html.*

Doering, L.V., Moser, D.K., Lemankiewicz, W., Luper, C., Khan, S. (2005) Depression, healing, and recovery from Coronary Artery Bypass Surgery. *American Journal of Critical Care, 14(4),* 316-324.

Doliszny, K.M., Luepker, R.V., Burke, G.L., Pryor, D.B., Blackburn, H. (1994) Estimated contribution of coronary arery bypass graft surgery to the decline in coronary heart disease mortality: The Minnesota Heart Survey. *Journal of American College of Cardiology, 24,* 95-103.

Duits, A.A., Duivenvoorden, H.J., Boeke, S., Taams, M.A., Mochter, B., Krauss, X.H., Passchier, J., Erdman, R.A.M. (1998) The course of anxiety and depression in patients undergoing coronary artery bypass graft surgery. *Journal of Psychosomatic Research, 45,* 127-138.

European Coronary Surgery Study Group (1979) Coronary Artery Bypass Graft Surgery in stable angina pectoris: survival at two years. *Lancet, 332,* 889-893.

Fava, G.A., Magnani, B. (1988) Quality of life: a review of contemporary confusion. *Medical Science Research, 16,* 1051-1054.

Ferguson, T.B., Coombs, L.P., Peterson, E.D. (2002) Pre-operative B-blocker use and mortality and morbidity following CABG surgery in North America. *Journal of American Medical Association, 287 (17),* 2221-2227.

Fitzgibbon, G.M., Kafka, H.R., Leach, A.J., Keon, W.J., Hooper, D., Burton, J.R. (1996) Coronary bypass graft fate and patient outcome: angiographic follow-up of 5,065 grafts related to survival and reoperation in 1,388 patients during 25 years. *Journal of American College of Cardiology, 28,* 616-626.

Fitzsimons, D., Richardson, S.G., Scott, M.E. (2000) Prospective study of clinical and functional status in patients awaiting Coronary Artery Bypass Graft Surgery. *Coronary Health Care, 4 (3),* 117-122.

Fletcher, A. Gore, S., Jones, D., Fitzpatrick, R., Spiegelhalter, D., Cox, D. (1992). Quality of life measures in health care II: Design, analysis and interpretation. *British Medical Journal, 305,* 1145-1148.

Ford, D.E., Mead, L.A., Chang, P.P., Cooper-Patrick, L., Wang, N., Klag, M.J. (1998) Depression is a risk for coronary artery disease in men. *Archives in Internal Medicine, 158,* 1422-1426.

Frasure-Smith, N., Lesperance, F., Juneau, M., Talajic, M., Bourassa, M.G. (1999) Gender, depression and one-year prognosis after myocardial infarction. *Psychosomatic Medicine, 61,* 26-37.

Fruitman, D.S., MacDougall, C.E., Ross, D.B. (1999) Cardiac surgery in octogenarians: can elderly patients benefit? Quality of life after cardiac surgery. *Annals of Thoracic Surgery, 68 (6),* 2129-2135.

Gallagher, D., Nies, G., Thompson, L.W. (1982) Reliability of the Beck Depression Inventory with older adults. *Journal of Consulting and Clinical Psychology, 50,* 152-153.

Garces, K. (2002) Drug eluting stents: managing coronary artery stenosis following PTCA. *Issues in Emergency Health Technology, 40,* 1-6.

Gavaghan, T.P., Gebski, V., Baron, D.W. (1991) Immediate post-operative aspirin improves vein graft patency early and late after coronary bypass graft surgery: a placebo-controlled, randomized trial. *Circulation, 83,* 1526-1533.

Gill, R., Murkin, J.M. (1996) Neuropsycholgic dysfunction after cardiac surgery: what is the problem? *Journal of Cardiothoracic and Vascular Anesthesia, 10,* 91-98.

Glassman, A.H., O'Connor, C.M., Califf, R.M., Swedberg, K., Schwartz, P., Bigger, J.T., Krishman, K.R., van Zyl, L.T., Swenson, J.R., Finkel, M.S., Landau, C., Shapiro, P.A., Pepine, C.J., Mardekian, J., Harrison, W.M., Barton, D., McIvor, M; Sertaline Antidepressant Heart Attack Randomised Trial (SADHEART) Group. Sertaline treatment of major depression in patients with acute MI or unstable angina. *Journal of American Medical Association*, 288, 701-709.

Glassman, A.H., Shapiro, P.A. (1998) Depression and the course of coronary artery disease. *American Journal of Psychiatry, 155,* 4-11.

Goldman, L., Cook, E.F., Mitchell, N., Flatley, M., Sherman, H., Cohn, P.F. (1982) Pitfalls in the serial assessment of cardiac fuctional status. *Journal of Chronic Disease,35 (10),* 763-771.

Goldsmith, I., Lip, G.Y., Kaukuntla, H., Patel, R.L. (1999). Hospital morbidity and mortality and changes in quality of life following mitral valve surgery in the elderly. *Journal of Heart Valve Disease, 8 (6),* 702-707.

Goyal, T.M., Idler, E.L., Krause, T.J., Contrada, R.J. (2005) Quality of life following cardiac surgery: impact of the severity and course of depressive symptoms. *Psychosomatic Medicine, 67 (5),* 759-765.

Goyal, A., Alexander, J.H., Hafley, G.E., Graham, S.H., Mehta, R.H. et al. (2007) Outcomes associated with the use of secondary prevention medications after coronary artery bypass graft surgery. *The Annals of Thoracic Surgery, 83 (3),* 993-1001.

Greenland, P., Knoll, M.D., Stamler, J.D., Dyer, A.R., Garside, D.B., Wilson, P.W. (2003) Major risk factors as antecedents of fatal and nonfatal coronary heart disease events. *Journal of American Medical Association, 290,* 891-897.

Grundy, S.M., Pasternak, R., Greenland, P., Mith, S., Fuster, V. (1999) American Assessment of cardiovascular risk by use of Multiple-Risk-Factor Assessment Equations. *Journal of American College Cardiology;* 34: 1348-1359. Available from URL:*http://www.acc.org/ clinical/consensus/risk/risk1999.pdf.*

Gundle M.J., Reeves, B.R., Tate, S., Raft, D., McLaurin, L.P. (1980) Psychosocial outcome after coronary artery surgery. *American Journal of Psychiatry, 137,* 1591-1594.

Hannan, E.L., Racz, M.J., Walford, G., Jones, R.H., Ryan, T.J., Bennett, E., Culliford, A.T., Isom, O.W., Gold, J.P., Rose, E.A. (2005) Long-term outcomes of coronary-artery bypass grafting versus stent implantation. *New England Journal of Medicine, 352,* 2174-2183.

Hannan, E.L., Wu, C., Smith, C.R., Higgins, R.S.D., Carlson R.E., Culliford, A.T., Gold, J.P., Jones, R.H. (2007) Off-pump versus on-pump coronary artery bypass graft surgery: Differences in short-term outcomes and in long-term mortality and the need for subsequent revascularisation. *Circulation, 116,* 1145-1152.

Hawkes, A.L., Nowak, M., Bidstrup, B., Speare, R. Outcomes of coronary artery graft surgery. *Vascular Health Risk Management, 2 (4),* 477-484.

Herlitz, J., Wiklund, I., Caidahl, K., Karlson, B.W., Sjoland, H., Hartford, M., Haglid, M., Karlsson, T. (1999) Determinants of an impaired quality of life five years after Coronary Artery Bypass Surgery. *Heart, 81,* 342-346.

Herlitz, J., Wiklund, I., Sjoland, H., Karlson, B.W., Karlsson, T., Haglid, M., Hartford, M., Caidahl, K. (2000a) Impact of age on improvement in health-related quality of life five years after coronary artery bypass grafting. *Scandinavian Journal of Rehabilitative Medicine, 32,* 41-48.

Herlitz, J., Wiklund, I., Sjoland, H., Karlson, B.W., Karlsson, T., Haglid, M., Hartford, M., Caidahl, K. (2000b) Relief of symptoms and improvement of quality of life five years after coronary artery bypass grafting in relation to preoperative ejection fraction. *Quality of Life Research, 9,* 467-476.

Hofer, S., Doering, S., Rumpold, G., Oldridge, N., Benzer, W. (2006) Determinants of health-related quality of life in patients with coronary artery disease. *European Journal of Cardiovascular Preventive Rehabilitation, 13 (3),* 398-406.

Holahan, C.J., Moss, R.H., Holahan, C.K., Brennan, P.L. (1996) Social support, coping strategies, and psychosocial adjustment to cardiac illness: Implications for assessment and prevention. *Journal of Prevention and Intervention Community, 13,* 33-52.

Huber, C.H., Goeber, V., Berdat, P., Carrel, T., Eckstein, F. (2007) Benefits of cardiac surgery in octogenarians – a postoperative quality of life assessment. *European Journal of Cardio-thoracic Surgery,* 31, 1099-1105.

Hyland, M.E. (1992) A reformulation of quality of life for medical science. *Quality of Life Research, 1,* 267-272.

Inouye, S.K., Peduzzi, P.N., Robinson, J.T., Hughes, J.S., Horwitz, R.I., Concato, J. (1998) Importance of functional measures in predicting mortality among older hospitalised patients. *Journal of American Medical Association, 279 (15),* 1187-1193.

Inouye, S.K., Wagner, D.R., Acampora D. (1993) A predictive index for functional decline in hospitalised elderly medical patients. *Journal of General Internal Medicine, 8,* 645-652.

Irvine, J., Basinski, A., Baker, B., Jandciu, S., Paquette, M., Cairns, J., Connolly, S., Roberts, R., Gent, M., Dorian, P. (1999) Depression and risk of sudden cardiac death after myocardial infarction: testing for the confounding effects of fatigue. *Psychosomatic Medicine, 61,* 729-737.

Ivanov, J., Weisel, R.D., David, T.E., Naylor, D. (1998) Fifteen-year trends in risk severity and operative mortality in elderly patients undergoing coronary artery bypass graft surgery. *Circulation, 97,* 673-680.

Jenkinson, C., Layte, R., Wright, L., Coulter, A. (1996) *The UK SF-36: An analysis and interpretation manual.* Oxford: Health Services Research Unit, University of Oxford.

Jenkinson, C., Layte, R., Lawrence, K. (1997) Development and testing of the medical outcomes study 36-item short form health survey summary scale scores in the United Kingdom. *Medical Care, 35 (4),* 410-416.

Khatri, P., Babyak, M., Clancy, C., Davis, R., Croughwell, N., Newman, M., Reves, J.G., Mark, D.B., Blumenthal, J.A. (1999) Perception of cognitive function in older adults following Coronary Artery Bypass Graft Surgery. *Health Psychology, 18 (3),* 301-306.

Kirklin, J.W., Naftel, D.C., Blackstone, E.H., Pohost, G.M.(1989) Summary of a consensus concerning death and ischaemic events after coronary artery bypass grafting. *Circulation, 79* (supp I), 81-91.

Koch, C.G., Li, L., Sabik, J., Starr, N.J., Blackstone, E.H. (2007) Effect of functional health-related quality of life on long-term survival after cardiac surgery. *Circulation, 115,* 692-699.

Koivula, M., Tarkka, M.T., Tarkka, M., Laippala, P., Paunonen-Ilmonen, M. (2002) Fear and anxiety in patients at different time-points in the coronary artery bypass process. *International Journal of Nursing Studies, 39(8),* 811-822.

Kubo, S.H., Schulman, S., Starling, R.C., Jessup, M., Wentworth, D., Burkhoff, D. (2004) Development and validation of a patient questionnaire to determine New York Association classification. *Journal of Cardiac Failure, 10 (3),* 228-235.

Kulik, J.A., Mahler, H.J.M. (1989) Social support and recovery from surgery. *Health Psychology,* 8, 221-238.

Laghrissi-Thode, F., Wagner, W.R., Pollock, B.G., Johnson, P.C., Finkel, M.S. (1997) Elevated platelet factor 4 and beta-thromboglobulin plasma levels in depressed patients with ischaemic heart disease. *Biological Psychiatry, 42,* 290-295.

Lavie, C.J., Milani, R.V. (2004) Prevalence of anxiety in coronary patients with improvement following cardiac rehabilitation and exercise training. *American Journal of Cardiology, 93(3),* 336-339.

Lazar, H.L., Fitzgerald, C.A., Ahmad, T., Bao, Y., Colton, T., Shapira, O.M., Shemin, R.J. (2001) Early discharge after coronary artery bypass graft surgery: are patients really going home earlier? *Journal of Thoracic and Cardiovascular Surgery, 121 (5),* 943-950.

Lear, S.A., Spinelli, J.J., Linden, W., Brozic, A., Kiess, M., Frohlich, J.J., Ignaszewski, A. (2006) The Extensive Lifestyle Management Intervention (ELMI) after cardiac rehabilitation: a 4-year randomised controlled trial. *American Heart Journal, 152 (92),* 333-339.

Lesperance, F., Frasure-Smith, N, Theroux, P., Irwin, M. (2004) The association between major depression and levels of soluble intercellular adhesion module 1, interleukin-6 and C-reactive protein in patients with recent acute coronary syndromes. *American Journal of Psychiatry, 161 (2),* 271-277.

Lett, H.S., Blumenthal, J.A., Babyak, M.A., Sherwood, A., Straumann, T., Robins, C., Newman, M.F. (2004) Depression as a risk factor for coronary heart disease: evidence, mechanisms, and treatment. *Psychosomatic Medicine, 66 (3),* 305-315.

Lindal, E., Haroarson, P., Magnusson, J., Alfreosson, H. (1996) A 5-Year psycho-medical follow-up study of coronary bypass artery graft patients. *Scandinavian Journal of Rehabilitation Medicine, 28,* 27-31.

Lindsay, G. and Gaw, A. (eds) (2004) *Coronary Heart Disease Prevention.* 2nd Ed. London: Churchill Livingstone.

Lindsay, G.M., Hanlon, P., Smith, L.N., Wheatley, D.J. (2000) Assessment of changes in general health status using the short-form 36 questionnaire 1 year following coronary artery bypass grafting. *European Journal of Cardiothoracic Surgery,* 18, 557-564.

Loponen, P., Taskinen, P., Laakkonen, E., Nissinen, J., Luther, M., Wistbacka, J.O. (2003) Perioperative stroke in coronary artery bypass patients. *Scandanavian Journal of Surgery, 92 (2),* 148-155.

Lukkarinen, H. (2005) Methodological triangulation showed the poorest quality of life in the youngest people following treatment of coronary artery disease: a Longitudinal study. *International Journal of Nursing Studies, 42,* 619-627.

McCrone, S., Lenz, E., Tarzian, A., Perkins, S. (2001) Anxiety and depression: Incidence and patterns in patients after coronary artery bypass graft surgery. *Applied Nursing Research, 14 (3),* 155-164.

McKhann, G.M., Goldsborough, M.A., Borowicz, L.M., Selnes, O.A., Mellits, E.D., Enger, C., Quaskey, S.A., Baumgartner, W.A., Cameron, D.E., Stuart, S., Gardner, T.J. (1997b)

Cognitive outcome after coronary artery bypass: A one-year prospective study. *Annals of Thoracic Surgery, 63,* 510-515.

Mahanna, E.P., Blumenthal, J.A., White, W.D., Croughwell, N.D., Clancy, C.P., Smith, R., Newman, M.F. (1996) Defining neuropsychological dysfunction after coronary artery bypass grafting. *Annals of Thoracic Surgery, 61,* 1342-1347.

Malinowski, M., Mrozek, R., Twardowski, R., Biernat, J., Deja, M.A., Widenka, K., Dalecka, A.M., Kobielusz-Gembala, I., Janusiewicz, P., Wos, S., Golba, K.S. (2006). Left internal mammary artery improves 5-year survival in patients under 40 subjected to surgical revascularisations. *Heart Surgery Forum, 9 (1),* E493-498.

Mallick, S., Krumholz, H.M., Lin, Z.Q., Kasl, S.V., Mattera, J.A., Roumains, S.A., Vaccarino, V. (2005) Patients with depressive symptoms have lower health status benefits after Coronary Artery Bypass Graft Surgery. *Circulation, 111,* 271-277.

Mayou, R. (1990) Quality of life in cardiovascular disease. *Psychotherapy Psychosomatics, 54,* 99-109.

Mayou, R., Gill, D., Thompson, D.R., Day, A., Hicks, N., Volmink, J., Neil, A. (2000) Depression and anxiety as predictors of outcome after myocardial infarction. *Psychosomatic Medicine, 62,* 212-219.

Mensah, G.A., Brown, D.W., Croft, J.B., Greenlund, K.J. (2005) Major coronary risk factors and death from Coronary Heart Disease. *American Journal of Preventive Medicine, 29(5S1),* 68-74.

Michalopoulos, A., Tzelepis, G., Dafni, U., Geroulanos, S. (1999) Determinants of hospital mortality after coronary artery bypass grafting. *Chest, 115,* 1598-1603.

Murkin, J.M., Newman, S.P., Stump, D.A., Blumenthal, J.A. (1995) Statement of consensus on assessment of neurobehavioural outcomes after cardiac surgery. *Annals of Thoracic Surgery, 59 (5),* 1289-1295.

Musselman, D.L., Evans, D.L., Nemeroff, C.B. (1998). The relationship of depression to cardiovascular disease. *Archives of General Psychiatry, 55,* 580-592.

Nathoe, H.M., van Dijk, D., Jansen, E.W.L., Suyker, W., J.L., Diephuis, J.C., van Boven, W., de la Riviere, A., Borst, C., Kalkman, C.J., Grobbee, D.E., Buskens, E. and de Jaegere, P.P.T. (2003) A comparison of on-pump and off-pump coronary bypass surgery in low-risk patients. *New England Journal of Medicine, 348,* 394-402.

National Cholesterol Education Program Expert Panel (2002) Third Report of the National Cholesterol Education Program Expert Panel on detection, evaluation and treatment of high blood cholesterol in adults final report. *Circulation, 106,* 3143-3373.

National Diabetes Statistics. National Estimates on Diabetes. Available from URL: *http://diabetes.niddk.nih.gov/dm/pubs/statisitcs/.*

National Institute for Health and Clinical Excellence [n.d.]. Available from URL: *http://www.nice.org.uk/page.aspx?0=244129.*

National Institute of Health (2001). *Strong Heart Study Data Book.* US: National Institute of Health.

National Lipid Association [n.d.] Clinical article: New ATP III guidelines, opportunities and challenges. Available from URL: *www.lipid.org/clinical/articles/1000006.php.*

Newman, M.F., Croughwell, N.D., Blumenthal, J.A., White, W.D., Lewis, J.B., Frasco, P., Towner, E.A., Schell, R.M., Hurwitz, B.J., Reves, J.G. (1994) Effect of aging on cerebral autoregulation during cardiopulmonary bypass. *Circulation, 90 (II)*, 243-249.

Newman, M.F., Kirchner, J.L., Philips-Bute, B., Gaver, V., Grocott, H., Jones, R.H., Mark, D.B., Reves, J.G., Blumenthal, J.A. (2001a) Longitudinal assessment of neurocognitive function after Coronary Artery Bypass Graft Surgery . *New England Journal of Medicine, 344 (6)*, 395-402.

Newman, M.F., Grocott, H., Matthew, J.P., White, W.D., Landolfo, K., Reves, J.G., Laskowitz, D.T., Mark, D.B., Blumenthal, J.A. (2001b) Report of the substudy assessing impact of neurocognitive function on quality of life 5 years after coronary surgery. *Stroke, 32*, 2874-2881.

Newman, S., Smith, P., Treasure, T., Joseph, P., Ell, P., Harrison, M. (1987) Acute neuropsychological consequences of Coronary Artery Bypass Graft Surgery . *Current Psychological Research and Reviews, 6 (2)*, 115-124.

Newman, S., Stygall, J. (1997) Neuropsychological and psychological changes following cardiac surgery. *Proceedings of the American Academy of Cardiovascular Perfusion, 17,* 14-21.

Nordenfelt, L. (1994) *Concepts and measurement of quality of life in health care*. London: Kluwer Academic Publishers.

Pai, J.K., Pischon, T., Ma, J., Manson, J.E., Hankinson, S.E., Joshipura, K., Curhan, G.C., Rifai, N., Cannuscio, C.C., Stampfer, M.J., Rimm, E.B. (2004) Inflammatory markers and the risk of coronary heart disease in men and women. *New England Journal of Medicine, 351,* 2599-2610.

Orth-Gomer, K., Rosengren, A., Wilhelmsen, L. (1993) Lack of social support and incidences of coronary heart disease in middle-aged Swedish men. *Psychosomatic Medicine, 55,* 37-43.

Pande, R.U., Nader, N.D., Donias, H.W., D'Ancona, G., Karamanoukian, H.L. (2003) Review: Fast-tracking cardiac surgery. *Heart Surgery Forum, 6 (4),* 244-248.

Paoletti, R., Gotto, A., Hajjar, D.P. (2004) Inflammation in atherosclerosis and implications for therapy. *Circulation, 109 (23)* Supplement III, 20-26.

Parisi, A.F., Khuri, S., Deupree, R.H., Sharma, G.V.R.K., Scott, S.M., Luchi, R.J. (1989) Medical compared with surgical management of unstable angina. *Circulation, 80,* 1176-1189.

Pearson, S., Stewart, S., Rubenbach, S. (1999) Is health-related quality of life among older, chronically ill patients associated with unplanned readmission to hospital? *Australian and New Zealand Journal of Medicine, 29,* 701-706.

Phillips Bute, B., Mathew J., Blumenthal, J.A., Welsh-Bohmer, K., White, W.D., Mark, D., Landolfo, K., Newman, M.F. (2003) Female gender is associaited with impaired quality of life 1 year after Coronary Artery Bypass Graft Surgery . *Psychosomatic Medicine, 65 (6),* 944-951.

Plomondon, M.E., Cleveland, J.C., Ludwig, S.T., Grunwald, G.K., Kiefe, C.I., Grover, F.L., Shroyer, A.L. (2001) Off-pump coronary artery bypass is associated with improved risk-adjusted outcomes. *Annals of Thoracic Surgery, 72 (1),* 114-119.

Pocock, S.J., Henderson, R.A., Rickards, A.F., Hampton, J.R., King, S.B., Hamm, C.W., Puel, J.,Hueb, W., Goy, J.J., Rodriguez, A. (1995) Meta-analysis of randomised trials comparing coronary angioplasty with bypass surgery. *Lancet, 346,* 1184-1189.

Possati, G., Gaudino, M., Prati, F., Alessandrini, F., Trani, C., Glieca, F., Mazzari, M.A., Luciani, N., Schiavoni, G. (2003) Long-term result of the radial artery used for myocardial revascularisation. *Circulation, 108 (11),* 1350-1354.

Pugsley, W. (1989) The use of doppler ultrasound in the assessment of microemboli during cardiac surgery. *Perfusion, 4,* 115-122.

Pugsley, W., Klinger, L., Paschalis, C., Aspey, B., Newman, S. Harrison, M., Treasure, T. (1990) Microemboli and cerebral impairment during cardiac surgery. *Vascular Surgery, 24,* 34-43.

Pugsley, W., Klinger, L., Paschalis, C., Treasure, T., Harrison, M., Newman, S. (1994) The impact of microemboli during cardiopulmonary bypass on neuropsychological functioning. *Stroke, 25,* 1393-1399.

Radley, A., Green, R., Radley, M. (1987) Impending surgery: the expectations of male coronary patiens and their wives. *International Rehabilitation Medicine, 8 (4),* 154-161.

Rogers, W.J., Coggon, J., Gersh, B.J., Fisher, L.D., Myers, W.O., Obermann, A., Sheffield, L.T. (1990) Ten-Year follow-up of quality of life in patients randomised to receive medical therapy or coronary artery bypass graft surgery. *Circulation, 82,* 1647-1658.

Rothenhausler, H.B., Grieser, B., Nollert, G., Reichart, B., Schelling, G., Kapfhammer, H. P. (2005) Psychiatric and psychosocial outcome of cardiac surgery with cardiopulmonary bypass: a prospective 12-month follow-up study. *General Hospital Psychiatry, 27 (1),* 18-28.

Rumsfeld, J.S., Ho, P.M. (2005) Depresison and cardiovascular disease: A call for recognition. *Circulation, 111,* 250-253.

Rumsfeld, J.S., Mawhinney, S., McCarthy, M., Shroyer, A.L., Villaneuva, C.B., O'Brien, M., Moritz, T.E., Hederson, W.G., Grover, F.L., Sethi, G.K., Hammermeister, K.E. (1999) Health-related quality of life as a predictor of mortality following coronary artery bypass graft surgery. Participants of the department of Veterans Affairs Cooperative Study Group in processes, structures and outcomes of care in cardiac surgery. *Journal of American Medical Association, 281 (14),* 1298-1303.

Ruo, B., Rumsfeld, J.S., Hlatky, M.A., Liu, H., Browner, W.S., Whooley, M.A. (2003) Depressive symptoms and health-related quality of life: the Heart and Soul Study. *Journal of American Medical Association, 290 (2),* 215-221.

Rymaszewska, J., Kiejna, A., Hadrys, T. (2003) Depression and anxiety in coronary artery bypass grafting patient. *European Psychiatry, 18 (4),* 155-160.

Sandoe, K.L., Kappel, K. in Nordenfelt, L. (1994) *Concepts and measurement of quality of life in health care.* London: Kluwer Academic Publishers.

Sarason, I.G., Sarson, B.R., Potter, E.H., Antoni, M.H. (1985) Life events, social support and illness. *Psychosomatic Medicine, 47,* 156-163.

Savageau, J.A., Stanton, B., Jenkins, C.D., Klein, M.D. (1982) Neuropsychological dysfunction following elective cardiac operation. *Journal of Thoracic and Cardiovascular Surgery, 84,* 585-594.

Schulz, R., Beach, S.R., Ives, D.G., Martire, L.M., Ariyo, A.A., Kop, W.J. (2000) Association between depression and mortality in older adults. *Archives of Internal Medicine, 160,* 1761-1768.

Seeman, J. (1989) Towards a model of positive health. *American Psychologist, 44,* 1099-1109.

Sellman, M., Holm, L., Ivert, T., Semb, B.K.H. (1992) A randomised study of neuropsychological function in patients undergoing Coronary Artery Bypass Graft Surgery. *Thoracic and cardiovascular surgeon, 41,* 349-354.

Selnes, O.A., Royall, R.M., Grega, M.A., Borowicz, L.M., Quakey, S., McKhann, G.M. (2001) Cognitive changes 5 years after coronary artery bypass grafting. *Archives of Neurology, 58,* 598-604.

Shen, B.J., Avivi, Y.E., Todaro, F.J. et al. (2008) Anxiety characteristics independently and prospectively predict myocardial infarction in men: The unique contribution of anxiety among psychologic factors. *Journal of American College of Cardiology, 51,* 113-119.

Sheps, D.S., Shepard, D. (2001) Depression, anxiety and cardiovascular system: the cardiologist's perspective. *Journal of Clinical Psychiatry, 62 (Suppl 8),* 12-16.

Shumaker, S.A., Naughton, M.J. (1995) in Shumaker, S.A., Naughton, M.J. (eds) *The International Assessment of Health-Related Quality of Life: Theory, translation, measurement and analysis.* Oxford: Rapid Communications.

Simons-Morton, B.G., Pate, R.R., Simons-Morton, D.G. (1988) Prescribing physical activity to prevent disease. *Postgraduate Medicine, 83 (1),* 165-166

Sjoland, H, Wiklund, I., Caidahl, K., Haglid, M., Westberg, S., Herlitz, J. (1996) Improvement in quality of life and exercise capacity after Coronary Artery Bypass Graft Surgery. *Archives of Internal Medicine, 156,* 265-271.

Smith, K.W., Avis, N.E., Assmann, S. F. (1999) Distinguishing between quality of life and health status in quality of life research: a meta-analysis. *Quality of Life Research, 8,* 447-459.

Society of Cardiothoracic Surgeons of Great Britain and Ireland [2001] National Adult Cardiac Surgical Database Report 1999-2000. Available from URL: *www.scts.org /file/NAGSDreport200parts.pdf.*

Sousa, K.H., Williamson, A. (2003) Symptom status and health-related quality of life: clinical relevance. *Journal of Advanced Nursing, 42 (6),* 571-577.

Spielberger, C.D., Gorsuch, R.L., Luchene, R.E. (1983) *Manual for the State-Trait Anxiety Inventory* (revised edn). Palo Alto, Ca: Consulting Psychologists Press.

Spilker, B. (1990) *Quality of Life Assessments in clinical trials.* New York: Raven Press.

Stafford, L., Berk, M., Reddy, P., Jackson, H.J. (2007) Comorbid depression and health-related quality of life in patients with coronary artery disease. *Journal of Psychosomatic Research, 62(4),* 401-410.

Stahle, E., Bergstrom, R., Holmberg, L., Edlund, S., Nystrom, O., Sjorgen, I., Hansson, H.E. (1994) Survival after coronary artery bypass grafting. *European Heart Journal, 15,* 1204-1211.

Steed, L., Kong, R., Stygall, J., Acharya, J., Bolla, M., Harrison, M.J., Humphreys, S., Newman, S.P. (2001) The role of apolipoprotein E in cognitive decline after cardiac operations. *Annals of Thoracic Surgery, 71 (3),* 823-826.

Stewart, A.L. and King, A.C. (1994) Conceptualising and measuring quality of life in older populations. In Abeles, R.P., Gift, H.C., Ory, M.G. (eds) *Aging and Quality of Life* (pp 27-53) New York: Springer Series.

Stewart, A.L., Ware, S.J., Sherbourne, Wells, K.B. (1992) Psychological distress, well-being and cognitive functioning measures. In Stewart, A.L., Ware, J.E. (Eds) *Measuring functioning and well-being: The medical outcomes study approach.* Durham, North Carolina: Duke University Press.

Stone, A.A., Broderick, J.E., Shiffman, A., Schwartz, B. (2004) Understanding recall of weekly pain from a momentary assessment perspective: absolute agreement, between-and within-person consistency, and judged change in weekly pain. *Pain, 107(1-2),* 61-69.

Strauss, B., Paulsen, G., Strenge, H., Graetz, S., Regensburger, D., Spiedel, H. (1991) Preoperative and late postoperative psychosocial state following Coronary Artery Bypass Graft Surgery. *Thoracic and Cardiovascular* Surgeon, 40, 59-64.

Stump, D. (1995) Selection and significance of neuropsychologic tests. *Annals of thoracic surgery, 59,* 1340-1344.

Stygall, J., Newman, S.P., Fitzgerald, G.A., Steed, L, Mulligan, K., Arrowsmith, J., Pugsley, W, Humphries, S., Harrison, M.J. (2003) Cognitive change 5 years after Coronary Artery Bypass Graft Surgery. *Health Psychology, 22 (6),* 579-586.

Sullivan, M.D., LaCroix, A.Z., Baum, C., Grothaus, L.C., Katon, W.J. (1997) Functional Status in Coronary Artery Disease: A One-Year Prospective Study of the Role of Anxiety and Depression. *American Journal of Medicine, 103,* 348-356.

Swenson, J.R., O'Connor, C.M., Barton, D., van Zyl, L.T., Swedberg, K., Forman, L.M., Gaffney, M, Glassman, A.H.,; Sertaline Antidepressant Heart Attack Randomised Trial (SADHEART) Group. Influence of depression and effect on treatment with sertaline on quality of life after hospitalisation for acute coronary syndrome. *American Journal of Cardiology, 92,* 1271-1276.

The Criteria Committee of the New York Heart Association (1974). *Diseases of the Heart and Blood Vessels: Nomenclature and Criteria for Diagnosis.* 6th ed. Boston, Mass: Little Brown.

The Multiple Risk Factor Intervention Trial Research Group (1996) Mortality after 16 years for participants randomized to the multiple risk factor intervention trial. *Circulation, 94,* 946-951.

Timberlake, N., Klinger, L., Smith, P., Venn, G., Treasure, T., Harrison, M., Newman, S.P. (1997) Incidence and patterns of depression following coronary artery bypass graft surgery. *Journal of Psychosomatic Research, 43 (2),* 197-207.

Todaro J.F., Shen, B.J., Raffa, S.D., Tilkemier, P.L., Niaura, R. (2007) Prevalence of anxiety disorders in men and women with established coronary heart disease. *Journal of Cardiopulmonary Rehabilitation and Prevention, 27(2),* 86-91.

Treat-Jacobsen, D (1998) *Quality of life five years post Coronary Artery Bypass Graft Surgery* . Minniosta University: Unpublished PhD.

Vaillant, G.E., Meyer, S.E., Mukamal, K., Soldz, S. (1998) Are social supports in late midlife a cause or a result of successful physical ageing? *Psychological Medicine, 28 (5),* 1159-1168.

Van Dam, F. (1986) Quality of life: methodological issues. *Bulletin Cancer, 73 (5),* 607-613.

Van Dijk, D., Keizer, A.M., Diephuis, J.C., Durand, C., Vos, L.J., Hijman, R. (2000) Neurocognitive dysfunction after Coronary Artery Bypass Graft Surgery: a systematic review. *Journal of Thoracic and Cardiovascular Surgery, 120 (4),* 632-639.

Vasan RS, Sullivan LM, Wilson PWF, Sempos, C.T., Sundstrom J., Kannel, W.B., Levy, D., D'Agnostino, R.B. (2005) Relative importance of borderline and elevated levels of coronary heart disease risk factors. *Archives of Internal Medicine, 142,* 393-402.

Vingerhoets, G., Van Nooten, G., Vermassen, F., De Soete, G., Jannes, C. (1997) Short-term and long-term neuropsychological consequences of cardiac surgery with extracorporeal circulation. *European Journal of Cardiothoracic Surgery, 11,* 424-431.

Walter, P. (ed) (1992) *Quality of Life after Open Heart Surgery.* London: Kluwer Academic Publishers.

Wang, M.Q., Eddy, J.M., Fitzhugh, E.C. (1992). Towards a standardisation of Measures in Health Assessments. *Health Values, 16 (1),* 52-56.

Ware, J.E., Kosinski, M., Keller, S.D. (1994) *The SF-36: Physical and mental health summary scores: a user's manual.* Boston, MA: The Health Institute.

Ware, J.E., Snow, K.K., Kosinski, M., (1988). *The SF-36 Health Survey: Manual and interpretation guide.* Boston: Health Institute, New England Medical Centre.

Ware, J.E., Kosinski, M., Keller, S. (1993) *SF-36 Physical and mental summary scores: A user's manual.* Boston: Health Institute, New England Medical Centre.

Wenger, N.K., Mattson, M.E., Furberg, C.D., Elinson, J. (eds). (1984) *Assessment of quality of life in Clinical Trials of Cardiovascular Therapies.* New York: LeJacq Publishing.

Williams, A. (1985) Economics of coronary artery bypass grafting. *British Medical Journal, 291,* 326-327.

World Health Organisation [n.d.]. *Cardiovascular diseases mortality rates.* Available from URL: *http://www.who.int/cardiovascular_diseases/en/index.html.*

World Health Organisation [n.d.] *Health Evidence Network.* Available from URL: *http://www.euro.who.int/eprise/main/WHO/Progs/HEN/Syntheses/depressmgt/20050523 _5.*

Yates, B. (1995). The relationships among social support and short- and long-term recovery outcomes in men with coronary artery disease. *Research in Nursing and Health, 18 (3),* 193-203.

Yuuf, S., Zucker, D., Reduzzi, P., Fisher, L.D., Takaro, T., Ward Kennedy, J., Davis, K., Killip, T., Passamani, E., Norris, R., Morris, C., Mathur, V., Varnauskas, E., Chalmers, T.C. (1994) Effect of coronary artery bypass graft surgery on survival: overview of 10-year results from randomised trials by the Coronary Artery Bypass Graft Surgery Triallists Collaboration. *Lancet, 344,* 563-570.

Zaidi, A.M., Fitzpatrick, A.P., Keenan, D.J.M., Odom, N.J., Grotte, G.J. (1999) Good outcomes from cardiac surgery in the over 70s. *Heart, 82,* 134-137.

Zimet, G.D., Dahlem, N.W., Zimet, S.G, Farley, G.K. (1988) The Multidimensional scale of perceived social support. *Journal of Personality Assessment, 52 (1),* 30-41.

In: Trends in Nursing Research
Editors: Adam J. Ryan and Jack Doyle
ISBN 978-1-60456-642-0
© 2009 Nova Science Publishers, Inc.

Chapter 5

Research to Support Data-Driven Decisions: The 3-D Health Services Research Model for Nursing

Mary Beth Zeni
Florida State University, College of Nursing

Abstract

This chapter describes a research model developed and used by the author, the 3-D Health Services Research Model (3-D HSR Model). The model provides a framework for the design and interpretation of research data to support evidence-based practice in community health settings. The model incorporates the following three research approaches: population-based data analysis, process evaluations, and outcome evaluations. The model consists of the following three aspects: 1) the interpretation of population-based data to identify major health issues affecting a defined community, 2) the selection of effective interventions to enhance the health of the community, and 3) the integration of evaluative research, specifically a process evaluation to ascertain the extent the intervention was delivered as intended and an outcome evaluation to determine the measurable impact the intervention had on the community's health issues. The 3-D HSR model includes key approaches from both epidemiology and health services research. For example, epidemiologic research approaches provide the foundation in the identification of major health issues in a community through the analysis of selected population-based datasets, data from state vital statistics, and mortality and morbidity data on communicable and other diseases collected and reported by county, state, national, and international public health agencies. The model is consistent with the concepts from health services research and Nursing-Health Services Research as described by Jones and Mark in 2005. In addition, the model supports the scope of nursing research as outlined in the 2006 American Association of Colleges of Nursing (AACN) Position Statement on Nursing Research.

A case example is included to illustrate the application of the model to a current national health issue: assuring that children have access to continuous, quality, primary health care. The case example, original research by the author as principle investigator, is an analysis of a population-based dataset, the National Survey of Children's Health, to identify factors through regression analysis of U.S. children at risk for not having access to continuous, quality primary health care.

Introduction

The impact of many major health conditions affecting people in the United States could have been lessened and even prevented through the selection and implementation of an effective health intervention. For example, in the past 20 years the US population has seen an untoward increase in obesity levels among children and adults. Co-morbidity is noted between obesity and other health conditions, such as Type II diabetes and hypertension. The emphasis on health prevention cannot be overlooked considering that one condition can result in the development of other serious health conditions and death. A recent study by Nolte and McKee found that the United States has the highest rates of preventable death each year compared to nineteen industrialized nations, accounting for more than 100,000 deaths annually (Nolte and McKee, 2008).

Previous effective health interventions resulted in improved health indicators and the prevention of life threatening illnesses. Numerous studies document the effectiveness of HIV prevention interventions with specific at-risk groups (e.g., Des Jarlais, Casriel, Friedman, and Rosenblum, 1992; Dicelmente and Wingood, 1995; Kelly, Murphy, Washington, Wilson, 1994; Kegeles, Hays, and Coates, 1996; Rotheram-Borus, Koopman, Haignere, and Davies, 1991). Effective campaigns against the use of tobacco products have resulted in the decreased use of tobacco among young adults. (e.g., Bruvold, 1993). Well-planned and employed interventions resulted in increased immunization rates (e.g., Briss, Rodewald, Hinman, Shefer, Strikas, Bernier, Carende-Kulis, Yusuf, Ndiaye, Williams, and The Task Force on Community Preventive Services, 2000). Even as we enter 2008 and both the World Health Organization and US Department of Health and Human Services prepare for the heightened probability of a pandemic influenza, recommended interventions to avoid the transmission of H5N1virus or another deadly virus include prevention efforts, such as hand hygiene and social distancing, until an effective vaccine is developed. One can refer to http://www.pandemicflu.gov/ for additional information.

A challenge facing practitioners, administrators, and educators is how to systematically study a health issue in a designated community. Specifically, how does one go about selecting and critiquing data sources, developing a plan to address the issues, selecting evidence-based interventions, and evaluating the implementation and overall effectiveness of the intervention.

The settings of this integration of research within practice can occur at national, regional, state, county, and community levels and is more encompassing than the traditional boundaries of public health. The term 'community health' is used in this chapter to designate the possible practice areas instead of the term 'public health'. Community health used in this context includes ambulatory and primary care sites, such as practitioners' office settings, which are usually not included within the traditional perception of public health. The process described in this chapter can occur outside the scope of a specific agency defined within a government bureaucracy. Acknowledging that community health includes key players outside of government agencies is consistent with the Institute of Medicine's report (2003) which called for "the creation of an effective intersectorial public health system" (p. 46).

The process addressed in this chapter is a research utilization model, the Data-Driven Decisions Health Services Research Model (3-D HSR Model). The model provides a framework for the selection, critique, and interpretation of research data to support and evaluate evidence-based practice in community health settings. The model encompasses the following four aspects: 1) the interpretation of population-based data to identify major health issues affecting a defined community; 2) the selection of effective interventions to enhance the health of the community; 3) the implementation of a process evaluation to ascertain if the implementation of the intervention was conducted as intended; and 4) the incorporation of an outcome evaluation to determine the measurable impact of the intervention on specific health indicators with a community.

These four aspects comprise the three stages of the model. Each of the three stages will be addressed in this chapter with a brief explanation of the model, an example, and potential implications for nursing research, education, and practice.

The Data-Driven Decisions Health Services Research Model

The Data-Driven Decisions Health Services Research Model, hereafter referred to as the *3-D HSR Model*, integrates key approaches from epidemiology and health services research to facilitate: 1) the identification of community health problems, 2) the selection and evaluation of evidence-based interventions, and 3) the integration of key evaluative research methods. Epidemiology research approaches provide the foundation in the identification of major health issues in a community through the analysis of selected national population-based datasets, data from state health departments, and other quality health-related data collected by various government and non-government agencies. Health services research specifically includes the incorporation of evaluative research methods. Two types of evaluative research, process and outcome evaluations, are integrated into the model to determine the effectiveness of the selected intervention.

The model is based on General Systems Theory as defined by Ludwig von Bertalanffy in the 1920s. The 3-D HSR Model emphasizes von Bertalanffy's concepts of interaction among the components of the model, nonlinear functioning, and feedback. The major components of the model are viewed as interconnected and interdependent systems which do not operate in isolation. The components influence each other. Viewing and interacting with only one part of the model leaves the outcome to chance while a holistic, or macro-level view, will support a more objective view of the interplay between and among the various components, inputs, and outputs of the model and aim for intended outcome. The model is considered dynamic, open, transparent, and vulnerable to various outside influences, implying a semi-permeable state (von Bertalanffy, 1968).

The following diagram illustrates the three major tiers of the 3-D HSR Model with emphasis on feedback and interrelated aspects of the tiers.

The model's lines are considered semi-permeable since various outside factors can influence the model and affect the intended outcomes, both in a positive and negative manner. Practitioners and administrators in the community health arena are familiar with the impact the following factors have on a well-intended and evidence-based program's outcomes: funding, technical resources, personnel resources, politics (including policies of elected officials and special interest groups), and personalities and operating paradigms (i.e., personal beliefs) of key players involved with the issue. The histories surrounding the implementation of two programs in the US community health arena can be examined to understand the influence of "outside factors": 1) needle exchange for injection drug users to prevent HIV/AIDS and serve as a linkage to rehabilitation services, and 2) abstinence only programs for adolescents to delay the onset of sexual intercourse. These two programs represent opposing political paradigms and have supporting and opposing points of view. The model also has an element of chaos theory in that "a small, but well-timed or well-placed jolt to a system can throw the entire system into a state of chaos" (Walonick, 2008). Often these "jolts" are not evidence-based but emotional-based, reinforcing the author's opinion that 'public health is a reflection of political health'.

The 3-D HSR Model includes the following assumptions: 1) consumer involvement through an authentic and welcomed partnership through the entire process; 2) the identification and inclusion of macro and micro-level strengths present in the community health setting; 3) a complete data review and interpretation process will identify and prioritize key health issues in the community; 4) the critique of evidence-based interventions will result in selection of best intervention for the community; and 5) evaluative research methods are integrated at the beginning of the model and feedback from the evaluations are utilized, resulting in needed changes.

There is an aspect that the model does not address and is more at the micro level of health care: the individual and the decision to participate in a health intervention. The focus of the 3-D HSR Model in relation to an individual is the ability of people in a community to *access* an effective, community-based intervention. Behavioral change models are available that address the individual level – both within nursing and in other fields – and it is recommended that one refer to these sources to study individual behavioral change. The intent of the 3-D HSR Model is to select, implement, and evaluate the best evidence-based intervention with a community.

Access to an effective intervention is needed before one can expect and measure changes in individuals. What good results in implementing an intervention that is not considered evidence-based or effective and then evaluating (or judging) individuals in meeting the expected results?

The inability to access quality services raises important ethical considerations. What are the ethical implications for expecting communities to embrace interventions that are not based on sound science? What are the ethical implications for labeling communities as "non-compliant" or "uncooperative" for not embracing interventions that may not fit the community's needs or culture? What are the ethical implications for withholding evidence-based interventions due to outside political forces when the community needs and wants the intervention? Although the model does not address individual behavioral change, aspects of the model can impact the individual. The model challenges us to look beyond and around the individual and immediate social support systems (including the individual's family as defined by the individual) to comprehend factors that can affect the individual, especially access to effective community-based interventions.

The next sections of this chapter discuss the three major aspects of the model. A case example follows to briefly illustrate an application of the model.

Identification, Interpretation, and Critique of Population-Based Health Datasets

The term population-based health data is intricately linked to the concepts population health and population-based research. Kindig and Stoddard (2003) defined population health as "the health outcomes of a group of individuals, including the distribution of such outcomes within the group" (p. 380). Population-based research "draws on populations or random samples of populations at national, state, or local level" (Institute of Medicine, 2003, p. 377). Population-based research acknowledges the numerous determinants of health and various levels of influence upon the health of a population – environmental (social and physical) to behavioral and individual (genetics and biological) (Institute of Medicine, 2003). Population-based research addresses disparities in health related to economic class, race, ethnicity, and gender.

Population-based research involves the collection and subsequent analysis of population-based health datasets, also referred to as health databases. Data collection and analysis will vary depending on the availability of datasets. Various agencies within the federal government plan, implement, collect, and organize a variety of population-based health datasets for researchers to use for analysis of original research questions.

A previously published article by the author and a co-author discuss the use and availability of select population-based health datasets for researchers (Zeni and Kogan,2007).

The analysis of population-based datasets is one aspect of public health research, especially epidemiology. Epidemiology is the foundation of the 3-D HSR Research Model. Epidemiology has traditionally been defined as "the study of how disease is distributed in populations and the factors that influence or determine this distribution (Gordis, 2004, p.3). As noted by Gordis (2004), a broader definition of epidemiology is widely accepted to encompass "'the study of distribution and determinants of health-related states or events in specified populations and the application of this study to health problems'" (Last, 1988, as cited by Gordis, 2004, p. 3). Further work of epidemiologists has emphasized the distribution of health among specific populations in relation to various social attributes. For example, Krieger and colleagues have and are studying the relationships between social inequalities (income, race, ethnicity, and gender) and health outcomes, documenting the importance of ecosocial inequalities in population health (e.g., Krieger, Williams, and Moss, 1997; Krieger, 2001; Mustillo, Krieger, Gunderson, Sidney, McCreath, and Kiefe, 2004; Krieger, Chen, Waterman, Rehkopf, and Subramanian, 2005; Subramanian, Chen, Rehkopf, Waterman, and Krieger, 2005; Krieger, Smith, Naishadham, Hartman, and Barbeau, 2005; Krieger, Waterman, Hartman, Bates, Stoddard, Quinn, Sorensen, and Barbeau, 2006)).

Gordis (2004), in his book *Epidemiology*, presented the utilization of epidemiology to evaluate health care services and screening programs. Contrary to the use of epidemiology to study disease etiology where the relationship between a possible cause (independent variable) and an adverse health effect (dependent variable) are studied, the emphasis in health services research is the relationship between the health service (the independent variable) and the reduction in adverse health effects (the dependent variable) (Gordis, 2004). The 3-D HSR Model encompasses this use of epidemiology with health services research, specifically evaluative research.

The main benefits of using population-based research methods, including analyses of population-based datasets, is representative sampling. Population-based research implies the use of carefully constructed and implemented sampling frames to assure representation and the ability to generalize findings to the population of interest. A major limitation is the level of analyses. Most federal health datasets are available only for analysis at the federal or state level. Most datasets are not available at the county level since it is too expensive.

Program planners and managers at a community level should be encouraged to examine population-based health datasets since the information may still provide a picture of major problems noted in their area. If national and state analyses note that children from lower income families lack continuous health insurance coverage, then wouldn't lower income children in a certain county within the state be just as vulnerable? Studies at the county level may not be needed.

Local planners can consider if and how a situation is different at the local level and utilize various community-based needs assessments to fine-tune the problem at the local level. These community-based needs assessments include models developed by the Centers for Disease Control and Prevention, such as Planned Approach to Community Health (PATCH), and models developed by public health nurses, which will be addressed later in this chapter. Local assessment models can incorporate qualitative methods and emphasize consumer involvement in the assessment and subsequent program delivery and evaluation stages.

Major epidemiology texts provide an overview of national and state datasets. For example, Jekel and colleagues in *Epidemiology, Biostatistics and Preventive Medicine* cited the following population-based data sources: US census data, US Vital Statistics System (i.e., birth and death data,) National Notifiable Disease Surveillance System, studies by National Center of Health Statistics (i.e., the National health Interview Survey and National Health Assessment and Nutrition NHANES), Behavioral Risk Facto surveillance System (BRFSS), Disease Registries, and data from third parties (insurance carriers, Veteran's Administration, and Medicare) (Jekel, Katz, Elmore, and Wild, 2007). A vast majority of these datasets have been analyzed by researchers and results published in leading peer-review journals. Federal and state agencies also list contact staff for each of the datasets for further questions and information specific to health indicators.

Any defined population provides an opportunity to select a representative sample and study a health issue, such as hospital and agency databases providing services to patients and clients. For example, hospital medication error and infectious disease reports are two data sets that could be used for analyses. The work of Fisher, Wennberg and colleagues at the Dartmouth Atlas Project is an excellent example of outcome evaluations based on population-based data from hospital markets as noted on the website http://www.dartmouthatlas.org/atlases. Wennberg reported variations between hospital markets in one state regarding the likelihood that a woman would undergo a hysterectomy by the age of 70; the likelihood in one hospital market was 20 percent vs. 70 percent in another market (Wennberg, 1984). Harrison and Aller discussed the importance of including clinical lab results in large databases for research (Harrison and Aller, 2008). Population-based data and representative sampling methods are not limited to datasets collected and maintained by public health agencies within federal and state governments.

Most government population-based health datasets include variables that address major health indicators of interest to community health. Data about major health indicators serve as the organizing framework for US public health goals. Major health goals for the nation are comprised and published on a regular basis, as in *Health People 2010* (U.S. Department of Health and Human Services, 2000). Incorporating the same health indicators and supporting data on the regional, state, and local levels supports consistency toward the attainment of public health goals for the nation.

A risk when analyzing a selected dataset is to jump to conclusions by focusing on a single aspect and misinterpretation data. It is beneficial to interpret a result in context of the environment and surrounding events that could influence a single indicator. A review team noted an increase in the number of reported cases of giardiasis among preschool-aged children and interpreted this finding as an epidemic in the county and concluded the county health department was not addressing an epidemic. The county epidemiologist explained that the increase was an expected outcome due to educational sessions held by epidemiology staff at day care settings. The focus of the educational sessions was to educate day care operators to report cases resembling giardiasis for epidemiology staff to validate. Data collected prior to and after the educational sessions ascertained anecdotal data that day care staff were seeing symptoms most likely associated with the disease, but were either not aware of reporting requirements or were not aware of the process to report symptoms for confirmation. What was interpreted as an ignored epidemic was really a favorable outcome variable to the county epidemiology unit since the data reflected increased reporting. The situation supported a well-known aspect in public health that effective, active surveillance results in an increased number of reported cases of a certain condition.

It is an important and worthwhile goal to view a complete picture when interpreting data. Examining and evaluating intervening factors is important. The 3-D HSR Model acknowledges that various factors will affect interpretation and outcome since the model is an open system.

The end result of the first stage of the model is the identification and prioritization of health issues. While this process is open to constant revisions depending on outside or environmental circumstances, it is imperative that health issues are identified and prioritized before going to the next stage of the model.

Selection of Effective Interventions to Enhance Health of Community

One of the most challenging aspects in the practice of community-based health is the selection of effective interventions. While the latest jargon in health care includes the term 'evidenced-based practice', the concept of evidence-based practice was developed in the early 1970s by Dr. Archie Cochrane, an epidemiologist, in relation birth outcomes. The work of Dr. Cochrane led to the establishment of an international collaboration supporting evidence-based practice initiatives, including systematic reviews of health interventions available online through The Cochrane Library. Detailed information about the Cochrane initiative can be found on the website http://www.cochrane.org.

Evidence-based practice in public health is supported in the 2003 Institute of Medicine's report *The Future of the Public's Health in the 21st Century*. Public health nurses have emphasized the importance of evidence in the selection of nursing interventions for a community. Two models were developed by public health nursing units: the *Los Angeles County Public Health Nursing Practice Model* and the *Intervention Wheel* developed by the Minnesota Department of Health, Section of Public Health Nursing (e.g., Smith and Bazini-Barakat, 2003; Keller, Strohschein, Lia-Hoagberg, and Schaffer, 2004). Both of these practice models emphasize population-based approaches and incorporate aspects of the nursing process. The 3-D HSR Model can be used in conjunction with these models to further strengthen the selection and critique of evidence-based interventions and the incorporation of evaluative research methods.

It is beneficial to examine how community health interventions are sometimes selected. The following examples are based on anecdotal information gathered through observations by the author during various community health meetings at county, state, and national levels.

- Historical Approach: What has been done in the past seemed to work for a particular health issue or a similar issue, so we might as well try the intervention for the current issue. The details may be vague regarding exact steps that were implemented to reach the previous outcome, but the group will attempt to reconstruct the process. Unfortunately, documents are usually not available to consult; people involved in the previous intervention are not available for consultation since they either left the agency due to retirement or different employment.

- Hysterical Approach: "Something" needs to be done now for some pressing reason. This urgent reason may be one or a combination of the following: 1) legislatures and/or powerful special interest groups are demanding quick action, 2) funding has just been released and if action does not follow, then the funding will be returned to its source, and 3) the work just did not get done and now the deadline is approaching and the funder is expecting the product. An intervention may be selected that is easy to implement and appealing to the groups advocating for action and/or a portion of the funding.

- Omnipotent (Divine Intervention) Approach: Just our presence alone improves a client's and family's outcome. We can just talk or be with a client and the client will decide to change risk behaviors. It is easy to distinguish this approach from others since people advocating this approach have a tendency to become very annoyed with a few basic questions from evaluators, such as: "What exactly did you do? How would you explain the intervention to people in another area of the state who want to do what you did?" The approach is usually claimed by one group (or profession) and used to eliminate competition from other groups for the same (limited) funding and client base.

- Magic Bullet Approach: Current health policy recommendations seem to cluster around one intervention. Everyone starts to jump on the bandwagon, promoting this one intervention as the cure-all for a challenging health issue, the new "magic bullet". An example is the focus on increasing knowledge of a health issue through the distribution of brochures and health fair events with little regard to factors such as the readability of the brochures, relevance to the community, and possibility of actual change in risk behaviors with communities. A benefit is providers feel a sense of satisfaction as they were busy doing something to address a health issue.

- Importation Approach: We heard at a conference, a meeting, or from a colleague that a certain intervention worked in another area for the same or a similar health issue. Perhaps the intervention could be used in this situation. The group delegates a member to find and contact the source and ascertain details of the intervention. Outcome will vary depending on the planning process of the group who reported intervention. It is usually unknown if the imported intervention was evaluated in a systematic way to determine effectiveness.

- Blame the Victim Approach: Blame for the health issue is assigned to certain groups, thereby serving as a mask for institutional racism, classism, and other "–isms". People employing this approach are resistant to evaluations and consumer involvement since they perceive themselves as the experts. This approach includes patronizing with undertones of paternalism.

- Political Approach: Regardless of the evidence and community's requests, political forces will block interventions that are not consistent with the party line and force the implementation of their selected interventions. The interventions most vulnerable to elimination are those who do not have the economic resources to have their voices heard. Action can be accomplished due to the organization of informed consumers, as noted during the early years of the HIV/ADIS epidemic among gay activists.

What can be done? What can groups do to identify and implement effective interventions in a community health setting? These questions have been addressed in reference to the HIV/AIDS epidemic and resulted in a process established by the Centers of Disease Control and Prevention (CDC) to evaluate and select evidence-based HIV behavioral interventions, the HIV/AIDS Prevention Research Synthesis (PRS) Project. An outcome of the PRS Project is the publication of a document consisting of a collection of HIV prevention interventions deemed effective and appropriate to specific risk groups. The document was first published in 1999 as the *Compendium of HIV Prevention Interventions with Evidence of Effectiveness* and was updated in 2001; the CDC continues to update and release a revised document on a regular basis, titled *Updated Compendium* (Centers for Disease Control and Prevention, 1999; Lytes, Kay, Crepaz, Herbst, Passin, Kim, Rama, Thadiparthi, DeLuca, and Mullins,

2007). Specific information about the compendiums can be found on the CDC website: http://www.cdc.gov/hiv/topics/prev_prog/rep/resources/initiatives/compendium.htm

The evidence-based interventions listed in the *Updated Compendium* were identified by PRS through a series of efficacy reviews, resulting in an intervention catalogued as either best-evidence or promising-evidence (Lytes et al., 2007). The studies published in the compendium are interventions that have been identified, through a systematic review process, "as having rigorous study methods and demonstrated evidence of effectiveness in reducing sex-and drug-related risk behaviors or improving health outcomes." (Centers for Disease Control and Prevention, 2008) The compendium can be used by HIV prevention providers in the community health setting to select appropriate, evidence-based interventions for groups at-risk for HIV/AIDS.

How are interventions reviewed and selected for publication in the Updated Compendium? The CDC's HIV/AIDS PRS Project established an efficacy review method for the selection and classification of interventions. The method, described in detail on the CDC website, consists of the following steps:

1. A *Search Strategy* is employed to identify relevant studies. This strategy includes both an automated search of four electronic bibliographic databases and a manual search. The manual search involves staff reviewing 35 journals not yet indexed in the electronic databases, reference lists of published articles, select listservs, and unpublished manuscripts. The staff then searches the CDC PRS cumulative databases to link studies in the database with the newly identified study.

2. A *Study Eligibility* screening is then done with each study identified through the Search Strategy to determine if the study should be included in an intervention efficacy review.

3. *Study Coding Procedures* are done with each study. Pairs of trained content analysts independently code the study using the PRS efficacy criteria. The authors of studies are contacted if additional information is needed. A final determination of the study's efficacy is made through PRS team consensus.

Only studies that meet Tier I (Best-evidence interventions) or Tier II (Promising-evidence interventions) are included in the compendium database. Tier I studies are defined as "interventions that have been rigorously evaluated and have been shown to have significant and positive evidence of efficacy" (Centers for Disease Control and Prevention, 2008). Tier I interventions are considered to be scientifically rigorous and provide the strongest efficacy; Tier II interventions may not meet the same rigor of a Tier I intervention but are still considered sound, providing sufficient evidence of efficacy (Centers for Disease Control and Prevention, 2008).

While it is beyond the scope of most groups to replicate the CDC PRS model to determine efficacy of an intervention, aspects of the model can be used in the determination and selection of an evidence-based intervention, including interventions outside of HIV/AIDS prevention. A set of questions were developed by the author to determine the feasibility of implementing an intervention in the community. The questions are the core components of *MAP* (*M*atch, *A*scertain, and *P*lan):

1. *M*atch the intervention to the health issue and community.
    - Has the intervention been used with the identified health issue? Is the identified intervention appropriate for the health issue?
    - Is the intervention appropriate for use with the intended community?
2. *A*scertain the intervention is effective and under what circumstances.
    - Has the intervention undergone an evaluation? If so, how rigorous was the evaluation? A quality design usually includes the following general components:
        o Prospective, longitudinal study design with a treatment and control group of an adequate sample size
        o Treatment and control groups were assigned randomly or through a carefully constructed and followed sampling plan. There was a low drop-out rate among participants
        o Valid and reliable instruments were selected to measure pre and post intervention differences. The same measurements were used for pre and post intervention measurements.
        o Appropriate statistical analyses were used at a standard, acceptable level of significance to measure any changes due to the intervention.
        o Study clearly presented limitations and discussed how limitations may affect findings.
        o Study clearly defined population and subsequent sample that received the intervention.
    - What are the key elements that contributed to the success of this intervention? What are the barriers to achieving the intended outcome? How would the success factors and barriers play out in the intended community?
3. *P*lan how to *start* implementing the intervention in the community.
    - Is the intervention clearly described in detailed steps to replicate without difficulty and error? If not, could the developers provide more detailed information?
    - Could the key components of the intervention be successfully implemented as intended in the community to assure similar outcomes?
    - Is technical assistance available from the developers of the intervention to advise regarding training, implementation, and evaluation?

The HIV/AIDS prevention area provides two more important concepts to consider in the selection of evidence-based interventions: intervention fidelity and technology transfer. Intervention fidelity refers to "the demonstration that an experimental manipulation is conducted as planned" (Dumas, Lynch, Laughlin, Phillips Smith, and Prinz, 2001, p. 38). Intervention fidelity implies that key components of a successful intervention were delivered correctly in a similar community setting per the intervention protocol. Any changes in the key components could result in an unexpected outcome. This concept is similar to a practitioner prescribing a course of antibiotics to a patient and expecting the patient to correctly take and finish the antibiotics. Not completing the prescription or taking the medication incorrectly could result in an adverse outcome, which is a serious concern in some diseases such as TB. The general focus of intervention fidelity is adherence to an established protocol and a method to determine adherence, usually through a process evaluation. Process evaluations are discussed in the next section of this chapter.

Technology transfer was a term utilized in the mid-1990s in HIV prevention to "encompass the translation, dissemination, and acquisition of information about interventions, the process of deciding whether to use an intervention, the tailoring of the intervention, and the provision of training and technical assistance (TA) – programmatic, scientific, or technical support to providers for planning and implementation" (Kraft, Morozoff, Sogolow, Neumann, and Thomas, 2000, p. 8). Technology transfer has resulted in the development of HIV prevention 'packages' or 'toolkits' for providers to use to aid in the correct implementation of an evidence-based intervention. An example of applications of technology transfer in HIV prevention can be found on two websites: Diffusion of Effective Behavioral Interventions (DEBI) at http://www.effectiveinterventions.org/ and Replicating Effective Programs Plus (REP) at http://www.cdc.gov/hiv/topics/prev_prog/rep/index.ht.

In summary, the 3-D HSR Model supports data-driven decisions, not dogma-driven directives. Evaluative research, discussed in the next section of this chapter, can assist in maintaining an objective focus.

Integration of Evaluative Research

An essential aspect of the model is the incorporation of evaluative research. Although evaluative research is the third stage of the model, research activities are integrated in the prior stages of the model. A feedback loop exists in the illustration of the model to symbolize the link between this third stage of the model and the prior stages. The implication is that data obtained through evaluative research will provide information to the selection and implementation of evidence-based interventions and the interpretation of population-based data. The links with the prior two stages are possible through two specific types of evaluative research, process and outcome evaluations.

The term evaluative research is preferred instead of evaluation as explained provided by Suchman (1967) in his seminal work, *Evaluative Research Principles and Practice in Public Service and Social Action Programs*:

In our approach, we will make a distinction between "evaluation" and "evaluative research". The former will be used in a general way as referring to the social process of making judgments of worth. This process is basic to almost all forms of social behavior, whether that of a single individual or a complex organization. While it implies some logical or rationale basis for making such judgments, it does not require any systematic procedures for marshaling and presenting objective evidence to support the judgment. Thus, we retain the term "evaluation" it its more common-sense usage as referring to the general process of assessments or appraisal of value.

"Evaluative research" on the other hand, will be restricted to the utilization of scientific research methods and techniques for the purpose of making an evaluation...evaluative research refers to those procedures for collecting and analyzing data which increase the possibility for "proving" rather than "asserting" the worth of some social activity. (p. 7-8).

Suchman (1967) emphasized the need for social science research methods to obtain an objective appraisal of a program and not a subjective opinion of the worthiness of an activity. He explained the focus of the evaluation process "as the determination (whether based on opinions, records, subjective or objective data) of the results (whether desirable or undesirable; transient or permanent; immediate or delayed) attained by some activity (whether a program, or part of a program, a drug or a therapy, an on-going or a one-shot approach) designed to accomplish some valued goal or objective (whether ultimate, intermediate, or immediate, effort or performance, long or short range)" (Suchman, 1967, pp. 31-32) He advocated the examination of specific program objectives and assumptions, the development of measurable criteria related to the objectives, and the determination of the extent of achieving the objectives through a controlled situation, including the development of any negative side effects (Suchman, 1967). It appears that Suchman would support the use of quantitative and qualitative research methods.

The depth of the research processes can vary and will vary depending on various factors, including the availability of resources. While it may be beyond the scope of most programs to incorporate evaluative research and the expertise of a researcher (whether on staff or as a consultant), the need for integrating evaluative research with the selection and implementation of interventions cannot be denied. Two types of evaluative research are valuable in this light: process and outcome evaluations.

Rossi, Lipsey, and Freeman (2004) noted that one type of process evaluation is ongoing, repeated measurements over time to determine program functioning, thus referred to as program process monitoring. (Rossi et al., 2004) Program process monitoring corresponds with the concept "intervention fidelity" discussed in the previous section since "program process monitoring is the systematic and continual documentation of key aspects of program performance that assesses whether the program is operating as intended or according to some appropriate standard" (Rossi et al., 2004, p. 171). Program process monitoring provides an historical record of any revisions to the intervention and changes during implementation that may have affected the overall outcome.

In contrast, outcome monitoring is defined as" the continual measurement and reporting of the status of the social conditions a program is accountable for improving" (Rossi et all, 2004, p. 201). The challenge facing researchers is to design a quality study with valid and reliable measurements to detect any changes that could significantly be attributed to the selected intervention. In evaluation terminology, one is determining a program's (or intervention's) impact. A quality study is based on sound research principles, whether quantitative, qualitative, or a mixed methods approach.

Clearly defined, realistic, measurable objectives are the foundation of both process and outcome evaluations. The objectives are ideally determined collaboratively between program planners, staff, consumers, and researchers prior at the start of the project and during this second stage of the 3-D HSR Model. Keeping overall goals and general objectives in focus assist with the selection of an effective intervention. Collaboration assists in integrating evaluation in the entire process. It also provides a two-way educational opportunity, meaning researchers can understand why and how an intervention was selected and planners, staff, and consumers can learn what evaluative research brings to the table. This education occurs if evaluation is presented in a non-threatening and non-punitive manner.

Many models and approaches are available regarding process and outcome evaluations. Resources on logic models are available at the CDC website: http://www.cdc.gov/eval/ resources.htm#logic%20model. It is not the intent of this chapter to teach how to develop evaluations or provide one-size-fits-all recipe format to conduct evaluations. The intent is to discuss evaluative research and how it is an integral part of the 3-D HSR Model.

Example

A goal of Healthy People 2010 is to "increase the proportion of persons who have a specific source of ongoing care." (U.S. Department of Health and Human Services, 2000). This document reports:

> More than 40 million Americans do not have a particular doctor's office, clinic, health center, or other place where they usually go to seek care pf health-related advice. Even among privately insured persons, a significant number lacked a usual source of care or reported difficulty in accessing needed care due to financial constraints of insurance problems. People aged 18 to 24 years were most likely to lack a usual source of ongoing primary care. Only 80 percent of individuals below the poverty level and 70 percent of Hispanic had a usual source of ongoing primary care. (http://www.healthypeople.gov/ document/html/uih/uih_4.htm# accesshealth).

Do US children have a medical home, or a particular health care provider, to receive regular and consistent health care? This question was addressed by the author as a principle investigator in a series of analyses conducted with the 2004 National Survey of Children's Health (NSCH). The NSCH is a population-based dataset and consists of a representative sample of US children ages birth through 17 years, including a representative sample of all states. Analyses could include the entire US and an individual state, such as Florida.

Analyses of the NSCH, using the Aday and Andersen Access to Medical Care Model, found that 53.9% of US children lacked a medical home and regression analysis found that the odds of lacking a medical home were significantly increased for parental assessment of child's health status as good (1.39) and fair or poor (1.28) (versus excellent/very good), age 1–4 (1.68), age 5–12 (2.79), age 13–17 (3.38) (reference for age is age < 1), Hispanics (1.25), primary household language Spanish (1.87), Blacks (1.28), below 100% poverty level (1.93), poverty 100–200% (1.60), poverty 200–400% (1.24), household education less than high school (1.31), and moderate-severe emotional/ behavioral condition (1.51). While health insurance and being in a 2 parent family reduced the risk of lacking a medical home, findings indicated that numerous factors need to considered regarding the achievement of the goal of comprehensive health care, a variety of factors need to be considered (Zeni, Thompson, and Kogan, 2006).

While the concept of medical home was derived form eight questions in the NSCH to represent the components of a medical home as defined by the American Academy of Pediatrics, an additional study focused on risks associated with not having a personal health provider, meaning a physician, nurse practitioner, or physician assistant, for consistent and regular health care. Analysis of the NSCH with Florida data found that 20.1% of Florida children (0–17 years of age) did not have a personal health care provider compared with 16.7% in the United States. Children at greatest risk are those without health insurance. Other significant risk factors include family poverty up to 100% of federal poverty level, poverty level 100% to 199%, poverty level unknown, poverty level 200% to 399%, children aged 5 to 12 years, children aged 13 to 17 years, and Hispanic ethnicity. All the factors in the Florida model were also significant in the national model (Zeni, Sappenfield, Thompson, and Chen, 2007).

The findings of these population-based studies note the risk associated with lack of insurance, various levels of poverty, and race/ethnicity for the US study and Hispanic ethnicity for the Florida study. What evidence-based interventions can be identified to assist vulnerable children to access health care, including health care programs such as the State Children's Health Insurance Program (SCHIP)? SCHIP is a special health insurance program for uninsured children who do not meet federal income guidelines for Medicaid and do not have private insurance; it is not an entitlement program so states can yearly cap SCHIP expenditures (Perrin, 2007). The federal government provides the states with funding for SCHIP and each state can contribute funds and develop its own program, including variations in enrollment. In 2006, Congress required states that do not spend their federal allocations to redistribute those funds to states with projected shortfalls; Florida did not spend all its federal dollars and was projected to lose $20 million dollars (Florida KidCare Coordinating Council, 2007).

SCHIP programs in other states used their allocations and underwent extensive evaluations. Recommendations from these evaluations can be used for the development and implementation of a successful SCHIP program (Flores, Abreu, Brown, and Tomany-Kroman, 2005; Damiiano, Willard, Momany, and Chowdhury, 2003; Szilagyi, Zwanziger, Rodewald, Holl, Mukamel, Trafton, Pollard Shone, Dick, Jarrell, and Raubertas, 2000).

SCHIP successes in other states need to be examined to replicate effective models in Florida and assure that children who qualify for this benefit have access to health insurance and a consistent health care provider. Evaluative research from an independent group is needed to determine both process and outcome measures. An independent group has more flexibility to objectively evaluate.

Conclusion

The 3-D HSR Model compliments and supports current models and frameworks in nursing, addressing evidence-based practice and translation research. The model's emphasis on the selection of effective interventions and integration of evaluative research supports national efforts in research, practice, and education. The Agency for Healthcare Research and Quality (AHRQ) called for the use of evidence-based information to reach the goal of effectiveness by transforming research into practice to enhance quality and address health disparities (Clancy, Sharp, and Hubbard, 2005). The 3-D HSR model supports this goal since one of the core values of the model is employing quality data to make sound decisions.

This core value is consistent with the definition of evidence-based practice as defined by Fineout-Overholt and Melvyn and Sackett, Strauss, Richardson, Rosenberg, and Haynes: "Evidence-based practice (EBP) is a problem-solving approach to clinical care that incorporates the conscientious use of current best evidence from well-designed studies, a clinician's expertise, and patient values and preferences" (Finehout-Overholt, Melynk, and Schultz, 2005, p. 335). The 3-D model is congruent with this definition and stresses the expectation and dependency upon the expertise and collaboration of an interdisciplinary team in selecting effective community-based interventions in conjunction with community members. Community members are welcomed and equal participant-partners at the planning table and are the true owners of the process.

The model further supports the scope of nursing research as outlined in the 2006 American Association of Colleges of Nursing (AACN) Position Statement on Nursing Research. The statement identifies health systems and outcomes research as one of three scopes of nursing research, noting "nursing research is integrated with health services research regarding issues of organization, delivery, financing, quality, patient and provider behavior, informatics, effectiveness, cost, and outcomes" (American Association of Colleges of Nursing, 2006, p. 3) The statement cites the large numbers of indigent and/or uninsured Americans who are unable to receive minimal health care as an example of the need for nurse researchers to develop knowledge and skills in health services research (American Association of Colleges of Nursing, 2006).

The 3-D HSR model supports the aim of health services research as defined by Academy Health, a professional association of researchers and policy experts in health services. The model enhances access to quality interventions and functions within two of the six research domains identified by AcademyHealth, communities and populations (AcadmyHealth, 2000). One mission of the group that coincides with a core value of the 3-D HSR model is the translation of research findings into information for clinical, management, and policy decisions (AcademyHealth, 2007).

Further consistency between health services and nursing research was discussed by Jones and Mark (2005) through their identification of five areas of importance where Nursing-Health Services Research (N-HSR) can provide research contributions: (1) access to and utilization of care; (2) health and health behaviors; (3) quality of care and patient safety; (4) cost and cost-effectiveness of care; and (5) organization and delivery of care (Jones and Mark, 2005, p. 224). They advocated that N-HSR can answer important questions that intersect both nursing and health services research, reporting on a N-HSR research agenda established at a May 2004 national conference (Jones and Mark, 2005).

Bowman and Gardner (2001) noted that even though nursing is the largest group of health professionals, it is only a minor, even absent, contributor to health services research and unable to play a role in shaping future policy. Based on interviews with nursing leaders, they recommended nurses become better collaborators with health services researchers and the inclusion of health services research in undergraduate and graduate curriculum (Bowman and Gardner, 2001). Jones and Mark (2005) emphasized the need for building capacity within nursing regarding interdisciplinary education about HSR methods, including postdoctoral training opportunities (Jones and Mark, 2005). Jones and Lusk outlined recommendations for incorporating HSR into nursing doctoral programs (Jones and Lusk, 2002).

The 3-D HSR Model supports population-based public health nursing. For example, the Intervention Wheel is a population-based public health nursing practice model consisting of three levels of practice and seventeen community nursing interventions with the overall goal of improving population health. (Keller et al, 2004) The 3-D HSR Model can be used concurrently with the Intervention Wheel to assist in the interpretation of population-based data, the selection of effective community-based interventions and the integration of quality evaluation.

The 3-D HSR Model is compatible with major public health nursing competencies and Association of Community Health Nursing Educators (ACHNE) essentials for undergraduate public health nursing curriculum as presented by Carter and colleagues (2006). Carter and colleagues prepared tables of each major competency with possible undergraduate learning activities listed for each one with an emphasis on population-focused public health practice (Carter, Kaiser, O'Hare, and Callister, 2006).

Incorporating the 3-D HSR Model with current public health nursing models can enhance the shared nursing and public health roles of promoting social justice and political advocacy. Nursing can identify barriers that prevent the implementation of needed, effective community-based interventions and advocate for the removal of these barriers. This process of identification and strategies to remove barriers can be analyzed within the framework of health care ethics and provide further pro-active learning activities for students from a variety of disciplines.

The 3-D Health Services Research Model is consistent with values of health services and nursing-health services research. The model provides a method for supporting evidence-based practice and utilizing translation research to ensure the implementation and evaluation of quality effective interventions in the community setting.

References

AcadmyHealth (2000). What is health services research? Washington, DC: AcademyHealth. Retrieved 11/30/2007 from *http://www.academyhealth.org/about/whatishsr.htm.*

American Association of Colleges of Nursing (2006). AACN position statement on nursing research. Washington, DC: American Association of Colleges of Nursing. Retrieved 7/17/2006 from *http:www.aacn.nche.edu/Publications/positions/NsgRes.htm.*

Bowman, C.C. and Gardner, D. (2001). Building health services research capacity in nursing: views from members of nursing's leadership. *Nursing Outlook, 49,* 187-192.

Briss, P. A., Rodewald, L.E., Hinman, A.R., Shefer, A.M., Strikas, R.A., Bernier, R. R., Carende-Kulis, V.G., Yusuf, H.R., Ndiaye, S.M., Williams, S.M. and The Task Force on Community Preventive Services (2000). Reviews of evidence regarding interventions to improve vaccination coverage in children, adolescents, and adults. *American Journal of Preventive Medicine, 18,* 97-140.

Bruvold, W.H. (1993). A meta-analysis of adolescent smoking prevention programs. *American Journal of Public Health*, 83, 872-880.

Carter, K.F., Kaiser, L.K., O'Hare, P.A., and Callister, L.C. (2006). Use of PNH competencies and ACHNE essentials to develop teaching-learning strategies for generalist C/PHN curricula. *Public Health Nursing, 23,* 146-160.

Centers for Disease Control and Prevention (1999). *Compendium of HIV Prevention Interventions with Evidence of Effectiveness,* revised. Atlanta, GA: U.S. Department of Health and Human Services, Centers for Disease Control and Prevention.

Centers for Disease Control and Prevention. *HIV Prevention Research Synthesis Project* Web site. Retrieved January 23, 2008 from *http://www.cdc.gov/hiv/topics/research/ prs/index.htm.*

Clancy, C., Sharp, B.A., and Hubbard, H. (2005). Guest editorial: Intersections for mutual success in nursing and health services research. *Nursing Outlook, 53,* 263-265.

Damiiano, P.C., Willard, J.C., Momany, E.T., and Chowdhury, J. (2003). The impact of the Iowa S-SCHIP program on access, health status, and the family environment. *Ambulatory Pediatrics, 3,* 263-269.

Des Jarlais, D.C., Casriel, C., Friedman, S.R., and Rosenblum, A. (1992). AIDS and the transition to illicit drug injection results of a randomized trial prevention program. *British Journal of Addiction, 87,* 593-498.

Dicelmente, R.J., and Wingood, G.M. (1995). A randomized controlled trial of an HIV sexual risk-reduction intervention for young African-American women. *Journal of the American Medical Association, 274,* 1271-1276.

Dumas, J.E., Lynch, A.M., Laughlin, J.E., Smith, E. P., and Prinz, R.J. (2001). Promoting intervention fidelity: conceptual issues, methods, and preliminary results from the EARLY ALLIANCE prevention trial. *American Journal of Preventive Medicine, 20,* 38-47.

Finehout-Overholt, E., Melynk, B., and Schultz, A. (2005). Transforming health care from the inside out: advancing evidence-based practice in the 21st century. *Journal of Professional Nursing, 21,* 335-344.

Flores, G., Abreu, M., Brown, V., and Tomany-Kroman, S.C. (2005). How Medicaid and the state children's health insurance program can do a better job of insuring uninsured children: the perspective of parents of uninsured Latino children. *Ambulatory Pediatrics, 5,* 332-340.

Florida KidCare Coordinating Council (2007). Kidcare report. Retrieved 1/30/2008 from *http://www.floridachain.org/website/KCC2007report-Web.pdf.*

Gordis, L. (2004). Epidemiology (3rd edition). Philadelphia: Elsevier Saunders.

Harrison J.H., and Aller, R.D. (2008). Regional and national health care data repositories. *Clinics in Laboratory Medicine, 28,* 101-117.

Institute of Medicine (2003). The future of the public's health in the 21st century. Washington, D.C.: The National Academies Press.

Jekel, J. F., Katz, D.L., Elmore, J.G., and Wild, D. (2007). *Epidemiology, Biostatistics, and Preventive Medicine* (3rd edition). Philadelphia: Saunders.

Jones, C.B., and Lusk, S.L. (2002). Incorporating health services research into nursing doctoral programs. *Nursing Outlook, 50,* 225-231.

Jones, C. B., and Mark, B.A, (2005). The intersection of nursing and health services research: an agenda to guide future research. *Nursing Outlook, 53,* 324-332.

Jones, C. B., and Mark, B.A, (2005). The intersection of nursing and health services research: overview of an agenda setting conference. *Nursing Outlook, 53,* 270-273.

Kegeles, S.M., Hays, R.B., and Coates, T.J. (1996). The MPowerment project: a community-level HIV prevention intervention for young gay men. *American Journal of Public Health, 86,* 1129-1136.

Keller, L.O., Strohschein, S., Lia-Hoagberg, B., and Schaffer, M.A. (2004). Population-based public health interventions: practice-based and evidence-supported. Part I. *Public Health Nursing, 21,* 453-468.

Kelly, J.A., Murphy, D.A., Washington, C.D., Wilson, T.S., Koob, J.J., Davis, D.R., Lezezma, G, and Davanter, B. (1994). The effects of HIV/AIDS intervention groups for high-risk women in urban clinics. *American Journal of Public Health, 84,* 1918-1922.

Kindig, D., and Stoddard, G. (2003). What is population health? *American Journal of Public Health, 93,* 380-383.

Kraft, J.M., Morozoff, J.S., Sogolow, E. D., Neumann, M.S., and Thomas, M.A. (2000). A technology transfer model for effective HIV/AIDS interventions: science and practice. *AIDS Education and Prevention, Supplement A,* 12, 7-20.

Krieger, N. (2001). Theories for social epidemiology in the 21st century: an ecosocial perspective. *International Journal of Epidemiology, 30,* 668-677.

Krieger, N., Chen, J.T., Waterman, P.D., Rehkopf, D.H., and Subramanian, S.V. (2005). Painting a truer picture of US socioeconomic and racial/ethnic health inequalities: the public health disparities geocoding project. American Journal of Public Health, 95, 312-323.

Krieger, N., Smith, K., Naishadham, D., Hartman, C., and Barbeau, E. M. (2005). Experiences of discrimination: validity and reliability of a self-report measure for population health research on racism and health. *Social Science and Medicine, 61,* 1576-1596.

Krieger, N., Waterman, P.D., Hartman, C., Bates, L.M., Stoddard, A.M., Quinn, M.M., Sorensen, G., and Barbeau, E.M. (2006). Social hazards on the job: workplace abuse, sexual harassment, and racial discrimination – a study of black, Latino, and white low-income women and men workers in the United States. *International Journal of Health Services, 36,* 51-85.

Krieger, N., Williams, D.R., and Moss, N.E. (1997). Measuring social class in the US public health research: concepts, methodologies and guidelines. *American Review of Public Health, 18,* 341-378.

Last, J.M. (1988). *A dictionary of epidemiology* (2nd edition). New York: Oxford University Press.

Lytes, C.M., Kay, L.S., Crepaz, N., Herbst, J. H., Passin, W. F., Kim, A. S., Rama, S. M., Thadiparthi, B.S., DeLuca, J. B., and Mullins, M.M., for the HIV/AIDS Prevention Research Synthesis Team (2007). Best-evidence interventions: findings from a systematic review of HIV behavioral interventions for US populations at high risk, 2000-2004. *American Journal of Public Health, 97,* 133-143.

Mustillo, S., Krieger, N., Gunderson, E.P., Sidney, S., McCreath, H., and Kiefe, C.I. (2004). Self-reported experiences of racial discrimination and black-white differences in preterm and low-birthweight deliveries: The CARDIA study. *American Journal of Public Health, 94,* 2125-2131.

Nolte, E., and McKee, L.M. (2008). Measuring the health of nations: updating an earlier analysis. *Health Affairs, 27,* 58-71.

Perrin, J.M. (2007). Letter from the editor: SCHIP, children, and families. *Ambulatory Pediatrics, 7,* 405-406.

Rossi, P.H., Lipsey, M.W., and Freeman, H.E. (2004). *Evaluation a systematic approach* (7th edition). Thousand Oaks, CA: SAGE Publications.

Rotheram-Borus, M., Koopman, C., Haignere, C., and Davies, M. (1991). Reducing HIV sexual risk behaviors among runaway adolescents. *Journal of the American Medical Association, 266,* 1237-1241.

Smith, K., and Bazini-Barakat, N. (2003). A public health nursing practice model: melding public health principles with the nursing process. *Public Health Nursing, 20,* 42-48.

Subramanian, S.V., Chen, J.T., Rehkopf, D. H., Waterman, P. D., and Krieger, N. (2005). Racial disparities in context: a multilevel analysis of neighborhood variations in poverty and excess mortality among black populations in Massachusetts. *American Journal of Public Health, 95,* 260-265.

Suchman E.A. (1967). *Evaluative Research Principles and Practice in Public Service and Social Action Programs.* New York: Russell Sage Foundation.

Szilagyi, P. G., Zwanziger, J., Rodewald, L. E., Holl, J.L., Mukamel, D.B., Trafton, S., Pollard Shone, L., Dick, A.W., Jarrell, L., and Raubertas, R.F. (2000). Evaluation of a state health insurance program for low-income children: implications for state child health insurance programs. *Pediatrics, 105,* 363-371.

U.S. Department of Health and Human Services. (2000). *Healthy People 2010.* Washington, DC: U.S. Government Printing Office. Available from *http://www.healthypeople.gov/ document/tableofcontents.htm.*

von Bertalanffy, L. (1968). Passages from general systems theory. Retrieved 12/28/2007 from *http://www.panarchy.org/vonbertalanfft/systems.1968.html.*

Walonick, D.S. (2008). General systems theory. Retrieved 1/2/2008 from http://www.survey-software-solutions.com/walonick/systems-theory.htm.

Wennberg, J.E. (1984). Dealing with medical practice variations: a proposal for action. *Health Affairs, 3,* 6-32.

Zeni, M.B., and Kogan, M.D. (2007). Existing population-based health databases: useful resources for nursing research. *Nursing Outlook, 55,* 20-30.

Zeni, M.B., Sappenfield, W., Thompson, D., and Chen, H. (2007). Factors associated with not having a personal health care provider for children in Florida. *Pediatrics (supplement), 119,* S61-S67.

Zeni, M.B., Thompson, D., and Kogan, M.D. (2006). Factors associated with not having a medical home among US children. *American Journal of Epidemiology (supplement), 163,* S1-S258.

In: Trends in Nursing Research
Editors: Adam J. Ryan and Jack Doyle

ISBN 978-1-60456-642-0
© 2009 Nova Science Publishers, Inc.

Chapter 6

Current Issues in Translation Science

*Laura Cullen[*1] and Susan Adams[2]*

[1]Quality and Outcomes Management, Department of Nursing Services and Patient Care, University of Iowa Hospitals and Clinics, 200 Hawkins Drive, Iowa City, IA 52242-1009
[2]Research Translation and Dissemination Core, National Nursing Practice Network, Gerontological Nursing Interventions Research Center University of Iowa College of Nursing4116 Westlawn, Iowa City, IA 52242

Abstract

Nurses value providing high quality care, and adoption of evidence-based practices offer opportunities to make measurable improvements in healthcare outcomes. For this reason, providing evidence-based care has become the standard for quality in our healthcare system, yet research shows that patients only receive evidence-based care about half the time (Asch et al., 2006; Clark, 2005; Mangione-Smith et al., 2007; McGlynn et al., 2003; McInerny, Cull, and Yudkowsky, 2005; Peterson et al., 2006; Shrank et al., 2006; Zuckerman, Stevens, Inkelas, and Halfon, 2004). While the body of research in this area is growing, a great deal of work is still needed to better understand how to improve use of evidence-based healthcare at the practitioner and organizational levels.

Expectation of Using Evidence-Based Practice in Nursing

Increased use of evidence-based practice results in improved care processes and measurable improvements in patient outcomes such as decreased death rates (AHRQ, 2005; Perencevich et al., 2007; Peterson et al., 2006; Titler, 2002; Woolf, Grol, Hutchinson, Eccles, and Grimshaw, 1999), decreased complications (AHRQ, 2003), optimized use of resources

---
[*] Tel: (319) 384-9144, (319) 356-4348, E-mail: laura-cullen@uiowa.edu

by elimination of unnecessary procedures and testing (AHRQ, 2000) and reduction of healthcare costs (Cullen, Greiner, Greiner, Bombei, and Comried, 2005). Federal regulatory agencies, accrediting bodies, and private payer insurance companies expect that health care organizations will provide services based on the best available evidence (Garber, 2001). In addition, the American Nurses Association (ANA) standards of practice, *Nursing: Scope and Standards* (American Nurses Association, 2004), emphasizes the need for individual practitioners' use of evidence-based practice. This requires a commitment from all health care professionals to integrate evidence-based practices into their daily professional practice, and a commitment by organizational leaders to build structures and processes facilitating delivery of evidence-based healthcare.

When using evidence-based practice, healthcare practitioners rely on the integration of the best research evidence available combined with their expertise, in accordance with the preferences of the patient and family (Sackett, Rosenberg, Gray, Haynes, and Richardson, 1996; Sackett, Straus, Richardson, Rosenberg, and Haynes, 2000). The process involves asking a question about a clinical issue; finding, critically appraising and synthesizing the evidence; and applying and evaluating the results in practice. Clinical expertise is needed to integrate and interpret information about patient and family preferences, clinical information, clinically relevant and robust evidence, and healthcare resources, when advising patients or making healthcare decisions (Cullen, 2007b; Dicenso and Cullum, 1998; McCormack, Rycroft-Malone, Cullen, Griffith, and DiCenso, under development). An additional step requires evaluation to determine the impact on quality care, cycling back to identifying other potential clinical issues to address (DePalma, 2000; Titler and Everett, 2001a; Titler et al., 2001b) in a circular continuous improvement process.

The increase in the quality and quantity of clinical research, increased availability of evidence-based practice guidelines and synthesis reports, and growing evidence of positive outcomes should assure an increase in use of evidence based healthcare practices, but the evidence does not support this (Clark, 2005; Mangione-Smith et al., 2007; McGlynn et al., 2003; Titler, 2006; Zuckerman, Stevens, Inkelas, and Halfon, 2004). Use of evidence-based practice remains inconsistent, with studies showing that it takes as long as two decades for research findings to become incorporated into everyday practice unless interventions are actively used to increase the rate and extent of adoption of evidence-based practice in the clinical setting (Agency for Healthcare Research and Quality (AHRQ), 2001).

The push for use of evidence-based practice leaves the clinician asking how best to implement practice changes, and more specifically, what implementation strategies will increase the rate of adoption of an evidence-based healthcare practice in their clinical setting, and leaves researchers wondering how to test multiple and overlapping implementation strategies (Titler, 2004a). Translation science, also known as implementation science, is a relatively new area of research which tests the effects of interventions aimed at improving the rate and extent of adoption of evidence-based practices by nurses, physicians, and other healthcare providers (Titler, 2005, 2007). The goal of implementation science is to identify interventions or factors that promote or hinder adoption of evidence-based health care practices by individuals and organizations, in order to improve clinical and operational decision making (Titler, 2004a; Titler, Everett, and Adams, 2007).

Evidence-Based Practice Models

Experts in translation science support the use of a theoretical model to guide implementation strategies as a way to explore possible relationships among concepts, reduce the likelihood of overlooking important factors that may influence the success or failure of practice change occurring and being sustained, and provide a guide when evaluating the results of the implementation strategies (Grimshaw, Eccles, Walker, and Thomas, 2002; ICEBeRG, 2006). The difficulty comes in choosing an appropriate theoretical model from the multitude available (Estabrooks, Thompson, Lovely, and Hofmeyer, 2006; Grol and Grimshaw, 2003; ICEBeRG, 2006). A review of all models is beyond the scope of this article; the reader is referred to Grol and colleagues' (2007) recent review of models relevant to quality improvement and implementation of change in healthcare, which includes cognitive, educational, motivational, social interactive, social learning, social network, social influence theories, as well as those models related to team effectiveness, professional development, and leadership (Grol, Bosch, Hulscher, Eccles, and Wensing, 2007).

One model, the Translation Research Model (Figure 1) has been used to guide implementation strategies in a series of multi-site experimental studies funded by the Agency for Healthcare Research and Quality (PI Titler, RO1 HS10482 and PI Titler, 2 RO1 HS010482) and the National Cancer Institute (PI Herr, R01-CA115363-01). This model provides a framework for development of an implementation plan using effective implementation strategies to promote adoption of evidence-based practices (Titler and Everett, 2001a). The Translation Research Model, which continues to be supported through growing research in this field, is based on the ground breaking work of Everett Rogers, who proposed that "diffusion is the process by which an innovation is communicated through certain channels over time among members of a social system" (Rogers, 2003).

Evidence based strategies are provided in the Translation Research Model to target areas of potential influence identified by Rogers, such as the characteristics of the innovation (e.g., the use of evidence-based practice guidelines, practice prompts) to make it more easily adaptable, the communication channels (e.g., use of opinion leaders, educational outreach or academic detailing), the social system (e.g., modifying policies and procedures, obtaining leadership support) and individual users (e.g., performance gap assessment, focus group).

Implementation of evidence-based practice is accomplished by combining strategies from each component of the model. Using interactive and reinforcing strategies can be most effective, when based on a solid foundation. For example, credible evidence to support the proposed change, and education about the change are fundamental and necessary, but not sufficient to promote adoption of evidence-based healthcare (Atkins, Fink, and Slutsky, 2005; Bellomo and Bagshaw, 2006; Bloom, 2005; Greenhalgh et al., 2003; Jain et al., 2006; Leeman, Jackson, and Sandelowski, 2006; Lohr, 2004; Mansouri and Lockyer, 2007; Marinopoulos et al., 2007; O'Brien et al., 2001; Perria et al., 2007).

We know from Rogers' work that while education raises awareness, education alone does little to change behavior (Rogers, 2003).

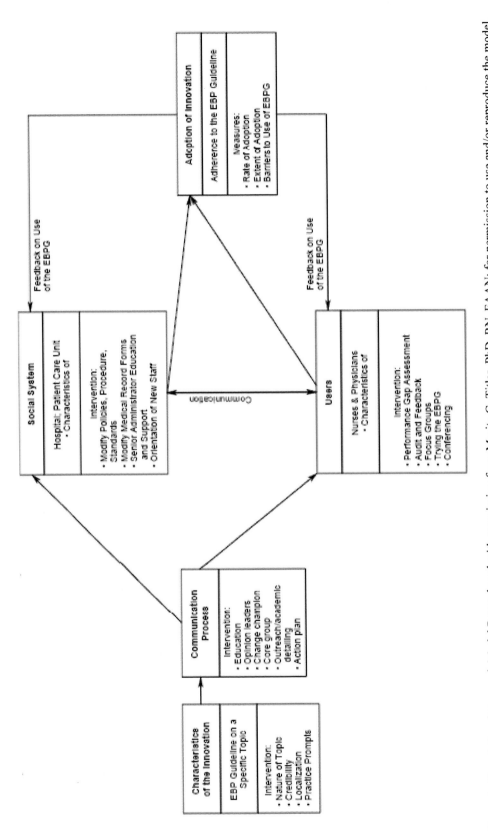

Figure 1. Translational Research Model Reproduced with permission from Marita G. Titler, PhD, RN, FAAN; for permission to use and/or reproduce the model, please contact Dr. Titler. Copyright will be retained by Dr. Titler and the University of Iowa Hospitals and Clinics. (Titler, M.G. and Everett, L.Q., 2001).

According to Rogers, peer influence is most effective in persuading people to adopt new practices. Indeed, empirical evidence suggests that information gained through social networks is highly influential in the spread of innovations, such as evidence-based healthcare practices (Greenhalgh, Robert, Macfarlane, Bate, and Kyriakidou, 2004; Rogers, 2003). While studies suggest that nurses prefer receiving information from other nurses they know personally (Adams, 2007; Estabrooks, Chong, Brigidear, and Profetto-McGrath, 2005; Estabrooks et al., 2005; Pravikoff, Tanner, and Pierce, 2005), a recent study by Adams (2007) indicates that while preferred, this source of information may not be associated with better practice. Therefore, integrity of the messenger, the validity of the message, and the channels used to transfer the message are all crucial components to the implementation plan. Using a core group or team with the same practice improvement goals, along with a knowledgeable opinion leader, increases the likelihood of promoting and sustaining the adoption of the evidence-based healthcare practice (Dopson, FitzGerald, Ferlie, Gabbay, and Locock, 2002; Nelson et al., 2002; Rogers, 2003; Titler, In press). This combination of implementation strategies allows nurses to continue to use their preferred approach of using the expertise of other nurse colleagues to address practice issues at hand, and still be assured of receiving accurate, evidenced-based information.

Hierarchy of Evidence

Credible evidence is fundamental for use of evidence-based practice (Rogers, 2003) yet there is continuing discussion about the most appropriate level and quality of evidence needed to support particular practice recommendations (Greenhalgh, 2002). The traditional research hierarchy using the medical model includes systematic reviews with a meta-analysis of randomized control trials as the highest level evidence with well conducted randomized controlled studies following next in line respectively. The lowest level of evidence is often expert opinion or case reports, with qualitative research designs excluded. These different levels are frequently schematically demonstrated using a pyramid structure (Health Links University of Washington, 2007). Nurses recognize that nursing research questions may be most appropriately answered using study designs other than randomized control trials (Brown, 2008; Goode, 2000; Stetler et al., 2006). It has been ten years since nurse leaders began expressing concern that traditional hierarchies of evidence ignore research designs central to certain nursing theoretical perspectives (Dicenso and Cullum, 1998; Greenhalgh, 2002; Mitchell, 1999). While nurses often still return to the traditional research hierarchy when evaluating and including evidence for systematic reviews (Thompson, Estabrooks, Scott-Findlay, Moore, and Wallin, 2007), in reality they often seek other forms of evidence to guide practice including qualitative studies and even quality improvement data (Goode, 2000; Stetler and Caramanica, 2007; Stetler et al., 2006).

Should practice be changed using anything less than randomized controlled trials and is other evidence acceptable? The answer is complex but large randomized control trial designed studies may be impractical, inappropriate, or unavailable for answering nursing practice questions. Nursing practice issues and nursing research often fit both within and between the highest and lowest levels of research posing distinct challenges to answering nursing questions using the traditional hierarchy.

Smith and Pell (2006) provide a humorous but thought provoking example when articulating the challenges of attempting to develop a systematic review of evidence addressing use of parachutes when jumping from an aircraft at elevated altitudes (Smith and Pell, 2006). They fail to develop a systematic review from a meta-analysis because of a lack of randomized control trials testing the efficacy of parachutes. The evidence supporting use of parachutes is merely observational; the inappropriateness of conducting a randomized control trial comes in finding participants to randomize to the "no parachute" group. In spite of the lack of "credible" evidence, few people would attempt a jump from a plane without a parachute. They clearly point out the problem that can arise when relying on randomized control trials as the exclusive design to use when addressing clinical issues. This illustrates the value of using other "lower level" forms of evidence to supplement randomized control trials when answering important clinical issues.

This bias toward randomized control trials carries over into implementation science. Strategies used for implementation of evidence-based practice are often discarded if not tested using a randomized control methodology, yet this method may not be appropriate for evaluating multifaceted strategies in a clinical setting with practitioners from various disciplines (Foxcroft and Cole, 2000; Thompson, Estabrooks, Scott-Findlay, Moore, and Wallin, 2007). Because of this some implementation strategies are well researched but in narrow application (e.g., academic detailing). Other implementation strategies have little research testing their effectiveness (e.g., action planning) (Shimizu and Shimanouchi, 2006). We are beyond the point of isolating individual strategies to test through randomized controlled trials. Differing research methods are needed to evaluate use of multifaceted strategies in complex clinical settings.

Academic detailing is an excellent example of an implementation strategy with a large body of evidence, but one of narrow focus. Academic detailing is an implementation strategy that has been used for decades but has been narrowly tested, often as a single intervention to promote adoption of evidence-based practice. Academic detailing, also called educational outreach visits, are presentations by a trained person who meets one-on-one with practitioners in their setting to provide information about the evidence-based practice and may include feedback on the provider's performance (Avorn and Soumerai, 1983; O'Brien et al., 2007; Sohn, Ismail, and Tellez, 2004; Titler, 2002). Academic detailing has long been used as a strategy by pharmaceutical representatives and pharmacists to influence physician prescribing practices in primary care settings (O'Brien et al., 2007). While a few studies evaluated using specialty nurses and general practitioners, testing beyond the primary care setting, on topics other than physician prescribing and with non-pharmacist detailers is limited. Research using this technique is limited in acute care, long-term care, home care, school nursing and other settings. In spite of its narrow focus, or perhaps because of it, the level of evidence supporting academic detailing is generally high on the traditional evidence pyramid. The vast majority of research supports the effectiveness of academic detailing (Cullen, 2007a; O'Brien et al., 2007), yet testing the use of academic detailing as a multifaceted strategy in clinical settings with various healthcare practitioners is needed. Despite the challenges involved in multisite clinical research, Titler, et al (AHRQ study) has expanded the evidence base by demonstrating that use of academic detailing increases use of evidence-based practice among staff nurses, when combined with other implementation techniques. Additional research is needed to determine how this implementation strategy can best be adapted for use by different roles, with different expertise and within other healthcare settings.

A great deal is both known and still not understood about academic detailing, indicating the need for more research on implementation strategies that are currently being used to increase the rate and extent of adoption of evidence-based healthcare practices. The paucity of evidence for use among staff nurses provides a call for research using various methodologies to evaluate implementation strategies with nurses as the end users in the varied settings within which they work. In addition, despite the large volume of studies on academic detailing, research is still needed in a number of areas (Box 1). It is clear that combining academic detailing with other strategies (Titler, In press) is important, as single interventions are less likely to successfully facilitate adoption of evidence-based practice recommendations, but it is not clear which other strategies and how those strategies should be used in combination for the greatest impact. Sustainability over time always remains an open question requiring additional research. Meta-analyses and multiple multi-site randomized controlled trials have demonstrated the effectiveness of academic detailing, yet multiple questions still need to be addressed. Academic detailing provides an additional example of the usefulness and limitations of evidence hierarchies.

Box 1. Issues related to use of academic detailing or educational outreach remaining to be addressed through conduct of research

- Clarifying the training needed for detailers.
- Determining how to measure and define the social interaction between detailers and practitioners.
- Determining how to identify or measure the differing communication skills of detailers.
- Clarifying who should do detailing (e.g., MD, RN, pharmD) and whether or not using different clinicians actually matters.
- Determining how to measure the appropriate dose of contacts, i.e, the effectiveness of academic detailing as individual or a series of sessions, or the frequency of follow-up needed.
- Testing in additional settings; the research is predominantly in primary care settings so it is unclear how system and user characteristics relate to the effectiveness of academic detailing.
- Determining how individual vs. group sessions may impact the effectiveness of academic detailing in different settings and
- Measuring the cost effectiveness of each approach is still needed.
- Determining how to effectively combine strategies
- Determining sustainability of the practice change

Priorities for Future Research:
A Call to Action

There is a growing recognition of the importance of organizational context on the rate, extent and sustainability of evidence-based healthcare practices (Dopson, FitzGerald, Ferlie, Gabbay, and Locock, 2002; Ferlie and Shortell, 2001; Rogers, 2003; Scott-Findlay and Golden-Biddle, 2005; Titler, 2002). Research to better understand and measure organizational context was rated the top priority by a leading group of translation scientists (Titler, 2005; Titler, Cullen, Buckwalter, and et al, In review). The organizational context consists of core elements that include culture and climate, interactive human relationships, and the measurement and evaluation processes specific to the organization. Yet, there is no general consensus on which core set of elements of the organization, or combination of elements, are key to promoting evidence-based practice. The challenge arises because the climate and culture of an individual practice environment is the combination and interaction of the characteristics of the organization and of the individuals working there, resulting in a complex and dynamic context that is unique to each practice setting. Dissemination strategies that focus primarily on the individual adopters or organizational structural change and minimize the importance of the dynamic, interactive organizational context may overlook key variables that influence adoption of evidence-based practice (Garside, 1998; Greenhalgh, Robert, Bate, Macfarlane, and Kyriakidou, 2005; Scott, Mannion, Davies, and Marshall, 2003).

A Cochrane systematic review done in 2000 (Foxcroft and Cole, 2000) on the impact of organizational infrastructures in promoting use of evidence-based practices reported locating no studies of sufficient quality, yet only RCT's, controlled clinical trials, and interrupted time series studies were included. It may be unrealistic to expect that these study designs could unravel the influences of organizational context due to its dynamic, fluid and interactive nature. Descriptive and qualitative studies, and case reports may provide more understanding of this interactive organizational context and its impact on the rate, extent and sustainability of evidence-based practice (Greenhalgh, 2002; Greenhalgh, Robert, Macfarlane, Bate, and Kyriakidou, 2004; Stetler, 2003; Stetler and Caramanica, 2007; Stetler et al., 2006).

Leadership is one important contextual factor impacting an organization's ability to consistently use evidence to inform practice (Aarons, 2006; Davies et al., 2006; Fleuren, Wiefferink, and Paulussen, 2004; Vaughn et al., 2002; World Health Organization, 2007). An exhaustive body of research on barriers consistently finds that leadership support is essential (Fink, Thompson, and Bonnes, 2005; Funk, Champagne, Wiese, and Tornquist, 1991a; Funk, Champagne, Wiese, and Tornquist, 1991b; Hutchinson and Johnston, 2006; Ring, Malcolm, Coull, Murphy-Black, and Watterson, 2005) and leaders have responsibility to provide resources, structures and processes (Fink, Thompson, and Bonnes, 2005; Hutchinson and Johnston, 2006; Pravikoff, Tanner, and Pierce, 2005). There is a call for research to better understand the impact of leadership on adoption of evidence-based practice and the impact on patient outcomes (Gifford, Davies, Edwards, Griffin, and Lybanon, 2007; Greenhalgh, Robert, Macfarlane, Bate, and Kyriakidou, 2004; Reeleder, Goel, Singer, and Martin, 2006; Shortell, 2004; Stetler, 2003). Expanding research to better understand organizational leadership was rated as very important (mean 4.2, 1-5 scale from not important to very important) for advancing our understanding of translation science (Titler, 2005; Titler, Cullen, Buckwalter, and et al, In review). More recent research has demonstrated the positive impact of leadership (Davies et al., 2006; Wallin, Rudberg, and Gunningberg, 2005) and a beginning understanding of how leaders can promote evidence-based practice (Newhouse, 2007; Udod, 2004). This early work remains relatively conceptual (Antrobus and Kitson, 1999; Davies et al., 2006; Gifford, Davies, Edwards, Griffin, and Lybanon, 2007; Gifford, 2006; Nagy, Lumby, McKinley, and Macfarlane, 2001; Newhouse, 2007) and continues to leave nursing leaders in the trenches without clear direction while juggling multiple completing demands.

Leading evidence-based practice changes can be difficult and nursing leaders have insufficient guidance from well developed research to guide use of specific leadership strategies and may have received insufficient tools or training to integrate the work and reap the benefits (Udod, 2004). A recent review by Gifford et al., (2007) provides beginning direction for leadership strategies that promote evidence-based care. Not surprisingly the roles are directed toward impacting the social system and organizational infrastructure (e.g., revising policies and capturing evidence-based practice work within the quality improvement systems) and expanding organizational capacity for innovation (Batalden, Nelson, Edwards, Godfrey, and Mohr, 2003; Cullen, Greiner, Greiner, Bombei, and Comried, 2005; Fleuren, Wiefferink, and Paulussen, 2004; Vaughn et al., 2002). Nursing leaders need additional leadership strategies to support clinicians' use of evidence. Despite early work identifying the importance of leadership, a great deal of research continues to be needed in this area.

Conclusion

It is clear that the use of evidence based practice is the expected standard of care both nationally and internationally, and will remain so because of its established impact on patient outcomes and the cost of care delivery. Not only do we need to use evidence in practice, we must use evidence-based (i.e., tested) strategies in promoting and implementing the evidence-based healthcare practices themselves. Use of a model, such as the Translation Research Model (Titler and Everett, 2001a) can guide the selection of strategies, but specific strategies may need further research using designs appropriate for nurses focusing on nurses as the end users and in various settings where nurses work. We need to recognize the potential pitfalls and limitations of using strategies tested in other settings, and of discarding studies that do not use randomized control trial designs. Many effective strategies are described in the Translational Research Model (e.g., academic detailing, audit and feedback, practice prompts or reminders). Despite the research supporting use of effective strategies for implementing evidence-based practice changes, use of ineffective implementation strategies persists (Bloom, 2005). In fact, Bloom (2005) states that use of these ineffective implementation strategies results in "reduced patient care quality and raises costs for all, the worst of both worlds" (Bloom, 2005). There is an evidence-base for implementing practice changes through translation research, and all levels of evidence should be evaluated for appropriateness for use. This is a call to action for research to better understand how implementation strategies used within organizational systems and leadership can promote provision of evidence-based healthcare by nurses in the multiple settings within which they work.

References

Aarons, G. A. (2006). Transformational and transactional leadership: Association with attitudes toward evidence-based practice. *Psychiatric Services, 57*(8).

Adams, S. (2007). *Understand the context for translation of evidence-based practice into school nursing.* Unpublished Dissertation, University of Iowa College of Nursing.

Agency for Healthcare Research and Quality (AHRQ). (2001). TRIP Fact sheet: Translating research into practice.

AHRQ. (2000). *Routine Preoperative Testing Before Cataract Surgery. Clinical Highlights.* Retrieved. From *http://www.ahrq.gov/clinic/precataract.htm.*

AHRQ. (2003). *Treatment to Prevent Sudden Cardiac Death. Clinical Highlights.* . Retrieved. From *http://www.ahrq.gov/clinic/suddcard.htm.*

AHRQ (Ed.). (2005). *Commitment to Respond to COMMIT/CCS-2 Trial Beta Blocker Use for Myocardial Infarction (MI) Within 24 Hours of Hospital Arrival.* Practice Advisory. Rockville, MD: Agency for Healthcare Research and Quality. *http://www.ahrq.gov/clinic/commitadvisory.htm.*

American Nurses Association. (2004). *Nursing: Scope and standards of practice.* Washington, DC: American Nurses Publishing.

Antrobus, S., and Kitson, A. (1999). Nursing leadership: influencing and shaping health policy and nursing practice. *Journal of Advanced Nursing, 29*(3), 746-753.

Asch, S. M., Kerr, E. A., Keesey, J., Adams, J., Setodji, C., Malik, S., et al. (2006). Who is at greatest risk for receiving poor-quality health care? *The New England Journal of Medicine, 354*(11).

Atkins, D., Fink, K., and Slutsky, J. (2005). Better information for better health care: The evidence-based practice center program and the agency for healthcare research and quality. *Annals of Internal Medicine, 142*(12).

Avorn, J., and Soumerai, S. B. (1983). Improving drug-therapy decisions through educational outreach. A randomized controlled trial of academically based "detailing". *The New England Journal of Medicine, 308*(24), 1457-1463.

Batalden, P. B., Nelson, E. C., Edwards, W. H., Godfrey, M. M., and Mohr, J. J. (2003). Microsystems in health care: Part 9. Developing small clinical units to attain peak performance. *Joint Commission Journal on Quality and Safety, 29*(11).

Bellomo, R., and Bagshaw, S. M. (2006). Evidence-based medicine: Classifying the evidence from clinical trials - the need to consider other dimensions. *Critical Care, 10,* 232.

Bloom, B. (2005). Effects of continuing medical education on improving physician clinical care and patient health: A review of systematic reviews. *International Journal of Technology Assessment in Health Care, 21*(3), 380-385.

Brown, S. (2008). *Evidence-Based Nursing.* Sudbury, Massachusetts: Jones and Bartlett Publishers.

Clark, A. (2005). Measuring quality of care nationwide. *Caring, 24*(3).

Cullen, L. (2007a). *Expert panel on implementation strategies: Focus on academic detailing.* Paper presented at the 14th National Evidence-Based Practice Conference, Iowa City, IA.

Cullen, L. (2007b). *Moving nursing's agenda forward into the 21st century: Sigma Theta Tau International's position on evidence-based practice.* Paper presented at the Sigma Theta Tau International 39th Biennial Convention, Baltimore, MD.

Cullen, L., Greiner, J., Greiner, J., Bombei, C., and Comried, L. (2005). Excellence in evidence-based practice: organizational and unit exemplars. *Critical Care Nursing Clinics of North America, 17*(2), 127-142.

Davies, B., Edwards, N., Ploeg, J., Virani, T., Skelly, J., and Dobbins, M. (2006). *Determinants of the sustained use of research evidence in nursing: Final Report.* Ottawa, Ontario, Canada: Canadian Health Services Research Foundation and Canadian Institutes for Health Research.

DePalma, J. A. (2000). Evidence-based clinical practice guidelines. *Seminars in Perioperative Nursing, 9*(3), 115-120.

Dicenso, A., and Cullum, N. (1998). Implementing evidence-based nursing: Some misconceptions. *Evidence-Based Nursing, 1*(2), 38.

Dopson, S., FitzGerald, L., Ferlie, E., Gabbay, J., and Locock, L. (2002). No Magic Targets! Changing Clinical Practice To Become More Evidence Based. *Health Care Management Review, 27*(3), 35.

Estabrooks, C. A., Chong, H., Brigidear, K., and Profetto-McGrath, J. (2005). Profiling Canadian nurses' preferred knowledge sources for clinical practice. *Canadian Journal of Nursing Leadership, 37*(2), 118-140.

Estabrooks, C. A., Rutakumwa, W., O'Leary, K. A., Profetto-McGrath, J., Milner, M., Levers, M. J., et al. (2005). Sources of practice knowledge among nurses. *Qualitative Health Research, 15*(4), 460-476.

Estabrooks, C. A., Thompson, D. S., Lovely, J. J., and Hofmeyer, A. (2006). A guide to knowledge translation theory. *Journal of Continuing Education in the Health Professions, 26*(1), 25-36.

Ferlie, E. B., and Shortell, S. M. (2001). Improving the Quality of Health Care in the United Kingdom and the United States: A Framework for Change. *Milbank Quarterly, 79*, 281.

Fink, R., Thompson, C. J., and Bonnes, D. (2005). Overcoming barriers and promoting the use of research in practice. *Journal of Nursing Administration, 35*(3).

Fleuren, M., Wiefferink, K., and Paulussen, T. (2004). Determinants of innovation within health care organizations. *International Journal for Quality in Health Care, 16*(2), 107-123.

Foxcroft, D., and Cole, N. (2000). Organisational infrastructures to promote evidence based nursing practice. *Cochrane Database of Systematic Reviews*(Issue 3), Art. No.: CD002212. DOI: 002210.001002/14651858.CD14002212.

Funk, S., Champagne, M., Wiese, R., and Tornquist, E. (1991a). Barriers: the barriers to research utilization scale. *Applied Nursing Research, 4*(1), 39-45.

Funk, S. G., Champagne, M. T., Wiese, R. A., and Tornquist, E. M. (1991b). Barriers to using research findings in practice: the clinician's perspective. *Applied Nursing Research, 4*(2), 90-95.

Garber, A. M. (2001). Evidence-based coverage policy. *Health Affairs (Millwood), 20*(5), 62-82.

Garside, P. (1998). Organisational context for quality: lessons from the fields of organisational development and change management. *Quality in Health Care, 7 (Suppl),* S8-S15.

Gifford, W., Davies, B., Edwards, N., Griffin, P., and Lybanon, V. (2007). Managerial leadership for nurses' use of research evidence: an integrative review of the literature. *Worldviews on Evidence-Based Nursing, 4*(3), 126-145.

Gifford, W. A. (2006). Nursing research: Leadership strategies to influence the use of clinical practice guidelines. *Canadian Journal of Nursing Leadership, 19*(4), 72-88.

Goode, C. J. (2000). What constitutes the "evidence" in evidence-based practice? *Applied Nursing Research, 13*(4), 222-225.

Greenhalgh, T. (2002). Integrating qualitative research into evidence based practice. *Endocrinology and Metabolism Clinical of North America, 31*(3), 583-601.

Greenhalgh, T., Robert, G., Bate, P., Macfarlane, F., and Kyriakidou, O. (2005). *Diffusion of innovations in health service organizations*. Massachusetts: Blackwell Publishing Ltd.

Greenhalgh, T., Robert, G., Macfarlane, F., Bate, P., and Kyriakidou, O. (2004). Diffusion of innovations in service organizations: systematic review and recommendations. *Milbank Quarterly, 82*(4), 581-629.

Greenhalgh, T., Toon, P., Russell, J., Wong, G., Plumb, L., and Macfarlane, F. (2003). Transferability of principles of evidence-based medicine to improve educational quality: systematic review and case study of an online course in primary health care. *British Medical Journal, 326.*

Grimshaw, J. M., Eccles, M. P., Walker, A. E., and Thomas, R. E. (2002). Changing physicians' behavior: what works and thoughts on getting more things to work. *The Journal of Continuing Education in the Health Professions, 22*(4), 237-243.

Grol, R., and Grimshaw, J. (2003). From best evidence to best practice: effective implementation of change in patients' care. *Lancet, 362*(9391), 1225-1230.

Grol, R. P., Bosch, M. C., Hulscher, M. E., Eccles, M. P., and Wensing, M. (2007). Planning and studying improvement in patient care: the use of theoretical perspectives. *Milbank Quarterly, 85*(1), 93-138.

Health Links University of Washington. (2007). Retrieved March 2007, from *http://images.google.com/imgres?imgurl=http://healthlinks.washington.edu/ebp/images/ pyramid_50_pct.gifandimgrefurl=http://healthlinks.washington.edu/ebp/ebptools.htmlan dh=317andw=318andsz=10andhl=enandstart=1andtbnid=AjvxRs4oSNJ2hM:andtbnh= 118andtbnw=118andprev=/images%3Fq%3Devidence%2Bpyramid%26gbv%3D2%26sv num%3D10%26hl%3Den*

Hutchinson, A., and Johnston, L. (2006). Beyond the BARRIERS scale. *Journal of Nursing Administration, 36*(4), 189.

ICEBeRG. (2006). Designing theoretically-informed implementation interventions. *Implementation Science, 1,* 4.

Jain, M. K., Heyland, D., Dhaliwal, R., Day, A. G., Drover, J., Keefe, L., et al. (2006). Dissemination of the Canadian clinical practice guidelines for nutrition support: Results of a cluster randomized control trial. *Critical Care Medicine, 34*(9).

Leeman, J., Jackson, B., and Sandelowski, M. (2006). An evaluation of how well research reports facilitate the use of findings in practice. *Journal of Nursing Scholarship, 38*(2), 171-177.

Lohr, K. N. (2004). Rating the strength of scientific evidence: relevance for quality improvement programs. *International Journal for Quality in Health Care, 16*(1), 9-18.

Mangione-Smith, R., DeCristofaro, A., Setodji, C., Keesey, J., Klein, D. J., Adams, J., et al. (2007). The quality of ambulatory care delivered to children in the United States. *The New England Journal of Medicine, 357*(15), 15-23.

Mansouri, M., and Lockyer, J. (2007). A meta-analysis of continuing medical education effectiveness. *Journal of Continuing Education in the Health Professions, 27*(1), 6-15.

Marinopoulos, S., Dorman, T., Ratanawongsa, N., Wilson, L., Ashar, B., Magaziner, J., et al. (2007). *Effectiveness of continuing medical education.* Evidence Report/Technology Assessment No. 149. AHRQ Publication No. 07-E006. Rockville, MD: Agency for Healthcare Quality and Research.

McCormack, B., Rycroft-Malone, J., Cullen, L., Griffith, R., and DiCenso, A. (under development). *Sigma Theta Tau International's position on evidence-based practice.*

McGlynn, E. A., Asch, S. M., Adams, J., Keesey, J., Hicks, J., DeCristofaro, A., et al. (2003). The quality of health care delivered to adults in the United States. *The New England Journal of Medicine, 348*(26), 35-45.

McInerny, T. K., Cull, W. L., and Yudkowsky, B. K. (2005). Physician reimbursement levels and adherence to American Academy of Pediatrics well-visit and immunization recommendations. *Pediatrics, 115*(4).

Mitchell, G. J. (1999). Evidence-based practice: critique and alternative view. *Nursing Science Quarterly, 12*(1), 30-35.

Nagy, S., Lumby, J., McKinley, S., and Macfarlane, C. (2001). Nurses' beliefs about the conditions that hinder or support evidence-based nursing. *International Journal of Nursing Practice, 7*, 314-321.

Nelson, E. C., Batalden, P. B., Huber, T. P., Mohr, J. J., Godfrey, M. M., Headrick, L. A., et al. (2002). Microsystems in health care: part 1. Learning from high-performing front-line clinical units. *Joint Commission Journal on Quality Improvement, 28*(9), 472-493.

Newhouse, R. P. (2007). Creating Infrastructure Supportive of Evidence-Based Nursing Practice: Leadership Strategies *Worldviews on Evidence-Based Nursing, 4*(1), 21-29.

O'Brien, M. A., Freemantle, N., Oxman, A. D., Wolf, F., Davis, D. A., and Herrin, J. (2001). Continuing education meetings and workshops: Effects on professional practice and health care outcomes. *The Cochrane Database of Systematic Reviews, 2*, Art. No.: CD003030. DOI: 003010.001002/14651858.CD14003030.

O'Brien, M. A., Rogers, S., Jamtvedt, G., Oxman, A., Odgaard-Jensen, J., Kristoffersen, D., et al. (2007). Educational outreach visits: effects on professional practice and health care outcomes. *Cochrane Database of Systematic Reviews*(4), No. CD000409. DOI.001002/14651858.CD14000409.pub14651852.

Perencevich, E. N., Stone, P. W., Wright, S. B., Carmeli, Y., Fisman, D. N., and Cosgrove, S. E. (2007). Raising standards while watching the bottom line: Making a business case for infection control. *Infection Control and Hospital Epidemiology, 28*(10).

Perria, C., Mandolini, D., Guerrera, C., Jefferson, T., Billi, P., Calzini, V., et al. (2007). Implementing a guideline for the treatment of type 2 diabetics: results of a Cluster-Randomized Controlled Trial (C-RCT). *BMC Health Services Research, 7*(79).

Peterson, E. D., Roe, M. T., Mulgond, J., DeLong, E. R., Lytle, B. L., Brindis, R. G., et al. (2006). Association between hospital process performance and outcomes among patients with acute coronary syndromes. *The Journal of the American Medical Association, 295*(16).

Pravikoff, D. S., Tanner, A. B., and Pierce, S. T. (2005). Readiness of U.S. nurses for evidence-based practice. *American Journal of Nursing, 105*(9), 40-51; quiz 52.

Reeleder, D., Goel, V., Singer, P. A., and Martin, D. K. (2006). Leadership and priority setting: The perspective of hospital CEOs. *Health Policy, 79*, 24-34.

Ring, N., Malcolm, C., Coull, A., Murphy-Black, T., and Watterson, A. (2005). Nursing best practice statements: an exploration of their implementation in clinical practice. *Journal of Clinical Nursing, 14*, 1048-1058.

Rogers, E. (2003). *Diffusion of innovations* (5th ed.). New York: Simon and Schuster, Inc.

Sackett, D. L., Rosenberg, W. M., Gray, J. A., Haynes, R. B., and Richardson, W. S. (1996). Evidence based medicine: what it is and what it isn't. *British Medical Journal, 312*(7023), 71-72.

Sackett, D. L., Straus, S. E., Richardson, W. S., Rosenberg, W. M., and Haynes, R. B. (2000). *Evidence-based medicine: How to practice and teach EBM* (2nd ed.). Edinburg: Churchill Livingstone.

Scott-Findlay, S., and Golden-Biddle, K. (2005). Understanding how organizational culture shapes research use. *Journal of Nursing Administration, 35*(7-8), 359-365.

Scott, T., Mannion, R., Davies, H., and Marshall, M. (2003). The quantitative measurement of organizational culture in health care: a review of the available instruments. *Health Services Research, 38*(3), 923-945.

Shimizu, Y., and Shimanouchi, S. (2006). Effective components of staff and organizational development for client outcomes by implementation of action plans in home care. *International Medical Journal, 13*(3), 175-183.

Shortell, S. M. (2004). Increasing value: A research agenda for addressing the managerial and organizational challenges facing health care delivery in the United States. *Medical Care Research and Review, 61*(3).

Shrank, W. H., Asch, S. M., Adams, J., Setodji, C., Kerr, E. A., Keesey, J., et al. (2006). The quality of pharmacologic care for adults in the United States. *Medical Care, 44*(10).

Smith, G. C., and Pell, J. P. (2006). Parachute use to prevent death and major trauma related to gravitational challenge: systematic review of randomised controlled trials. *International Journal of Prosthodontics, 19*(2), 126-128.

Sohn, W., Ismail, A., and Tellez, M. (2004). Efficacy of educational interventions targeting primary care providers practice behaviors: An overview of published systematic reviews. *Journal of Public Health Dentistry, 64*(3), 164-172.

Stetler, C. B. (2003). Role of the organization in translating research into evidence-based practice. *Outcomes Management, 7*(3), 97-103; quiz 104-105.

Stetler, C. B., and Caramanica, L. (2007). Evaluation of an evidence-based practice initiative: outcomes, strengths and limitations of a retrospective, conceptually-based approach. *Worldviews on Evidence-Based Nursing, 4*(4), 187-199.

Stetler, C. B., Legro, M. W., Rycroft-Malone, J., Bowman, C., Curran, G., Guihan, M., et al. (2006). Role of "external facilitation" in implementation of research findings: a qualitative evaluation of facilitation experiences in the Veterans Health Administration. *Implementation Science, 1*, 23.

Thompson, D. S., Estabrooks, C. A., Scott-Findlay, S., Moore, K., and Wallin, L. (2007). Interventions aimed at increasing research use in nursing: a systematic review. *Implementation Science, 2*, 15.

Titler, M. G. (2002). *Toolkit for promoting Evidence-based Practice*: Iowa City, Iowa: University of Iowa Hospitals and Clinics.

Titler, M. G. (2004a). Methods in Translation Science. *Worldviews on Evidence-Based Nursing, 1*, 38-48.

Titler, M. G. (2005). *Moving Evidence-Based Practice Forward: Priorities for Translation.* Paper presented at the 12th National Evidence-Based Practice Conference, University of Iowa Hospitals and Clinics, Iowa City, IA.

Titler, M. G. (2006). Developing an evidence-based practice. In G. LoBiondo-Wood and J. Haber (Eds.), *Nursing Research: Methods and critical appraisal for evidence-based practice* (6th ed.). St. Louis: Mosby.

Titler, M. G. (2007). *Moving Nursing's Agenda Forward into the 21st Century: Sigma Theta Tau International's Position on Translation Research.* Paper presented at the Sigma Theta Tau, International 39th Biennial Convention, Baltimore, MD.

Titler, M. G. (In press). The evidence for evidence-based practice implementation. In R. Hughes (Ed.), *Advances in patient safety and quality.* Rockville, MD: Agency for Healthcare Research and Quality.

Titler, M. G., Cullen, L., Buckwalter, K. C., and et al. (In review). Future research agenda for translation science.

Titler, M. G., and Everett, L. Q. (2001a). Translating research into practice. Considerations for critical care investigators. *Critical Care Nursing Clinics of North America, 13*(4), 587-604.

Titler, M. G., Everett, L. Q., and Adams, S. (2007). Implications for Implementation Science. *Nursing Research, 56*(4S), S53-S59.

Titler, M. G., Kleiber, C., Steelman, V. J., Rakel, B. A., Budreau, G., Buckwalter, K. C., et al. (2001b). The Iowa Model of Evidence-Based Practice to Promote Quality Care. *Critical Care Nursing Clinics of North America, 13*(4), 497-509.

Udod, S. A. C., W.D. (2004). Innovation in leadership. Setting the climate for evidence-based nursing practice: what is the leader's role? *Canadian Journal of Nursing Leadership, 17*(4), 64-75.

Vaughn, T. E., McCoy, K. D., BootsMiller, B. J., Woolson, R. F., Sorofman, B., Tripp-Reimer, T., et al., (2002). Organizational predictors of adherence to ambulatory care screening guidelines. *Medical Care, 40*(12), 1172-1185.

Wallin, L., Rudberg, A., and Gunningberg, L. (2005). Staff experiences in implementing guidelines for Kangaroo Mother Care--a qualitative study. *International Journal of Nursing Studies, 42*, 61-73.

Woolf, S. H., Grol, R., Hutchinson, A., Eccles, M., and Grimshaw, J. (1999). Clinical guidelines: potential benefits, limitations, and harms of clinical guidelines. *British Medical Journal, 318*(7182), 527-530.

World Health Organization. (2007). Practical guidance for scaling up health service innovations. Switzerland: World Health Organization.

Zuckerman, B., Stevens, G. D., Inkelas, M., and Halfon, N. (2004). Prevalence and correlates of high-quality basic pediatric preventive care. *Pediatrics, 114*, 1522-1529.

In: Trends in Nursing Research
Editors: Adam J. Ryan and Jack Doyle

ISBN 978-1-60456-642-0
© 2009 Nova Science Publishers, Inc.

Chapter 7

Chronic Pain among Older People

Ulf Jakobsson[*]

Department of Health Sciences, Faculty of Medicine, Lund University,
P.O. Box 157, SE-221 00 Lund, Sweden

Abstract

Age frequently carries the burden of diseases, many of which in turn are associated with discomfort and various complaints. Chronic pain is such a common complaint and is an important issue in the care of older people, and perhaps the most important problem in their daily lives. It is known to, alone or together with other factors, negatively affect an older person's quality of life. Examples of covariates to chronic pain are functional limitations, fatigue, sleeping problems, and depressed mood/depression. All these factors have been found to be more prevalent among people with chronic pain, but studies about these topics (in relation to pain) in older people are sparce, especially those focusing on fatigue and sleeping problems. Also the need for care and treatment is found to increase with increased degree of pain, especially among those with musculoskeletal pain. Despite this, studies focusing on chronic pain, pain management, and quality of life among older people (especially the oldest and frailest) are limited, and a pharmacological approach to diminishing pain dominates in the literature. A broad view is needed when studying pain as well as when caring for people in pain. This is especially important when the pain cannot be fully removed, and relief from suffering through other factors leading to increased quality of life is a more realistic option.

Ageing

The number of older people is increasing and hence age-related symptoms and diseases are also increasing. However, research regarding complaints, diseases and other health problems often does not include those over 65 and especially not the oldest and frailest. The

---

[*] E-mail: Ulf.Jakobsson@med.lu.se, Telephone: +46 46 222 19 24, Fax: +46 46 222 19 34

exclusion is often due to problems with co-morbidity, and hence the outcome may lack validity [1]. However, co-morbidity may be seen as more or less a habitual state for elderly people and should therefore be studied in this context.

The structure of the population is changing and people tend to live longer, leading to an increased number of very old people. For example, persons aged 65 years and above in Sweden have doubled their share of the population during the past forty years [2]. The large number of older people could be explained by the increase in average life expectancy. Additionally, when those who were born during and after World War II reach higher ages, the community will see an even larger growth in the elderly population in the future [2, 3]. With the increasing number of older people and hence age-related symptoms and diseases, health-care professionals need to know more about common health problems in older people. Thus, it seems urgent to gain knowledge about health problems such as chronic pain to meet the increasing demands in the health care of older people.

Older people do not seem to be a homogenous group, and the differences between the younger old and the oldest old tend to be great. There is, however, no consensus about how to categorise subgroups of older people. Therefore research about older people calls for definitions, e.g. of the meaning of being old and when a person becomes an older person. Previous research has made a division into younger old (65–74), old/mid-old (75–84) and oldest old (85+) [4]. A similar definition has been stated by Field and Minkler [5] as follows: young old (age 60–74), old old (75–84) and very old (85+). This division is often used in international literature, although it is based on chronological age and hence does not take, for example, social age, psychological age and biological age into consideration. Using categories other than chronological age raises methodological problems, and the division by chronological age in the older people may be the best option, especially if it is also combined with measures such as functional health status. Furthermore, chronological age makes it possible to make comparisons with other studies performed.

Ageing is a highly individualised process that affects each person in unique ways. It could be seen as the result of interaction between genetic factors, environmental influences, lifestyles and the effect of disease processes [6]. Ageing frequently carries the burden of chronic diseases, many of which are associated with pain and discomfort, as well as various other complaints [7]. Thus, it is highly important to gain knowledge and find solutions to actions that can be taken to ease such complaints. Research should especially focus on complaints/health problems common among older people, such as pain that may be caused by and lead to other complaints/health problems (e.g. functional limitations, fatigue) and decreased quality of life [8]. One of the challenges when studying ageing in the later years of adult life is differentiation of age-dependent biological changes from chronic illnesses and disease processes, because the probability of chronic health problems increases with age [9]. The distinction between "normal" and "abnormal", like the definitions of what is "normal", "abnormal" and "successful" ageing, is hard to make. The difference between successful and unsuccessful ageing is defined by most people as the difference between sickness and health [9].

Pain

The definition of pain, according to the International Association for Study of Pain (IASP), is an "unpleasant sensory and emotional experience associated with actual or potential tissue damage, or is described in terms of such damage" [10]. The definition also emphasises that pain is a subjective experience. The definition highlights various aspects of pain, e.g. that pain is a sensory as well as an emotional experience. However, pain is not only subjective but also a multidimensional phenomenon and some of the dimensions could be described as physical, psychological and social.

To understand pain and pain mechanisms, the gate-control theory was developed [11]. The theory proposes that the gate-control system modulates sensory input (pain) and that the transmission of the pain is not "all or nothing" but is modified by other phenomenon in the nervous system [11]. Nociceptive information is delivered from peripheral nerves through A-fibre and C-fibre to the dorsal horn (spinal cord). The nerve cells in the dorsal horn also receive sensory input other than pain signals from other nerves and this is said to be site of the "gate". If the dorsal horn is receiving information from a nociceptive and a non-nociceptive fibre at the same time, then the non-nociceptive input can moderate the nociceptive input [11]. This could explain the moderating effect on pain from, e.g. massage. The gate control theory is important for understanding pain, although the theory might be limited in that it overlooks the importance of environmental factors in the development of pain over time and the possible contribution of cognitive appraisal to the perception and the response to the pain.

Due to the limitations in the gate-control theory (i.e., its unidimensionality) Ronald Melzack developed a theory about the neuromatrix from the gate-control theory, and this meant a broader perspective on pain [12, 13]. The neuromatrix theory of pain proposes that the pain experience is determined by the synaptic architecture of the neuromatrix, which is produced by genetic and sensory influences [13]. It can be summarised as the brain generating perceptual experience even when no external inputs occur; the neural networks for perceiving the body and its parts are built into the brain. The brain is not passively receiving input from an active body but the brain itself generates the experience of the body, and sensory inputs merely modulate the experience, they do not directly cause it [12]. This theory could explain, e.g. phantom pain and a patient's experience of the pain in a missing limb [12]. Other phenomena such as distraction as a method for pain management may also be explained by this theory.

Pain can be divided into two different types of pain, acute and chronic [14]. *Acute pain* could be defined as pain with a well-defined time pattern of the beginning of the pain and with signs of hyperactivity in the autonomic nervous system often following [7]. Typical signs of this hyperactivity could be, e.g. perspiration and vasodilatation. However, these signs may not always be as obvious in older persons [7]. Acute pain also often responds well to treatment by analgesics and treatment for the reason behind the pain. *Chronic pain* is defined by IASP as the report of pain experience past expected healing time for particular tissue damage – usually operationalised as three months [15]. Chronic pain differs from acute pain in that the chronic pain generates changes in the central nervous system and is often more difficult to treat. There are adaptations in the autonomic nervous system leading to many symptoms that are frequent among those suffering from acute pain, diminish through time. This can make the observer (e.g., health-care professionals and relatives) doubt the genuineness of the patient's pain. However, it is of great important that the patient isn't mistrusted because it can lead to even worse pain and maybe also depressed mood/depression and other symptoms which in turn will make the pain even worse. Instead of signs of hyperactivity in the autonomic nervous system chronic pain causes changes in e.g., lifestyle, social relations, and functional and psychological health status.

Pain among Older People

Pain is an important issue in the care for older people, and perhaps the most important problem in their daily lives. It may, alone or together with other factors, negatively affect these people's quality of life [8]. Helme and Gibson [16] found in their review of studies focusing on older people that the prevalence of pain ranged from 29–86% among those aged 75–84 years and 40–79% among those aged 85 and above. A study in France showed a pain prevalence of 71.5% for people over 65 years and that 32.9% reported persisting pain [17]. Mobily et al. [18] found that 86% reported some type of pain for at least one year, and that 59% reported multiple pain locations. A study in Sweden showed a prevalence of chronic pain of about 68% for individuals over 85 years and 47.1% of the respondents reported pain in two or more locations [19]. Previous studies also show gender differences. The study also showed that musculoskeletal pain was more common among older men than among older women [19]. Magni et al. [20], in contrast, found when studying musculoskeletal pain in the USA that this type of pain was more common among old women than among old men. The results from various studies about how pain (non-disease-related) develops with age show inconsistency [21]. Brattberg et al. [22] found a slight decrease in the prevalence of pain after the age of 65. Brochet et al. [17] found the prevalence of pain among people over 65 years of age to be higher with increased age especially among women. Pain in older people is often musculoskeletal and common locations are limb, joints and back [17, 18]. For example, a study in Sweden showed that that the most common location of the pain was lower back (31.3%), shoulders/arms (30.7%), neck (26.2%), and legs (25.2%) [22].

Conclusions about whether pain, prevalence and the degree of the pain increase or decrease in old age differ between different studies [16, 21, 23]. A study in Sweden found that chronic pain was more common with higher age (age 75-79: 34.1%, age 80-84: 34.5%, age 85-89: 41.5%, and in the 90+ group: 50.1%) [8]. Grimby et al. [24] found no increase in pain with age but an increase in the use of minor analgesics. Brattberg et al. [22] found a slight decrease in the prevalence of pain after the age of 65. Brochet et al. [17] found the prevalence of pain among people over 65 years of age to be higher with increased age especially among women. Brattberg et al. [19] found a higher prevalence of chronic pain with age in men, but a lower prevalence with age was found among women. An explanation for the differences in prevalence could be differences in how large a share of the oldest old and the frailest was included in the studies. Another explanation for this could be that older people tend not to fully rate their pain and that they sometimes view pain as part of normal ageing and thus do not report it [21, 25]. Moreover, different use of designs, methods and ways of measuring pain could be other explanations. In any case, the results strongly indicate that pain is a common problem in old age and more so in the oldest age groups, hence the need for actions to be taken in the care of older people to ease their pain is obvious.

Rather few older people in chronic pain are diagnosed in terms of symptom-giving specific disorders/diseases. Various studies have shown that as many as 37-43% had not received any diagnosis/did not know the reason for the pain [c.f. 26]. This may cause problems when trying to cure or ease the pain because the cause behind the pain can then not be eliminated. Common causes of chronic pain among older people are e.g. osteoarthritis, various forms of arthritis, angina of effort/chest pain, arthralgia, herpes zoster, gout, and fractures [27, 28]. In nursing homes common causes of pain are reported to be various forms of arthritis, angina, cancer, atherosclerotic vascular disease, and herpes zoster [29]. Fractures are especially associated with increased morbidity and mortality among older people and are a considerable economic burden for the community [27]. Ferrell et al. [30] studied pain in nursing homes and found that most respondents reported the source of their pain (24% had constant pain, 47% had intermittent pain) as low-back pain (40%), previous fractures (14%), neuropathies (11%), leg cramps (9%), arthritic knee (9%). Persons with intermittent pain typically related their pain to movement, weight bearing, or overexertion [30].

Caring for people in pain can be a demanding task, and especially caring for older people in pain. One of the most important and maybe also the most difficult aspects of helping a person in pain is to accept and realise that only the person him-/herself can feel the pain, i.e. that the pain is completely subjective [31]. The patient's subjective reports are often used by health-care professionals to assess pain, but the reports are also judged against the patient's personality, past medical history and his/her own perceived notion of pain [32]. This may then result in poor agreement about the pain between the person in pain and the caregiver. A review of the literature shows that health-care professionals are often found to underestimate the pain, for various reasons, when performing clinical assessments [33]. Other problems that could appear, especially in the care of older people, may be related to the person in pain as well as to the caregiver. Examples of such hindrance are misconceptions that pain is a natural outcome of growing old, increased risks of side-effects related pharmacotherapy in older people, uncertainty about the effect of non-pharmacological methods, and the fact that older people may have e.g. hearing or vision problems that could complicate their ability to report pain or apply methods for pain management [31, 34]. In the care of older people in pain such hindrance to good care needs to be removed, and more research about pain and pain management among older people and well-educated caregivers may be some solutions. Further, the use of systematic assessment of the pain as well as pain management is a prerequisite for high-quality nursing care.

Factors Associated with Pain among Older People

Chronic pain should neither be studied nor treated in isolation. The individual will perceive pain based upon a range of physical, psychological and social factors, and hence the pain must be studied/treated from these perspectives. Furthermore, in the care of older people in pain, interventions such as reduced suffering by pain relief may not always be enough or possible, then interventions against coexisting complaints such as functional limitations, fatigue and sleeping problems are especially important. Below are some examples of factors that are related to chronic pain presented.

Functional Limitations

Chronic pain as well as increasing age has been associated with impaired functional abilities and performance of activities of daily living [8, 34, 35]. Scudds and Robertson [36] found in their study that those reporting musculoskeletal pain were three times more likely to have functional limitations. The ability to manage daily life independently may be crucial for older people's view of their daily life, health and quality of life. The impact of pain on functional health status may also lead people to avoid some movements and hence result in even more diminished performance of activities of daily living. The relationship seems to be even more important to consider for older people with a great need of help to manage activities of daily living, e.g. those in special accommodations. Increased functional limitations often lead to increased dependency, and this dependency on others because of the need for help to manage daily living could have a major effect on how people experience daily life and quality of life. Dependency could also lead to a feeling of helplessness and in turn helplessness is found to be strongly related to pain severity [37]. Thus, there is a complex interrelationship between these variables (pain, functional limitations, dependency, helplessness, and quality of life). It therefore seems important to consider such interrelationships in the care for older people.

Fatigue

Fatigue among older people in general is common and seems to be even more common with higher age as well as when in pain [8, 38, 39, 40]. Fatigue is a subjective feeling of tiredness that may or may not be related to physical activity, and becomes a major problem when it becomes interrupts daily life and when rest does not eliminate it [41]. The prevalence of fatigue has been found in previous research to be as high as 93–98% among older people in general [38, 42]. The high prevalence in these studies indicates the magnitude of the problem. In a Swedish study Jakobsson et al. [8] showed that the prevalence of fatigue was 24.2% for those not in pain and 56.8% for those in chronic pain. A systematic literature review found confirmed that the knowledge about fatigue among older are sparse, and that there was a disconcordance regarding the prevalence [40]. I the review the figures ranged from 30% to 98%. No articles were found focusing on interventions against fatigue among elderly in pain. Thus, despite the high prevalence of fatigue among elderly (especially among those in pain), fatigue seems to have been sparsely investigated, especially among those with chronic non-malignant pain [43, 44].

Fatigue may be difficult to intervene directly against (e.g. with rest and sleep), and actions that indirectly ease the impact of fatigue, such as interventions against other problems (e.g. pain and sleeping problems), could therefore be used instead. Fatigue has received more attention in cancer research, and various ways to support the person with fatigue have been recommended. For instance, information and assessment to increase the awareness of levels of fatigue and the factors that make it worse, and to recognise when rest and restoration are needed [45]. Adequate food-energy intake may also be considered. Such interventions are most likely also useful among older people, although there is no research to confirm this. Despite the amount of research about fatigue among cancer patients there are still few established nursing interventions [46]. Thus, there is an urgent need of further research about fatigue and interventions against fatigue among older people in pain as well as elderly in general.

Sleeping Problems

Sleeping difficulties are also common among older people [47, 48, 49], especially difficulties maintaining sleep [50]. A study of older people in Italy found a prevalence of insomnia for men of 36% and 54% for women [47]. Only 26% of the men and 21% of the women reported no sleeping problems [47]. In a multicentre study in the USA Foley et al. [51] found a prevalence of insomnia of 23–34%, and 7–15% rarely or never felt rested after waking up in the morning. Kim et al. [48] found in a general Japanese population that increased prevalence of insomnia was associated with e.g. older age, lack of habitual exercise, and poor perceived health. Pain has also been found to be associated with impaired sleep among older people [8, 49, 52]. Jakobsson et al. [8] found in their study that sleeping problems were significantly more common among those reporting chronic pain than those without, and more common with higher age among those in pain.

Social Network/Support

Pain appears to increase among older people at the same time as the social network seems to thin out in old age [53]. When a disease or other chronic condition affects a person the social network is often involved [54, 55]. Social as well as psychological factors are important to consider in nursing care because these factors seem to play a role in the genesis of pain [56]. Social network/support appears to be as valued a component of good quality of life as health status [57], and can buffer or reduce some of the negative effects on health [9] and quality of life [58, 59, 60]. Not all kinds of social support, however, may be beneficial, and no single type of support is uniformly effective for all people and all situations. The effectiveness of supportive actions depends on the situation, the person and his or her needs [9]. Unneeded or unwanted support can cause more harm than good, reducing older people's independence and self-esteem [9]. Waltz et al. [61] found that negative spouse behaviour, such as avoidance and critical remarks, increased pain among those with rheumatoid arthritis. Correspondingly, Cano et al. [62] found that more frequent negative spouse behaviour (negative responses to pain) were associated with increased pain severity and decreased marital satisfaction, which were linked to increased depressive symptoms. Thus, in most cases social network/support may buffer the negative effects of pain [56], but "negative social support" must be considered as well in the care of older people.

Pain Assessment

Pain is a subjective experience, a complex perceptual phenomenon and therefore, by its nature, pain can be assessed only indirectly. A common way of measuring pain is by a VAS scale [63], or similar tools such as verbal descriptor scale (VDS) and numerical rating scale

(NRS). When using this type of instruments only pain intensity is measured and not the entire multidimensional experience. The report of pain is related to several variables such as cultural background, past experience, the meaning of the situation, personality, attention, arousal level, emotions and reinforcement contingencies [64]. Therefore using only one dimension, such as intensity, will inevitably fail to capture the many qualities of pain and the pain experience. On the one hand, there is no single ideal pain assessment method for measuring pain in the clinic (and in general), and this is also true for pain assessment in elderly populations [23]. One explanation for this could be that instruments to measure pain have only begun to be validated for use among older people [34]. On the other hand, pain assessment in the clinic that works on younger people may also to some extent work rather well among older people, if they are not suffering from cognitive limitations. Herr and Mobily [65] found when studying various tools to assess pain (VAS, VDS, NRS) among elderly people (aged 65–93 years) that most respondents preferred the verbal rating scale because it was easy to complete and best described their pain. Unidimensional pain measuring tools may be useful to survey pain because they are easy to use and give a rough view of the prevalence and severity of the complaint. To measure pain fully, a wider view must be applied as in multidimensional instruments. Harkings and Price [23] stated examples of dimensions that especially need to be considered when measuring pain among older people: comorbidity, mental status, pain-independent functional status and activities of daily living, specification of pain-dependent limitations in instrumental activities of daily living, mood/emotional disorders (also including drug/alcohol abuse), and history of health-care utilisation. When measuring pain it is also important to consider that pain (especially pain intensity) is likely to vary over time and to depend on what the person is doing. Thus, a multidimensional pain instrument/measure is recommended to be used to capture as fully as possible the nature of the pain. However, a unidimensional measure, perhaps together with some additional questions about the effect of pain on daily life, may sometimes be more preferable when measuring pain among older people.

People in pain have to describe their pain experience to make pain visible to others. Problems in expressing and describing pain could be due to communicative problems such as reduced hearing, speech difficulties or cognitive impairment (e.g. dementia disease or acute confusion). Also cultural and contextual aspects can affect the way of expressing their pain. Pain is mostly reported verbally, but non-verbal reports must also be considered. Non-verbal reports of pain could be gestures and facial expressions [64]. Thus, pain measurement must also consider the problems of expressing the pain that could appear. Some attempts have been made to develop pain measurements based on verbal language or a combination of verbal and body expressions, but much work still remains to be done in this area.

Pain Management

Under-treatment of pain among older people is known to be common [52, 66] and one reason for this may be lack of systematic pain assessment [67]. For example, Allcock [67] found in a study performed in the United Kingdom that 69% of the nursing homes did not have a written policy regarding pain management and 75% did not use a standardised pain assessment tool. Another reason could be insufficient use of pain-relieving methods. A study in Sweden showed that although a high proportion (67%) of older people in nursing homes residents were estimated (by family members) to have physical pain, some (28.6%) of the residents with moderate to severe pain did not receive any analgesics [68].

Despite the development of different methods to manage pain, the use of the methods among older people has only been studied to some extent [26, 32, 69, 70]. Various methods for relieving pain are described in the literature, and are often categorised as either pharmacological or non-pharmacological [71, 72, 73]. Analgesic medication is the most commonly used method to relieve pain [70, 72]. For example, a study in Sweden showed a use of analgesic medication in 40% of older people with musculoskeletal pain [24]. However, the person in pain may not always consider commonly used pain management methods, such as medication, helpful [67, 74]. One reason to this could be that the analgesic medication does not fully relieve the pain due to that wrong type of medication/dose is prescribed. Another reason could be problems related to prescription of multiple drugs, which is common among older people, and may result in unwanted interactions such as lowered effect of the pain medication and/or unwanted side-effects [75]. Interactions and adverse side-effects of medication can also cause other problems among older people [69, 76]. For example, if the dose of the drug is lowered, by the older person as well as by the care provider, as a result of fear of addiction to the drugs (e.g. morphine) or side-effects, hence the effect is lowered too. The population is heterogeneous and the optimum dose as well as the side-effects are hard to predict, but unwanted side-effects could be reduced by dosing the patients with careful titration, frequent assessment and dose adjustments [77].

Also non-pharmacological methods have been developed and examples of this are TENS (Transcutaneous Electrical Nerve Stimulation), massage, rest, applying heat or cold [73]. These methods could be used, either alone or as a complement, to increase the pain-relieving effect and/or reduce adverse drug interactions [32, 71, 72, 75]. Studies about non-pharmacological treatments among older people are sparse, and the effect of such treatments may be unclear [78]. Some studies of older people with chronic pain have shown that the most commonly used methods to relieve pain were prescribed medicine, rest and distraction [26, 70, 74]. The fact that older people often choose pain relief methods that are convenient, inexpensive, easy to access/handle, and well known [79] may explain choice of methods reported in these above mentioned studies. Davis and Atwood [80] found in a sample of people with rheumatoid arthritis/osteoarthritis that exercise and rest were the most commonly used methods. Another study studying people with chronic pain in hip and knee, showed that hot bath/shower (used by 77% of the respondents), distraction (used by 72%), and exercise (64%) were the most commonly used methods [81]. However, combinations of both pharmacological methods and non-pharmacological methods are most likely the best way to ease the pain [75, 82], but the tricky part is find the combination that suites the individual and his/hers needs.

Conclusion

There is an inconsistency regarding both the prevalence of chronic pain and whether the pain increases or decreases with higher age. This means that no firm conclusions from the different studies can be drawn. Despite this, the results from the existing studies clearly indicate that chronic pain is common in old age and often results in other health complaints. Several coexisting complaints such as functional limitations, fatigue and sleeping problems are known to both be worsened and make the pain even worse, hence must be considered and treated together with the pain. Some other important variables such as various coping strategies and social network/support are also pointed out in the literature, but then as moderating factors. Thus, the need for actions to be taken in the care of older people to ease their pain is obvious. Research about pain management among older people is also rather sparse, especially regarding non-pharmacological methods. Both the use and effect of these methods needs to be further assessed. Thus, the knowledge, about older people with chronic pain is still rather sparse and further research is needed, especially focusing on the oldest old. However, in spite of the sparse knowledge it seems justified to state that pain and its impact on quality of life should be especially focused in everyday care for older people.

References

[1]   Grimley Evans J, Bond J. (1997). The challenges of age research. *Age and Ageing* 26 (Suppl. 4): 43-46.
[2]   Swedish Institute. (2003). *The Swedish population.* (Fact sheets on Sweden). Internet: *www.si.se.*
[3]   Easton KL. (1999). *Gerontological rehabilitation nursing.* Philadelphia, Pennsylvania: WB Saunders Company.
[4]   Given B, Given W. (1989). Cancer nursing for the elderly. A target for research. *Cancer Nursing* 12: 71-77.
[5]   Field D, Minkler M. (1988). Continuity and change in social support between young-old and old-old or very old age. *Journal of Gerontology* 43: 100–106.
[6]   McConnell ES. (1997). Conceptual bases for gerontological nursing practice: models, trends and issues. In Matteson MA, McConnell ES, Linton AD. (eds.). *Gerontological nursing. Concepts and practice* (2nd ed.). Philadelphia, Pennsylvania: WB Saunders Company.
[7]   Gibson SJ, Katz B, Corran TM, Farrell MJ, Helme RD. (1994). Pain in older persons. *Disability and Rehabilitation* 16: 127–139.
[8]   Jakobsson U, Klevsgård R, Westergren A, Hallberg IR. (2003). Old people in pain: a comparative study. *Journal of Pain and Symptom Management* 26: 625-636.
[9]   Rowe JW, Kahn RL. (1999). *Successful ageing.* New York: Dell Publishing.
[10]   IASP. (1979). Subcommittee on taxonomy: pain terms. A list with definitions and notes on usage. *Pain* 6: 249–252.
[11]   Melzack R, Wall PD. (1965). Pain mechanisms: a new theory. *Science* 150: 971–979.

[12] Melzack R. (1993). Pain: past, present and future. *Canadian Journal of Experimental Psychology* 47: 615–629.

[13] Melzack R. (1999). From the gate to the neuromatrix. *Pain* (Suppl. 6): 121–126.

[14] Wall PD, Melzack R. (eds.) (1999). *Textbook of pain* (4th ed.). Edinburgh: Churchill Livingstone, UK.

[15] Merskey H. (ed.) (1986). IASP subcommittee on taxonomy. Classification of chronic pain: Descriptions of chronic pain syndromes and definition of pain terms. *Pain* (Suppl. 3): 1–225.

[16] Helme RD, Gibson SJ. (2001). The epidemiology of pain in elderly people. *Clinics in Geriatric Medicine* 17: 417–431.

[17] Brochet B, Michel P, Barberger-Gateau P, Dartigues J-F. (1998). Population-based study of pain in elderly people: a descriptive survey. *Age and Ageing* 27: 279–284.

[18] Mobily PR, Herr KA, Clark KM, Wallace RB. (1994). An epidemiologic analysis of pain in the elderly. *Journal of Ageing and Health* 6: 139–154.

[19] Brattberg G, Parker MG, Thorslund M. (1996). The prevalence of pain among the oldest old in Sweden. *Pain* 67: 29-34.

[20] Magni G, Marchetti M, Moreschi C, Merskey H, Luchini SR. (1993). Chronic musculoskeletal pain and depressive symptoms in the National Health and Nutrition Examination I. Epidemiologic follow-up study. *Pain* 53: 163-168.

[21] Gagliese L, Melzack R. (1997). Chronic pain in elderly people. *Pain* 70: 3-14.

[22] Brattberg G, Thorslund M, Wikman A. (1989). The prevalence of pain in a general population. The results of a postal survey in a county of Sweden. *Pain* 37: 215–22.

[23] Harkins SW, Price DD. (1992). Assessment of pain in the elderly. In Turk DC, Melzack R. (eds.). *Handbook of pain assessment.* New York: The Guildford Press.

[24] Grimby C, Fastbom J, Forsell Y, Thorslund M, Claesson CB, Winblad B. (1999). Musculoskeletal pain and analgesic therapy in a very old population. *Archives of Gerontology and Geriatrics* 29: 29–43.

[25] Klinger L, Spaulding S. (1998). Chronic pain in the elderly: Is silence really golden? *Physical and Occupational Therapy in Geriatrics* 15: 1–17.

[26] Jakobsson U, Hallberg IR, Westergren A. (2004). Pain management in elderly persons who require assistance with activities of daily living: a comparison of those living at home with those in special accommodations. *European Journal of Pain* 8: 335-344.

[27] Harkins SW. (1996). Geriatric pain. Perceptions in the old. *Clinics in Geriatric Medicine* 12: 435–459.

[28] Jacobs JM, Hammerman-Rozenberg R, Cohen A, Stessman J. (2006). Chronic back pain among the elderly: prevalence, associations, and predictors. *Spine* 31: E203-E207.

[29] McCaffery LR, Beebe A. (1994). *Pain: Clinical manual for nursing practice.* London: Mosby.

[30] Stein WM, Ferrell BA. (1996). Pain in the nursing home. *Clinics in Geriatric Medicine* 12: 601–613.

[31] Ferrell BA, Ferrell BR, Osterweil D. (1990). Pain in the nursing home. *JAGS: Journal of the American Geriatric Society* 38: 409–414.

[32] Wallace M. (1994). Assessment and management of pain in the elderly. *MEDSURG Nursing.* 3: 293–298.

[33] Solomon P. (2001). Congruence between health professionals and patients pain ratings: a review of the literature. *Scandinavian Journal of Caring Sciences* 15: 174–180.

[34] Gagliese L, Katz J, Melzack R. (1999). Pain in the elderly. In Wall, PD., Melzack R. (eds.). *Textbook of pain* (4th ed). Edinburgh: Churchill Livingstone, UK.

[35] Jylhä M, Jokela J, Tolvanen E, Heikkinen E, Heikkinen R-L, Koskinen S, Leskinen E, Lyyra A-L, Pohjolainen P. (1992). The Tampere longitudinal study on ageing. *Scandinavian Journal of Social Medicine* (Suppl. 47): 1–51.

[36] Scudds RJ, Robertson JM. (1998). Empirical evidence of the association between the presence of musculoskeletal pain and physical disability in community-dwelling senior citizens. *Pain* 75: 229–235.

[37] Creamer P, Lethbridge-Cejku M, Hochberg MC. (1999). Determinants of pain severity in knee osteoarthritis : effect of demographic and psychosocial variables using 3 pain measures. *Journal of Rheumatology* 26: 1785-1792.

[38] Liao S, Ferell BA. (2000). Fatigue in an older population. *Journal of American Geriatric Society* 48: 426–430.

[39] Fishbain DA, Cole B, Cutler RB, Lewis J, Rosomoff HL, Rosomoff RS. (2003). Is pain fatiguing? A structured evidence-based review. *Pain Medicine* 4: 51–62.

[40] Jakobsson U. (2006). A literature review on fatigue among older people in pain: prevalence and predictors. *International Journal of Older People Nursing* 1: 11-16.

[41] Hawley D, Wolfe F. (1997). Fatigue and musculoskeletal pain. *Physical Medicine and Rehabilitation Clinics of North America* 8: 101–109.

[42] Belza BL, Henke CJ, Yelin EH, Epstein WV, Gilliss CL. (1993). Correlates of fatigue in older adults with rheumatoid arthritis. *Nursing Research* 42: 93–99.

[43] Leveille SG, Fried L, Guralnik JM. (2002). Disabling symptoms. What do older women report? *Journal of General Internal Medicine* 17: 766–773.

[44] Hellström Y, Persson G, Hallberg IR. (2004). Quality of life and symptoms among older people living at home. *Journal of Advanced Nursing* 48: 584–593.

[45] Wilson-Barnett J, Richardson A. (1993). Nursing research and palliative care. In Doyle D, Hanks GWC, MacDonald N. *Oxford textbook of palliative medicine.* Oxford: Oxford University Press.

[46] Magnusson K, Karlsson E, Palmblad C, Leitner C, Paulson A. (1997). Swedish nurses' estimation of fatigue as a symptom in cancer patients – report of a question-naire. *European Journal of Cancer Care* 6: 186–191.

[47] Maggi S, Langlois JA, Minicuci N, Grigoletto F, Pavan M, Foley DJ, Enzi G. (1998). Sleep complaints in community-dwelling older persons: prevalence, associated factors, and reported causes. *JAGS: Journal of American Geriatric Society* 46: 161–168.

[48] Kim K, Uchiyama M, Okawa M, Liu X, Ogihara R. (2000). An epidemiological study of insomnia among the Japanese general population. *Sleep* 23: 41–47.

[49] Byles JE, Mishra GD, Harris MA, Nair K. (2003). The problems of sleep for older women: changes in health outcomes. *Age and Ageing* 32: 154–163.

[50] Doi Y, Minowa M, Okawa M, Uchiyama M. (2000). Prevalence of sleep disturbance and hypnotic medication use in relation to sociodemographic factors in the general Japanese adult population. *Journal of Epidemiology* 10: 79–86.

[51] Foley DJ, Monjan AA, Brown L, Simonsick EM, Wallace RB, Blazer DG. (1995). Sleep complaints among elderly persons: an epidemiologic study of three communities. *Sleep* 18: 425–432.

[52] Ross MM, Crook J. (1998). Elderly recipients of home nursing services: pain, disability and functional competence. *Journal of Advanced Nursing* 27: 1117–1126.

[53] Persson G, Boström G, Allebeck P, Andersson L, Berg S, Johansson L, Thille A. (2001). Elderly people's health – 65 years and after. *Scandinavian Journal of Public Health* (Suppl. 58): 117–131.

[54] Rolland JS. (1994). *Families, illness and disability.* New York: Basic Books.

[55] Nolan M, Grant G, Keady J. (1996). *Understanding family care.* Buckingham: Open University Press.

[56] Roy R. (2001). *Social relations and chronic pain.* New York: Kluwer Academic/-Plenum Publishers.

[57] Farquhar M. (1995). Elderly people's definitions of quality of life. *Social Science and Medicine* 41: 1439–1446.

[58] Lambert VA, Lambert CE, Klipple GL, Meshaw EA. (1989). Social support, hardiness and psychological well-being in women with arthritis. *Image: Journal of Nursing Scholarship* 21: 128-131.

[59] Bowling A, Browne PD. (1991). Social networks, health and emotional well-being among the oldest old in London. *Journal of Gerontology: Social Science* 46: S20-S32.

[60] Kendig H, Browning CJ, Young AY. (2000). Impacts of illness and disability on the well-being of older people. *Disability and Rehabilitation* 22: 15-22.

[61] Waltz M, Krigel W, Van't Pad Bosch P. (1998). The social environment and health in rheumatoid arthritis: marital quality predicts individual variability in pain severity. *Arthritis Care and Research* 11: 356-374.

[62] Cano A, Weisberg JN, Gallagher RM. (2000). Marital satisfaction and pain severity mediate the association between negative spouse responses to pain and depressive symptoms in a chronic pain patient sample. *Pain Medicine* 1: 35–43.

[63] Huskisson EC. (1974). Measurement of pain. *The Lancet* 9: 1127–1131.

[64] Turk DC, Melzack R. (eds.) (1992). *Handbook of pain assessment.* New York: The Guildford Press.

[65] Herr KA, Mobily PR. (1993). Comparison of selected pain assessment tools for use with the elderly. *Applied Nursing Research* 6: 39–46.

[66] Blomqvist K, Hallberg IR. (1999). Pain in older adults living in sheltered accommodation – agreement between assessments by older adults and staff. *Journal of Clinical Nursing* 8: 159–169.

[67] Allcock N. (2002). Management of pain in older people within the nursing home: a preliminary study. *Health and Social Care in the Community* 10: 464–471.

[68] Hall-Lord ML, Johansson I, Schmidt I, Larsson BW. (2003). Family members perceptions of pain and distress related to analgesics and psychotropic drugs, and quality of care of elderly nursing home residents. *Health and Social Care in the Community* 11: 262–274.

[69] Novy CM, Jagmin MG. (1997). Pain management in the elderly orthopedic patient. *Orthopedic Nursing* 16: 51–57.

[70] Jakobsson U. (2004). Pain management among older people in need of help with activities of daily living. *Pain Management Nursing* 5: 137-143.

[71] Closs SJ. (1994). Pain in elderly patients: a neglected phenomenon? *Journal of Advanced Nursing* 19: 1072–1081.

[72] American Geriatric Society, AGS panel on chronic pain in older persons. (1998). The management of chronic pain in older persons (Clinical practice guidelines). *JAGS: Journal of American Geriatric Society* 46: 635–651.

[73] Carr ECJ, Mann EM. (2000). *Pain. Creative approaches to effective management.* London: Macmillan Press Ltd.

[74] Blomqvist K, Hallberg IR. (2002). Managing pain in older persons who receive home-help for daily living. Perceptions by older persons and care providers. *Scandinavian Journal of Caring Sciences* 16: 319–328.

[75] Helme RD. (2001). Chronic pain management in older people. *European Journal of Pain* 5 (Suppl. A): 31-36.

[76] Ferrell BA. (1995). Pain evaluation and management in the nursing home. *Annals of Internal Medicine* 123: 681–687.

[77] Ruoff GE. (2002). Challenges of managing chronic pain in the elderly. *Seminars in Arthritis and Rheumatism* 32: 43-50.

[78] Sindhu F. (1996). Are non-pharmacological nursing interventions for the management of pain effective? – A meta-analysis. *Journal of Advanced Nursing* 24: 1152–1159.

[79] Lansbury G. (2000). Chronic pain management: a qualitative study of elderly people's preferred coping strategies and barriers to management. *Disability and Rehabilitation* 22: 2–14.

[80] Davis GC, Atwood JR. (1996). The development of the pain management inventory for patients with arthritis. *Journal of Advanced Nursing* 24: 236–243.

[81] Hopman-Rock M, Kraaimaat FW, Bijlsma JWJ. (1997). Quality of life in elderly subjects with pain in the hip or knee. *Quality of Life Research* 6: 67–76.

[82] Miaskowski C. (2000). The impact of age on a patient's perception of pain and ways it can be managed. *Pain Management Nursing* 1 (Suppl.): S2-S7.

In: Trends in Nursing Research
Editors: Adam J. Ryan and Jack Doyle

ISBN 978-1-60456-642-0
© 2009 Nova Science Publishers, Inc.

Chapter 8

Nursing Education in Spain

A. Zabalegui and E. Cabrera
Universitat Internacional de Catalunya, Spain

Abstract

Nursing education in Spain is developing rapidly in accordance with the European Union growth and within an international globalization movement. The purpose of this chapter is to provide an overview of nursing education in Spain. A brief history of modern nursing education is presented together with its recent reform and a view of recent developments.

Since nursing education was integrated at the university level in 1977, the only academic recognition for this education in Spain was the three year diploma degree. Nurses had to move to other disciplines in order to achieve academic growth or forward their nursing studies abroad. Over these years, there have been numerous attempts to achieve the Bachelor in Nursing Science.

In 1998 eight Nursing Universities of Spain began to offer graduated –level advanced programs of 2 academic years, 120 European Credit transfer System (ECTS) . The degree upon completion of this advanced program is the master of nursing science. This program includes nursing research, teaching, management, and advanced care.

Recently in January 2005, the Spanish Government published the guidelines for undergraduate, master's and doctoral levels (BOE, 55/2005). Finally, as a result of the Bologna Process, nursing is being fully recognized as a higher education discipline, and its curriculum is being organized within the framework of undergraduate and graduate education.

At the same time, in May 2005, the Ministries of Health and Education approved the proposal of the specialities in Nursing (BOE,450/2005). These specialities determined the areas of Nursing care; family and community health nursing, nursing midwifery, mental health nursing, elderly nursing, health work nursing, medical care nursing and paediatric nursing. These specialities will improve patient care as well as the continuing education already available.

Introduction

Nursing education and practice in Spain is influenced by health care changes. The most important health-related factors that impact health care are: demographic changes such population aging and cultural diversity such as immigration, technology growth, economical and sociopolitical globalization, increased level of patient's knowledge and decision making, increased complexity of care, policies of health cost maintenance and reduction, new health care procedures, quality improvement, nursing evidence-based practice and advances in health and nursing science.

During the past 10 years nursing in Spain has gone through a great transformation, from an only university diploma program to a full academic development with a degree or bachelor, master and doctoral nursing programs. Now, nurses in Spain are allow to gain all knowledge, attitudes and skills required to effectively cope with present health care challenges and changes. Recently (July 3rd of 2006) the Spanish Government has recognized nursing as a science with its own right, and give to our profession a full academic pathway within the European framework of the Bologna agreement (bachelor, masters and doctoral education) (BOE,2006).

Historical Review of Nursing Education in Spain

The first Spanish Nursing School, Santa Isabel de Hungria, was created in 1898 with a religious and technical orientation. Later on, in 1917 another School of Nursing of Santa Madrona was created in Barcelona, with a focus on biology and techniques and in 1933, the Government of Catalonia created its own School of Nursing outside the religious arena and nursing was considered a health occupation devoted to care for sick people. Alter the Spanish civil war the nurse's formation was inspired more in the technocracies than religious philosophy. Later on in 1944 a law stated that nurses were subordinated to medical personnel, relegating to nurses a dependent role. In 1953 the three different programs for nursing professionals: nurses, midwives and practitioners were unified under a single title "Health Technical Helpers or *Ayudantes Tecnicos Sanitarios* (ATS)". These new professionals, ATS, had a great impact in the development of a public health care system in the 1960's that generated new hospitals and therefore a need for more nurses and new nursing schools. ATS were educated outside the universities, mainly in hospital schools of nursing. The characteristics of the ATS technical nurses were to focus on hospital care rather than on community care. Their main emphasis was on technical care lacking a scientific view. ATS lacked professional identity and autonomy, since they were subordinated to other health professionals, mainly physicians. Their care was based on a positivistic medical approach, which lacked the holistic perspective of nursing.

Since the early seventies different groups of nurses, influenced by international nursing movements, especially from USA and Canada, started working towards the development of nursing as a discipline. During this period, the Spanish General Education Law , allowed the integration of nursing studies into the University system, giving them the category of Nursing

School and offering a Diploma program and on July 1977, the law was passed (BOE 2128,1977). The Diploma was issued by the Ministry of Education and the requirements for admission were high school accreditation (12 years of formal pre-university education) and a national university entrance examination called *"Selectividad"*.

The general functions of the diploma nurse were to provide general nursing care to healthy or sick persons, families and communities, focusing care towards health promotion, disease prevention, health recovery and rehabilitation. Besides, nurses were expected to collaborate with other health care professionals and to contribute to student nursing education. Following the instructions of the EU Advisory Committee on Training Nurses a minimum of 4.600 hours of theory and practice or three years of education is required to work as a nurse in the EU countries (Council Directives for Nurses, 1977) . Although the number of hours is not a good indicator of goal accomplishment, this number of hours was established for the Diploma program to satisfy the requirements of European Directives. Moreover, it was established that theory would occupy 50% of the hours of study, whereas the other 50% would be devoted to practice. The rational for maintaining this proportion was to assure enough clinical training so that the students would incorporate the theoretical knowledge into practice at the same time that they would get the necessary attitudes and skills by direct observation and repetition. This approach put an emphasis on professionalism. Although, it can be said that, in general, the contents have maintained the original philosophy, since 1977 nursing curricula have evolved and changed to adjust to the new social and university demands. The main change was undertaken in 1990 to incorporate the recommendation of the Alma Ata conference (1978) that emphasized contents of primary health care, geriatric nursing and behavioral science (BOE 1466/1990).

Recent Transformation of Nursing Education in Spain

The biggest change in Spanish Nursing Education is due to the Bologna Declaration signed by the EU Ministries of Education on the 19 of June 1999 to re-structure university education. This agreement describes the framework of the European Higher Education Area and has the following objectives to be reach by October 1st 2010:

1. Adoption of a system of easily readable and comparable degrees.
2. Adoption of a system based on two main cycles: undergraduate (degree) and graduate (Master and Doctorate).
3. Establishment of a common system of credits "European Credits Transfer System (ECTS)" to promote student mobility.
4. Promotion of mobility for students, teachers, researchers and administrative staff.
5. Promotion of European co-operation in quality assurance with a view to developing comparable criteria and methodologies.
6. Promotion of the necessary dimensions in higher education, particularly with regards to curriculum development, inter-institutional co-operation, mobility schemes and integrated programs of study, training and research.

Until now, nurses in Spain were unable to acquire a doctoral degree in nursing. Nursing faculty were forced to obtain their bachelor and doctorate degrees in disciplines other than nursing (e.g., psychology, sociology, anthropology) or to enroll in universities abroad. Now nursing programmes are under a great transformation from a biomedical model to a nursing paradigm, from a focus on professors teaching to student learning, from a lecture classroom teaching to active cooperative and problem-based learning, from curriculum subject and grades to student competences as outcomes, from a Diploma to a Bachelor degree, from a minimum of 205 credits (1 credit represents 10 hours of classroom teaching or 15 hours of seminars or 35 hours of clinical practice) to a 240 European Credits Transfer System, ECTS (1 credits represent about 25 hours of student work that includes classroom teaching and other leaning activities). In Spain there are about 130 nursing Schools and these transformations are being piloted with Governmental support in a few Universities like the International University of Catalonia in Barcelona and the University of Girona.

The university structure for nursing education includes the following alternatives:

1. Nursing basic education, granted by the Ministry of Education: Diploma nursing program (3 university academic years) being transformed to Bachelor degree (4 academic years at full time with 240 ECTS credits, where each year will have 60 ECTS).
2. Master programs: Master of Nursing Science, granted by the Ministry of Education.
3. Doctoral program, granted by the Ministry of Education.
4. Specialities. By now, there are only two specialities accredited by the Ministry of Health. Midwifery, approved in 1992, is a program of two full time years with a total of 3.534 hours theoretical and-practical experience, and mental health nursing approved in 1999 with one year of clinical practice. The access to these two specialities is through a National Examination, a system similar to that used by medical residents. Each Spanish Autonomic Community negotiates with the Ministry of Health the number of positions available every year. Out of the 15.000 new nurse graduates every year from the basic program, only about 300 may undertake one of these two specialties. Recently five more specialties (family and community health nursing, elderly nursing, health work nursing, medical surgical nursing, and paediatric nursing) have been approved by our Government (BOE, 2005); but, so far these new specialties have not been offered because they are under study in terms of curriculum development, number of specialists needed, seats offered, teaching units, employment outcomes, and so on. Besides, all nursing specialties do not have academic credentials so are not recognized as Master degrees (BOE, 44/2003 and BOE 450/2005).
5. Post graduate continuing education. There are many post diploma course in all types of specific nursing areas (oncology, cardiology, surgical, intensive care, nutrition, palliative nursing care), or human being development (child, elderly) or nursing management. This type of education is certificated by the organization that offers it (university, hospital or a nursing association). (See Figure 1).

Graduate Nursing Education

The Real Decretory published in January 21st 2005 (BOE, 55/2005) has established the structure of official university education for the graduate level or Degree. Based on this framework, all nursing schools together have developed a bachelor of nursing science curricula after receiving a grant from the Ministry of Education (Agencia Nacional de Evaluacion de la Calidad, ANECA) and under the support of the Conference of Nursing School Directors. First, an analysis of nursing studies in all EU countries was done to identify the number of years, hours, and ECTS required, the type of academic institution, and the degree awarded upon graduation. Second, we analyzed the demand for nursing studies in Spain, evaluated the number of enrolees in each nursing school and the number of applicants. This second phase also included a national nursing survey to determine the level of employment satisfaction.

The third phase was the evaluation of generic and specific competencies needed for graduation at the bachelor's degree level. Based on previous Tuning methodology and results about nursing competencies, this analysis was done with a national survey of nursing students, professors, professional nurses, nursing administrators, and professional nursing associations. In the final phase, participants in the ANECA nursing project reported to the Spanish government on the degree curriculum, including its objectives, teaching strategies, structure of mandatory courses, and ECTS. Moreover, the competencies required for each course were identified and defined (Zabalegui A. *et al*, 2005).

Although the bachelor program is being piloted in a few universities our government still requires the universities to comply with mandatory subjects for the Diploma program (BOE, 1466/1990). However, the Degree curriculum to be implemented in 2008 will have a minimum 240 ECTS distributed in the following way:

A. 60 ECTS from health related sciences: Basic sciences, humanities, social, behavioral sciences, technology, computer sciences, foreign languages, etc. These credits will be generally included in the first academic year and will vary among universities.

B. 120 ECTS common for all the universities:

   –   Basic sciences (15 ECTS): Anatomy and physiology, pharmacology, microbiology.

   –   Nursing sciences (105 ECTS): Fundamentals of nursing (10), Clinical nursing (40), Psychosocial and mental health nursing (9), Community nursing (20 ECTS), Nursing along the life cycle (15), ethics, legislation and administration (5), and other nursing related subjects (6 ECTS) such as bioethics or communication. These credits will include theory and practice nursing and will be completed mainly in the second and third academic years.

C. Clinical practicum (60 ECTS) that will be done at the forth academic year.

Clinical Practice

Clinical learning is an essential part of nursing education. The clinical setting provides nursing education with the opportunity to transfer theoretical learning to professional practice. Through working with patients, families and communities the student makes sense of theory, applies it to practice and begins to recognize the problems and rewards inherent in nursing practice. The amount of time that nursing students spend on clinical placements is significant. In Spain nursing students start their clinical practice early in the program. Approximately 50% of the program is divided between simulation laboratories, clinical practice and post clinical seminars. The clinical practice lasts about 10 months of full time experience. The distribution of the clinical practice varies among university programs. Some divide the total practice in equal periods every year; while others accumulate it to the end of the program. Whether it is better to arrange the clinical experiences in a concentrated manner, or to spread it throughout the entire duration of the program is currently under debate among Spanish nursing educators (Zabalegui, 2005).

The different areas of practice include: nursing homes, hospitals outpatients units, critical care units, emergency units, surgical and medical floors, community health, palliative care units, maternal-child floors, drug abuse unit and home care. This practice is still heavily focused on acute-care facilities (Zabalegui, 1999). The process of clinical teaching includes:

- Simulation laboratories organized with small student groups.
- University teachers are responsible for planning clinical assignments, stating objectives clearly and selecting the experiences which are appropriate in achieving these objectives. They are also in charge of coordinating clinical with laboratory simulation and theoretical learning.
- Clinical practice follow up, control, supervision and evaluation are undertaken by a teacher collaborator. A teacher collaborator is usually a professional nurse employed by the hospital where the clinical practice is being done. The collaborator is responsible for matching each student with a registered nurse, to act as a mentor. The student works alongside their mentor undertaking the same hours of duty and caring for the same patients.
- Clinical Post-Conference Learning seminars.

The students in clinical practice assume responsibility for their own learning. They are encouraged to have a high degree of autonomy, choice and freedom in negotiating their learning needs, not only with the tutor, but also with the practical placement (reference/mentor) nurse, and with peers. The purpose of this is to allow the student to establish the sequence to achieve the competency (knowledge, skills and attitudes) according to individual needs. The trend to contain health care cost puts pressure on teachers and students since Human resources managers assume that upon graduation nursing students of the basic program will be safe and competent practitioners so they could be offered to work immediately on specialized units like intensive care units or emergency room or chemotherapy administration units.

Once the student finishes the basic university program the nurse automatically obtains nursing registration, which allows him or her to practice in Spain as well as in the EU. There are no Licensure National Examination Tests or further continuing education requirements since no relicensing policy has been established. However, out of the almost 200,000 nurses with diploma program, about 60% are in programs of continuing education. A possible explanation to the high level of enrollment in these programs is that nurses feel the need to further their education to enhance their curriculum vitae and provide a more qualified and excellence professional practice.

Postgraduate Master and Doctoral in Nursing Sciences Program

In Spain, a legislative norm (BOE 56/2005) published in January 25th of 2005 has laid down the guidelines for the degree, master and doctoral academic levels. Nursing as a higher education discipline is finally being recognized and its curricula is organized within the new framework of reference for the bachelor, master and doctoral degrees.

The Master's degree course in Nursing Sciences is an officially recognized inter-university programme given by a network of eight universities in Spain and one in Belgium (The Catholic University of Leuven). Its aim is to train researchers and specialists in Nursing Sciences to carry out research into the physical, social, cultural, political and psychological dimensions of care in the context of the health/illness of individuals, families and communities and the dynamics of the different healthcare systems.

Since 1998 the Universities of Alicante, International of Catalonia, Huelva, Almeria, Rovira i Virgili of Tarragona, Autonoma of Madrid, Lleida and Zaragoza and have been offering an advanced nursing program as a second cycle post basic education. The program focuses on nursing research, teaching, management and advanced care. More than 1500 Spanish nurses have completed this program. Some of these students on graduation have assume faculty and administrative roles across the country. Once the program was approved by our government (BOE, 2006) some of these students are enroll in doctoral nursing programs. The objectives of the Master in Nursing Science program are:

1. Develop and analyze the historical, theoretical and philosophical bases of nursing science.
2. Develop teaching programs for all nursing areas of knowledge.
3. Apply the scientific method to increase nursing body of knowledge and to solve health related problems of persons, families and communities.
4. Assume nursing leadership to manage resources and promote nursing changes towards professional development.
5. Gain the new scientific and technologic knowledge necessary to cope with health care demands.

The programme's ultimate objective is to offer training that prepares the ground for adapting healthcare services and quality of life to the 21st century. It is also designed to provide new theoretical and methodological healthcare tools in this changing, complex society, while contributing to improve people's health and quality of life in all its dimensions. Upon completion of this official Master's degree course, students are qualified to submit a thesis for a doctoral degree. See table 1.

Recently, these eight universities have signed an agreement creating a network for inter-university cooperation in nursing research, teaching and student exchange. This network hopes to incorporate other Universities from EU countries to enhance student outcomes and to implement future and collaborative doctoral programs. Some of the research areas included in this program are: oncology care (stress, coping, adaptation and cancer prevention); quality of life; ageing; self-care; caregivers; dependence; educational methodologies(cooperative learning); gender and health and organizational cultures in hospitals.

Doctoral Program

To enter into a doctoral program the candidate has to have 300 ECTS with at least 60 credits from a official master program. This program may have courses and the doctoral candidate has to public present his or her research work. Therefore, the doctoral programs include research lines supported by consolidated groups of researchers.

Nursing Professors Education

Nursing teachers should be the leaders making decisions about the future of the profession, planning new education, and implementing innovations based on their nursing research. In order to do this nurse teachers should have a higher education level, a minimum of master degree. In Spain, many nursing faculty members are moving from a diploma to a bachelor and doctoral degree programmes in other subjects other than nursing (for example anthropology, humanities, history, psychology). So far the only requirement to be a nursing teacher at the basic program was to have a Diploma degree in Nursing; however the new university structure requires to have a doctoral degree in order to be a University professor. Therefore, many nursing school teachers are undertaking their doctoral courses and nursing schools are threaten to loose their nursing staff.

In order to have a teaching position at the university, the candidates have to pass an oral examination were curriculum vitae and academic degree are key aspects. If nurses do not have doctoral degrees the teaching position could be given to other professionals with this academic credentials. Besides, the process of teacher selection is being evaluated under the criteria of bioscience impact factor of publications where most nursing journals are not included. Therefore, this new university structure brings a great opportunity for nursing development but at the same time bring a great challenge in terms of nursing school control.

Besides, to face the challenges of the new nursing academic levels we must also consider nursing student profile and global nursing mobility. Today, there is an increasing diversity in nursing student population. Students enter into university at the age of 18, although there is an increased in the number of mature students. This new population is characterized by including more males (13%), older females, students transferred from other sciences, self-paying tuition cost, and therefore combining the studies with work and family roles. Besides, every year some of our nursing students take part of their program in other EU universities and at the same time we receive students from other European universities as part of the Erasmus programs that promotes university student mobility.

Conclusion

Nursing education in Spain is being upgraded to international standards:

- Developing the Bachelor degree with four academic years (240 ECTS).
- Implementing a Master of Nursing Science with two academic years (120 ECTS).
- Implementing Doctoral Nursing programs.
- Developing specialist education programs.
- Developing collaborative inter-university agreements within Spain and the EU.

These transformations are contributing to nursing in Spain as an independent discipline, with its identity and self sufficiency. This new structure for higher education in Spain should enhance Spanish nursing competitiveness and promote the roles and influence of nurses on health status of individuals, families, and communities in Spain.

References

Council Directives 77/452/EEC and 77/453/EEC 1977. *Official Journal of the European Communities*, 20 no. L176, 15 July.

European Higher Education Area. 1999. Joint declaration of the European Ministers of Education. *European Higher Education*. Bologna.

Ley 14/1986, de 25 de Abril, General de Sanidad. 1986. (*Boletín Oficial del Estado*, número 102, de 24-04-86).

Ley 44/2003, de 21 de noviembre, de ordenación de las profesiones sanitarias. 2003.(*Boletín Oficial del Estado*, número 280 de 22-11-03).

Ministerio de Educación. Agencia Nacional de Evaluación de la Calidad (*ANECA*) Libro blanco de título de grado en enfermería. Madrid, 2005. www.aneca.es (February 16th 2006).

Orden de 31 de Octubre de 1977, por la que se dictan directrices para la elaboración de Planes de Estudios de la escuelas Universitarias de Enfermería. 1977.(*Boletín Oficial del Estado*, número 283, de 26 -11-77).

Real decreto 1466/1990, de 26 de Octubre de 1990, por el que se establece el título universitario de Diplomado de Enfermería y las directrices generales propias de los estudios conducentes a la obtención de aquél. 1990. (*Boletín Oficial del Estado*, número 278 de 20-11-90).

Real Decreto 2128/1977, de 23 de Julio de 1977, sobre integración en la Universidad de las Escuelas de Ayudantes Técnicos sanitarios como Escuelas Universitarias de Enfermería.1977. (*Boletín Oficial del Estado*, número 200 de 22-08-77).

Real Decreto 450/2005, de 22 de Abril, sobre especialidades de Enfermería. 2005. (*Boletín Oficial del Estado*, número 108, de 06-05-05).

Real Decreto 55/2005, de 21 de enero, por el que se establece las estructura de las enseñanzas universitarias y se regulan los estudios oficiales de Grado.2005. (*Boletín Oficial del Estado*, número 21, de 25-01-05).

Real Decreto 56/2005, de 21 de enero, por el que se regulan los estudios universitarios oficiales de Postgrado; Master y Doctorado. 2005.(*Boletín Oficial del Estado*, número 21,de 25-01-05).

Resolución de 22 de junio de 2006, de la Secretaría General del Consejo de Coordinación Universitaria, por la que se da publicidad a la relación de los programas oficiales de posgrado y de sus correspondientes títulos, cuya implantación ha sido autorizada por las comunidades autónomas.2006. (*Boletín Oficial del Estado*, número 157, de 03-07-06).

Roode J., Leino-Kilpi H, Zabalegui A, Begley C and Buscher A. 2001. The process of implementing the bolognia agreement in the EU countries. *Sigma Theta Tau International*. 12th International Nursing Research Congress. Copenhagen.

Tuning. Final Report and Conclusions of Tuning Phase I, Brussels. May 2002. Retrieved (February 16th 2006) from www.relint.deusto.es/TunningProject/index.htm Zabalegui. A. 1999. Practicas clínicas en enfermería: métodos docentes. *Educación Médica*, 2:4, 161-166.

Zabalegui A. 2002. Nursing education in Spain- past, present and future. *Nurse Education Today* 22, 1-9.

Zabalegui A. Changes in Nursing Education in the European Union. 2006. *Journal of Nursing Scholarship*, 38:2,1-5.

In: Trends in Nursing Research
Editors: Adam J. Ryan and Jack Doyle

ISBN 978-1-60456-642-0
© 2009 Nova Science Publishers, Inc.

Chapter 9

Nurse - Physician Communication: The Impact of Disruptive Behaviors on Factors Affecting Decision Making Affecting Patient Outcomes of Care

Alan H. Rosenstein and Michelle O'Daniel
VHA West Coast, CA, USA.

Abstract

Disruptive behaviors can have a profound effect on staff perceptions, attitudes and reactions that affect decision making and communication flow. Feelings of anger, hostility and frustration lead to impaired relationships, confused expectations, and unclear roles and responsibilities which can impede the transfer of vital information that can adversely affect patient outcomes of care. Health care organizations need to be aware of the significance of disruptive behaviors and develop appropriate policies, standards and procedures to effectively deal with this serious issue.

Introduction

Medical care is a complex system with multiple different parties interfacing and exchanging tasks and information important for patient care. When things go well, everyone benefits. But when things don't go well, the unintended consequences can be severe. Reports from the Institute of Medicine state that nearly 100,000 deaths each year occur because of preventable medical errors [1-3]. The Joint Commission on Accreditation of Hospitals (JCAHO) states that nearly two- thirds of sentinel events (an unexpected medical event that has serious medical consequences) can be traced back to a communication error [4]. The newest initiative from the Institute for Healthcare Improvement (IHI) is unveiling its five million lives saved from harm campaign that focuses on interventions that reduce the likelihood of patient harm [5].

Traditional approaches adopted by the patient safety movement have focused more on improving system related issues than people related issues. While the introduction of new technologies and redesigned safety processes and procedures have made a significant impact, there is still a large opportunity for improvement [6]. But in order to get to the next level, organizations need to be willing and able to address the human factor issues affecting emotions, attitudes and capability to perform the necessary functions needed to provide optimal patient care.

Background

For several years we have been conducting research on the frequency and significance of physician disruptive behaviors in the hospital sector. The research was originally conducted to see if there were a link between disruptive physician behaviors and nurse satisfaction and turnover as a contributing factor to the hospital nursing shortage. Review of the literature at that time revealed no conclusive findings so we decided to develop our own research survey tool. For the survey instrument disruptive behavior was defined as any inappropriate behavior, confrontation or conflict ranging from verbal abuse to physical or sexual harassment. Results from this research showed a significant linkage between physician disruptive behavior, nurse dissatisfaction and nursing turnover [7,8]. Not only did the research study quantify the frequency, significance and impact of disruptive physician behaviors, it also opened up a series of other important questions around the occurrence of nurse and other staff disruptive behaviors and the overall impact of disruptive behaviors on patient outcomes of care.

The second phase of research built on the findings of the previous research and added questions on the incidence and impact of nurse disruptive behaviors as well as other hospital staff employees. We were also intrigued about concerns raised about the impact of disruptive events on patient outcomes of care [9,10]. When we researched the literature, we could find references attesting to the benefits of more nurse time being spent at the patient's bedside and the lower likelihood of adverse clinical events (adverse clinical events are defined as any unexpected undesirable clinical patient experience, adverse occurrence or medical error that occurred during the hospitalization), and the benefits of good team collaboration on improving patient outcomes of care [11]. Other than a few anecdotal stories, we could not find any data supported evidence of poor clinical outcomes related to disruptive behaviors, poor communication or ineffective teamwork and collaboration [12-14]. With this objective in mind we added a series of questions to the phase two survey which were specifically designed to focus on the impact of disruptive behaviors on human factor issues and behaviors affecting patient outcomes of care.

Findings

To date our research database has results from over 5,000 participants from more than 150 hospitals across the United States. Overall, 75% of the respondents witnessed disruptive behavior in physicians. The most frequently mentioned medical specialties included General Surgery, Cardiovascular Surgery, Cardiology, Neurosurgery, Neurology, Anesthesiology and Orthopedics. 65% of the respondents witnessed disruptive behaviors in nurses. Most interestingly, more nurses witnessed disruptive behaviors in their peers than other groups witnessing disruptive behaviors in nurses. We also noted a significant concern about disruptive behaviors in respiratory therapists, lab technologists, pharmacists and physical therapists. The current stage (phase three) of the survey focuses on high intensity areas. The first special study was conducted specifically on peri-operative services. The surgical environment represents a rather unique micro chasm of medical care in that it is a high intensity service, conducted in a relatively small spatial confine with strong interdependence on team collaboration and assistance. Our results showed that the frequency and seriousness of disruptive events were more intensified in the surgical setting [10]. Special studies on the Intensive Care units (ICUs) and Emergency Departments (EDs) are planned for the near future.

The phase two and phase three surveys also contained a series of questions designed to assess the association between disruptive behaviors and adverse events. 38% of the respondents reported that they were aware of a potential adverse event that could have occurred as a result of disruptive behavior. 14% reported that they actually witnessed an adverse event as a direct result of disruptive behaviors. No one ever wants an adverse event to occur. The average occurrence rate of adverse events in US hospitals is 2-3%. This makes the 14% occurrence rate even more striking. Some of the comments provided in Table I highlight some of the critical concerns raised by some of the survey participants. The good news is that 80% of the respondents felt that these events could have been prevented.

In an effort to determine if there were a linkage between disruptive behaviors and psychological factors known to impede decision making, we asked a series of questions on the impact of disruptive behaviors on stress, frustration, loss of concentration, reduced team collaboration, reduced information transfer, reduced communication, and impaired nurse physician relations. Responses were recorded on a 10 point Likert scale. The results showed a significant impact of disruptive behaviors on all factors surveyed (see Figure I). Stress and frustration lead to loss of focus and impaired concentration which can lead to problems with communication and transfer of vital information which can ultimately result in a compromise in patient care.

In an effort to assess the relationship between disruptive behaviors and clinical outcomes of care, we asked a question about the perceived linkage between disruptive behaviors and the occurrence of adverse events, medical errors, compromises in patient safety, quality and patient mortality. Responses were recorded on a 10 point Likert scale. The results showed a significant impact of disruptive behaviors on all of the surveyed factors (see Figure II)

The concern raised by these findings is the significant impact disruptive events can have on behavioral factors known to increase stress, anxiety and frustration, which can impair focus and concentration. Reactions stimulated by these events can either directly or indirectly impair needed exchange of information and carrying out of responsibilities so important for patient care [15].

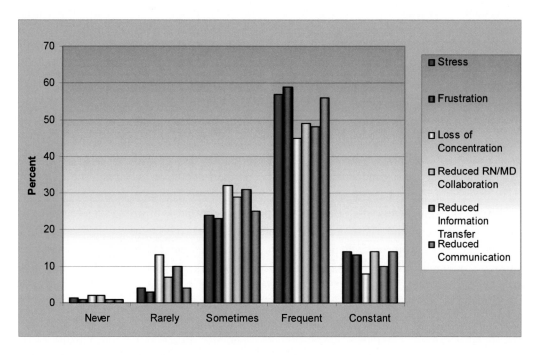

Figure I. How Often Does Disruptive Behavior Result in the Following?

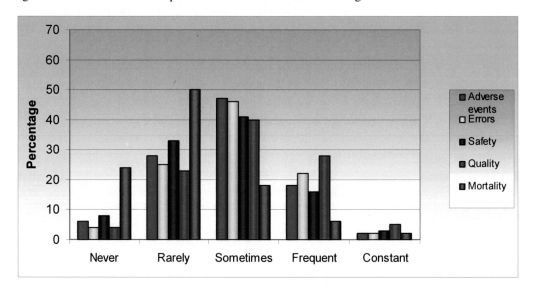

Figure II. Is How Often Do you Think There is a Link Between Disruptive Behaviors and the Following Clinical Outcomes of Care?

Table I. Selected Comments

- Most nurses are afraid to call Dr. X when they need to, and frequently won't call. Their patient's medical safety is always in jeopardy because of this.
- Staff was afraid to approach MD despite fact order was clearly incorrect. Disruptive behavior policy "wildly ineffective" Complaints delivered to a "black hole:"
- Cardiologist upset by phone calls and refused to come in. RN told it was not her job to think, just to follow orders. Rx delayed. MI extended
- MD became angry when RN reported decline in patient's condition and did not act on information. Patient required emergency intubation and was transferred to ICU. This caused the family much unnecessary heartache and disruption in family grieving process
- Poor communication post-op because of disruptive reputation resulted in delayed treatment, aspiration and eventual demise
- MD was told twice that sponge count was off. She said "they will find it later". Patient had to be re-opened.
- Dr. X has the social skills of a two year old
- The disruptive behavior from nurses is much more upsetting because I expect that behavior from the surgeons NOT the nurses b/c I rely on them as my peers (RN)
- When patient brought to unit for GI bleeding patient saw MD yelling at nurses. Patient asked if that was his doctor. Yes. Patient refused treatment and was transferred to another hospital. I am retiring early and never recommend someone becoming a nurse
- Disruptive behavior results in medication errors, slow response times and treatment errors!
- Specific group of MDs with poor communication habits which adversely affect patient care and nurse role
- Dr. X is so condescending to nurses that we are very reluctant to call him on patient's behalf.
- My concern is that the new nurses are afraid to call about patient problems and issues that truly need to be addressed in a timely manner impacting outcomes.
- It seems there is an increasing lack of respect by nurses and other ancillary caregivers toward practicing clinicians in the hospital environment. Decisions by clinicians are frequently challenged and some orders are flatly disobeyed or at least not carried thru with almost reflexive propensity, and with little or no forethought
- "Are you aware of any specific adverse events ....?" Yes. Death as a result of disruptive behavior. Staff nurses advocated for better patient care but MD would not willing to listen to reason. As a result patient died. The doctor chose to undo all the help that various staff had been working on for weeks to get this patient the help so badly needed.
- Yes, many incidents are preventable if both parties are willing to listen to each other, but many doctors are unwilling to accept a nurse's opinion just as some nurses are unwilling to listen to the opinions of LVNs, techs or CNAs, and it may have to do with the entrenched pecking order that exists at most hospitals.

Causative Factors

Human nature is complex, health care is a complex science and the health care environment functions in a bed of complexity. This implies that there are multiple factors involved in causing or stimulating disruptive events, none of which are mutually exclusive. Highlighted below are a series of factors known to contribute to disruptive behaviors (see Table II). Causative factors become particularly important when trying to develop and implement programs and strategies that will reduce the likelihood of disruptive behaviors and the resulting downside effects.

Table II. Factors Contributing to Disruptive Behaviors

- Setting
- Personality
- Gender
- Generation
- Culture and Ethnicity
- Life experiences
- Training
- Stakeholder interest

Setting

Disruptive events are inappropriate regardless of the cause or stimulating factor and there is never an excuse or rationalization for sanctioning such events as excusable. We noted that many of the disruptive events were evoked during a stressful situation. A common background would be a patient suddenly taking a turn for the worse or a procedure not going as planned. Another situation leading to a disruptive response is the unexpected call to the physician for clarification of orders or a discussion around plans for treatment or disposition, especially if calls occurred at night and/ or were directed at a physician covering for another physician.

Another factor contributing to the likelihood of occurrence of a disruptive event is either previous experience with the person or place and/ or reputation. Having had a previous bad experience with the individual or place or having prior knowledge of a bad reputation sets the stage for bad expectations which can increase the risk of a disruptive response.

The setting may play a role in setting up the potential for a disruptive outburst, but in most cases the potential lies more in the behind the scenes makeup of the individuals involved.

Personality

Suggestions have been made that disruptive events are more likely to occur from inherent personality traits than as a result of a specific inciting event. There are many different categorizations of personality classifications including Myers- Briggs, Personalysis, and others. For sake of discussion, we will break the personality types into four main groups: Directors, Socializers, Thinkers and Relaters [16].

Directors are described as being very task and results oriented, direct and to the point, demanding, and have a predilection for working independently. Under pressure they become more intense, demanding and controlling, and get results more by applying pressure and bullying than listening.

Socializers are described as being warm and sensitive, more people oriented, have a greater need for recognition and being appreciated, and value communication and collaboration. Under pressure they may become more dramatic, insistent and overbearing in their need to discuss and have their opinions heard.

Thinkers are intelligent, very systematic in their approach to a problem, are very precision and detail oriented, are slow, deliberate and meticulous in their methods, and with enough time, come up with well thought out analytical solutions. Under stress they tend to withdraw, work more independently and will lose interest in outside input.

Relaters are people oriented, tend to get along with everyone, are very agreeable, they don't want to rock the boat, and want to be liked. They shy away from confrontation and prefer to communicate more indirectly. Under pressure they may become more submissive, emotional or act in a passive- aggressive manner.

Gender

There has been a lot of research on gender characteristics and the role they play in influencing intention, action and reaction behaviors. If we follow the classic descriptions provided by John Gray PhD. in his text "Men are From Mars Woman are From Venus" we can use his assessment of male and female traits as a point for discussion and relate this to the health care environment [17]. We fully recognize that these are stereotypic descriptions and should not be the basis of conclusion, but our experience has shown us that these characteristics do play out in the medical arena.

Males are described as being very focused, task and goal driven, time dependent, power hungry, self-achievers, who tend to work in an autonomous independent fashion. They look for competency and efficiency in their co-workers. When under stress they either become more dominating and authoritative or withdraw to work things out on their own.

Females are described as being more social minded and communicative, interested in developing relationships, are more accepting and willing to listen and to share, are more sensitive and caring, and they value group consensus and companionship. When under stress they look more to group input and discussion as a way of solving the crisis.

In the health care environment, most of the physicians are male and most of the nurses and other clinical support staff are female. Under stressful situations, you can see how these traits may put males and females at odds [18].

Generation

There are several different classes of generation styles, attitudes and preferences based on a person's age [18]. For purposes of this discussion we will divide these generations into four different categories: Veterans (1900-1945), Boomers (1946-1964), Generation X (1965-1980) and Generation Y (1981-1999).

Veterans are known at the "conformists". They are typically very loyal employees, ardent rule followers, they don't challenge the system or the organizational hierarchy and take pride and satisfaction in doing good work,

Baby Boomers are known as "the me" generation. They are loyal hard workers, high achievers, very competitive, self absorbed workaholics who pride themselves on individual accomplishment and personal goal achievement. They want to be the star of the show.

The Generation Xers are referred to as "the survivors". They are self reliant more independent thinkers who value friends and family over work, are more skeptical and less impressed by authority and title, and seek a positive work-life balance.

The Generation Yers are referred to as "the loved ones". They maintain strong family ties, are more comfortable with diversity, are more interested in informal team collaboration than traditional structure, are very confident, possess strong technology savvy and look at life as fun, fast and interactive.

Every generation emerges with a different set of values and experiences as compared to the generation before and after them. One set of values is not better than another, they're just different. These differences can be a real barrier to effective communication. In order to maximize communication and team collaboration efficiency, we need to be conscious of other people's values, styles and priorities and work with them to support a process that maximizes their talents and preferences in a way that results in the best possible outcomes.

Culture/ Ethnicity

The United States is one of the most ethnically and culturally diverse countries in the world and many clinicians come from a variety of cultural backgrounds.

Culture, ethnicity, traditions, family values, political and religious beliefs all mold our thoughts, perceptions and interactions with society [20-22]. These values affect ones perceptions, viewpoints and opinions which influence specific actions and reactions to different situations. These values reflect views related to power and authority, roles and responsibilities of men and women, approach to conflict and confrontation and physical and emotional self confidence.

In all interactions, cultural differences can exacerbate communication problems. For example, in some cultures, individuals do not like to be assertive or challenge opinions openly, as loss of face is considered. As a result, it is very difficult for some nurses to speak up if they see something wrong. They often will communicate their concern in very indirect ways, which can inhibit important information transfer. Culture barriers can be furthered hindered by nonverbal communication. For example, some cultures have particular ideas about physical space, the meaning of eye contact, specific facial expressions, touch, tone of voice, and nods of the head. Potential misinterpretation of intentions is a set up for ineffective communication, and is compounded in emergent or stressful situations.

Other Life Experiences

In addition to the value set, beliefs and perceptions molded by the factors discussed above, real time life experiences can set the mood for the day. Recent arguments, conflicts, illness, financial troubles, substance abuse or any other disturbance can affect the way we approach and interact with others and influence the final outcome.

Training

If one looks at the process involved in training a physician, you will note it encompasses the full gamut of emotions from early training insecurities and abuse to having to make critical life and death decisions under extremely stressful situations.

When one starts out in medical school everyone is very quick to let you know that you don't know anything and your opinions are not wanted or valued. Your job is to do all the "scut work" that no one else wants to do. At the bottom of the chain of command you're abused by staff and as a result feel very isolated and insecure. The training period requires long hours of work and dedication, and the associated stress and fatigue doesn't help the situation. The training itself is focused on technical competency rather than personal interactions or leadership development skills. When you do reach a point of responsibility, you need to make immediate authoritative decisions which have a profound effect on patient care. This breeds a composite picture of dominating, autocratic, controlling behavior which lies on top of the insecurity, isolation and independency fostered by earlier conditions. What suffers is the lack of communication, people and team collaboration skills so important for patient care.

Stakeholder Interest

There are many participants in the health care delivery process, and they each have their own values and interests.

Nurses want to be respected. They want to feel like they're part of the health care team and are able to have input into the patient care process. They want to feel that their contributions make a difference in quality patient care. Other members of the health care team have similar values.

Physicians want to get the best possible outcome. They want staff to be responsive to their demands and they want to feel that the staff are trustworthy and competent to carry out all their duties.

Table III. Recommendations

1. Organizational awareness
   a. Internal assessment
   b. Business case
   c. Motivation and accountability
2. Organizational support and commitment
   a. Culture
   b. Leadership
   c. Champions
3. Meetings, discussion groups, education
   a. Informal get togethers
   b. Committees
   c. Department presentations
   d. Focus groups
   e. Training programs
4. Educational training seminars and workshops
   a. Diversity management
   b. Anger management
   c. Conflict management
5. Communication training
   a. Phone etiquette
   b. Scripting
   c. SBAR
6. Team training
   a. Crew resource management
   b. Pit crew management
   c. Lean process/ Six Sigma
7. Competency training
   a. Technical competency
   b. Language competency
8. Intervention strategies
   a. Assertiveness training
   b. De-briefings
   c. Code White
9. Behavior policies and procedures
   a. Zero tolerance policy
   b. Code of Conduct policy (credentialing)
   c. Disruptive Behavior policy
10. Reporting mechanisms
    a. Incident Reporting
    b. Incident evaluation
    c. Follow up plan

Assessment, Strategies and Recommendations:

Given the multiplicity of interacting factors, there is no canned set of strategies or recommendations that can be applied as a cookie cutter solution to the problem. Individual solutions will depend upon the scope of the problem, the underlying culture, leadership and organizational dynamics, and the current status and success of programs already in place. The overall goal is (1) to prevent these types of episodes from occurring, (2) to address acute events in real time to avoid a compromised result, and (3) to develop policies that set appropriate standards of behavior with follow up procedures when these standards are not met. Recommended steps are listed in Table III.

1. Organizational Awareness

The first step in the process is to assess the current state of affairs. One way to assess the situation is to review complaints and incident reports and/ or listen to the hallway or coffee lounge gossip. Another way to assess the situation is to force the issue with an internal survey. We recommend a combination of these approaches. The added value of the dedicated survey is that it not only gives you an objective assessment of what your staff sees and feels at the organization, it also allows you to pinpoint areas of concern. Our survey tool specifically addresses the frequency of disruptive behaviors by discipline, medical specialty and service unit, the impact of disruptive behaviors on behavioral factors affecting levels of stress, concentration, communication and information transfer, and the linkages of disruptive behavior to adverse events, medical errors, patient safety, quality, mortality, and staff satisfaction. The survey also adds a comments section where participants can go into more detail about their observations, experiences and surrounding issues (see example Table I). As mentioned earlier, these comments provide significant insight into the nature and extend of the problem. The two most important caveats are (1) the assurance that all results will be held confidential and (2) that actions will be taken and follow up feed back is provided.

Once the survey results are accumulated, they are analyzed and compared to other results in the database. The next step is to share the results with the staff at the hospital. The goal is to motivate action and responsibility by making a strong business case that this is an important issue that has series implications and repercussions. The business case developed around phase one of our research focused on the impact of disruptive behaviors on nurse satisfaction, retention and turnover and its contribution to the hospital nursing shortage. This may or may not have had a big impact on the physician audience. Phase two of the research focused on the impact of disruptive behaviors on patient care and this affects everyone in the health service industry. The business case for physicians is that poor patient outcomes may occur because of disruptive events that lead to communication mishaps and /or serious errors resulting in a potentially preventable adverse event and that you have accountability in this process.

2. Organization Commitment and Support

The organization itself sets the stage for expectations in regard to staff roles, responsibilities, behaviors and performance outcomes. Culture is defined as the integrated pattern of human knowledge, belief, and behavior that depends upon man's capacity for learning and transmitting knowledge to succeeding generations [24]. The organization needs to set the priorities by being committed to providing and supporting a culture that demands and reinforces appropriate professional behavioral standards. This needs to be is a top down bottom up commitment. Administrative leaders, Clinical Leaders, Directors, Line Managers, Hospital Employees and Physicians all have responsibilities for supporting this standard and everyone needs to be held accountable for adhering to these cultural and behavioral expectations as a way of doing business.

One of the key successes on the clinical side has been the enthusiasm and advocacy of a clinical champion. For physicians, the clinical champion could be a salaried physician executive (Chief Medical officer (CMO), Vice President of Medical Affairs (VPMA) or Medical Director), the Chief of Staff, or a physician who so believes in the importance of enforcing appropriate behavioral standards that he or she drives the process on their own. From the nursing side the champion could be the Chief Nursing Officer (CNO), the Vice President of Patient Care Services, a Department Director, or any other nursing staff advocate who is passionate about this issue. For a champion to be successful they must be respected, have a good rapport and reputation with the medical and nursing staff, and be eloquent and persuasive in their actions. The clinical champion usually works in conjunction with the administrative and clinical leadership staff. Some organizations have developed programs that are part of their patient safety, quality, risk management and accelerated performance initiatives.

3. Meetings and Discussions

One of the key principles in issue resolution is to have individuals address issues and concerns with the people involved. The earlier on in the evolutionary course of the disturbance, the greater the opportunity for clearing up expectations, assumptions and misperceptions that led to the problem.

One simple step is to encourage contact. Physicians can do a better job in making efforts to establish a positive nurse- physician relationship. Our research has shown us that while only 2-3% of physicians are overtly disruptive (this 2-3% can have profound effects on the entire organization), another 30-50% have poor communication and social interaction skills. In the hospital environment, physicians appear to often be stressed, hurried and pre-occupied, and want to get in and get out so they can get on to the next thing. If the physician would just take a step back and smile at the nurse or ask a question about how their patient was doing, this would do a lot in improving nurse- physician relations.

Another way to get physicians and nurses together is to set up task forces or committees where they work on mutually important topics. Some organizations have even set up department or town hall meetings where nurses and physicians can address issues of concern in a collaborative manner.

Some organizations have developed dedicated committees to address nurse physician relations. They are responsible for setting policy and addressing issues as they rise.

The topic of disruptive behaviors and its impact on organizational dynamics and patient care need to be discussed as part of the ongoing staff educational process. Topics can be presented at general sessions or ground rounds, at specific department meetings or at off- site events. More in-depth discussions can be conducted as specific focus groups, particularly in areas where problems are more evident. As mentioned previously, there is a growing need to introduce these discussions at the medical school and nursing school level to better prepare and equip students to be knowledgeable about the potential consequences of disruptive behaviors and impaired communication.

4. Educational Seminars and Workshops

In order to address some of the causative factors discussed previously, organizations need to provide more comprehensive educational seminars, workshops and training programs to improve staff skill sets so they can better address these issues. These programs could include a number of different topics such as diversity training, sensitivity training, anger management, conflict management, stress management, or any other topic appropriate for the situation.

5. Communication Training

Special efforts need to be made to improve staff communication skills. We don't think that anyone intentionally plans on being a poor communicator, but some are better than others. Communication is a two way street. The initiator has a specific intent or message that requires a response. The receiver processes the request and gives a response. As discussed previously, the intent and response may be influenced by emotions and attitudes related to events surrounding the current situation and the values already established via gender, age, culture, personality, and life experiences that influence thoughts and actions. Perceptions override reality. It is also important to remember that body language, verbal tone and presentation style have more of an influence on messaging than the actual content of the message itself.

There are a series of tools that have been designed to improve communication efficiency. Equally important are tools that specifically address language capacity and these will be discussed later on under competency.

Scripting is a very efficient way of organizing priorities into a series of straightforward questions designed to achieve desired objectives. One example would be a list of questions originally put together by the Quint Studer Group designed to prepare nurses when making a call to a physician [24]. The basic tenets are to identify who you are, identify the patient, state the problem, be familiar with the patient's chart including a thorough review of the orders, testing results and progress notes, and treat the physician with respect.

Another recently introduced tool that has become very popular is the SBAR tool ((Situation, Background, Assessment, and Recommendation). This tool has been successfully implemented at Kaiser and many other facilities where nurses, physicians and other staff members are trained simultaneously on tool purpose and utility. The tool provides a clear concise consistent process to exchange relevant information needed to make a decision about patient care [26,27].

6. Team Training

Another new innovation recently introduced into healthcare under the umbrella of patient safety and the importance of team collaboration is the adoption of crew pit management techniques as used in the aviation industry. The focus of these types of team training programs is to highlight the importance of understanding your role and everyone else's roles and responsibilities, increasing awareness and anticipation of upcoming events, trusting your team, avoiding conflict and confusion, and speaking up if something appears to be wrong or not proceeding as planned [28-30]. A recent extension of the cockpit crew management technique has been the adoption of the pit crew techniques used by the Ferrari team in the NASCAR races [31].

Many organizations are embracing Lean process design and Six Sigma techniques in an effort to improve efficiency, reduce errors and remove waste in their processes and procedures as a way to accelerate organizational performance. This requires both system redesign and human factor re-engineering which calls for meeting compliance standards around human behaviors.

7. Competency Training

Assuring competency, trust and respect is a key factor in communication efficiency and effectiveness. On one side physicians need to feel confident that nursing and other supporting staff are well trained, knowledgeable and technically competent in handling and carrying out appropriate patent care directives. Likewise, nurses and other clinical staff want to feel that the physician is able and competent in carrying out their duties. Many of these knowledge and technical competencies are mandated through accreditation, training verification and credentialing requirements.

A second area of competency is what we call communication competency. A person could have great knowledge and technical skills but through either a language barrier or an ineffective communication style, there is a risk to communication efficiency and effectiveness. In the previous section we addressed the use of certain tool kits designed to improve communication proficiency. In regard to language, our experience has shown us that in many of the organizations who participated in the survey, in a large percentage of both the clinical (particularly nursing) and medical staff English is a second language. In this regard, some of the organizations have provided specific courses on communication applications and techniques for those individuals where English is not the primary language [32].

8. Intervention Strategies

One of the biggest concerns is to get people to speak up in real time during the time in which a disruptive event is in the process of unfolding. As mentioned before, many individuals are reluctant to speak up because of issues related to personality, gender, culture, organizational hierarchy, reputation, personal experience, or other influencing factors. Think of the case of a new entry female nurse from the orient who is shy and respectful of position faced with an angry domineering foreign trained male physician who is yelling and screaming about an issue of concern.

There was a recent white paper published called "Silence Kills" which highlights the problems that occur when people don't speak up when they see a problem developing [33]. In their book titled *Crucial Conversations* the authors go into detail about the problems that occur from not speaking up and use role play examples to provide techniques that instill confidence on the why, how and when to speak up in an appropriate manner [34]. Another technique is to provide basic assertiveness training classes to all involved staff members.

Some organizations have utilized a briefing/ debriefing technique in an effort to either prevent an event from occurring by upfront discussion, or to address an event that did occur in a post-briefing session. For scheduled encounters the pre-briefing session can discuss objectives, clarify roles and responsibilities and can bring forward any issues of relevance prior to the scheduled event such as surgery, a procedure or group meeting. If someone is having a rough day, they can bring this out up front so people will understand and be more accepting or tolerant of the situation. The post event briefing can do the same. In crisis time some organizations have implemented a "Code White" policy. When a disruptive event is occurring, a call goes out to a team of individuals who then come to the scene to help intervene [35].

9. Behavior Policies and Procedures

Specific policies and procedures need to be developed to support behavioral standards of care. These policies come under the umbrella of Zero Tolerance, Code of Conduct, Code of Ethics or Standard Behavior policies which should outline appropriate behavior standards, expectations and ramifications if these standards are not followed. These policies and procedures need to be applied organization wide. Rather than one policy for physicians, another for nurses, and another for other employees, these policies need to be consistently and equitably applied across all levels of the organization. Staff employees and physicians must agree to abide by these policies as a condition of employment or acceptance of a new position or appointment and/or as part of the privileging and credentialing process.

There also needs to be a distinct Disruptive Behavior policy which includes specific criteria and procedures for handling disruptive individuals. There should a specific committee or group of individuals with representation from all involved disciplines (medical staff, nursing, administration, human resources other ...) who participate in a consistently applied process that evaluates issues and makes recommendations for appropriate action, follow up and feed back.

10. Reporting

Incident reporting is a vital issue. Our research has shown us that more than 50% of the respondents stated that they were reluctant to report in fear of concerns about confidentiality, retaliation, the fact that no one listens, no actions are taken and/ or they never get any feedback about recommendations or resolution.

In order to address these issues, the organization must support a confidential non-punitive reporting policy. Rather than depending upon specific incident reports, written or verbal reports to CMOs, CNOs, supervisors, directors or mangers or other formal or informal documentation streams, it would be preferable to have a consistent process for handling and responding to complaints.

Some organizations have implemented a process where they have one designated committee responsible for receiving and addressing all relevant complaints. The committee has a multidisciplinary composition that as a group (rather than an individual) is responsible for investigating each individual complaint and coming up with an appropriate action and follow up plan. The advantages of using this type of reporting system is that the process is straight forward, all inputs and outputs are held confidential, there is consistency and equity in the review process and decisions are made by a group process.

Conclusions

Disruptive behaviors are a common occurrence across all industries, but in health care the risks are more acute as it can adversely affect patient outcomes of care. Until recently, health care as an industry has been reluctant to deal with the issue as they were politically and financially reluctant to confront a high profile physician who voluntarily brings his or her patients to the hospital and is a main source of hospital revenue. Recent issues around workforce shortages, workplace safety, liability and bad patient outcomes have brought new fuel to the system where organizations can no longer afford to look the other way.

Of particular concern is the effect of disruptive relationships on increasing feelings of frustration, anger and antagonism, and its negative impact on willingness to communicate, collaborate and exchange information necessary for patient care. Disruptive relationships can heighten stress, increase distraction and impede concentration, all of which results in a higher likelihood of medical errors. Overall there is a strong linkage between disruptive relationships and the occurrence of adverse events and compromises in patient safety, quality and clinical outcomes of care.

Disruptive behaviors occur for a multitude of reasons. Some of the behaviors are based on deep seated values influenced by gender, age, ethnicity, religious beliefs, family values, training, personal experiences and personality. Some disruptive behaviors are provoked because of real time stresses that affect emotions and disposition.

In developing a program to address these behaviors the focus is to try to prevent such outbursts from occurring, minimizing the impact if they do occur, and taking action on any events which have significant consequences. While it may be difficult to change personalities or personal values, you can change situational awareness, perceptions and reactions through appropriate training and education.

In order to achieve desired results the organization must be committed to a zero tolerance policy, develop and support a professional behavior policy with the commitment to enforce desired standards consistently across all disciplines, provide education and appropriate support services and be prepared to take appropriate action as necessary.

References

[1]   Institute of Medicine Report To Err is Human: Building a Safer Health System. Washington (DC): National Academy Press; 2000.

[2]   Institute of Medicine Report "Crossing the Quality Chasm: A New Health System or the 21st Century" Washington (DC): National Academy Press; March 2001

[3]   Institute of Medicine Report "Preventing Medication Errors" Washington (DC): National Academy Press; July 2006

[4]   "The Joint Commission Guide to Improving Staff Communication" Joint Commission Resources Oakbrook Terrace, IL 2005

[5]   IHI 5 Million Lives Saved Campaign *www.IHI.org*

[6]   Longo, D., Hewett, J., Ge, B., Schubert, S. "The Long Road to Patient Safety: A Status Report on Patient Safety Systems*" JAMA Vol.294* No.22 December 14, 2005 p. 2858-2865

[7]   Rosenstein, A. "The Impact of Nurse-Physician Relationships on Nurse Satisfaction and Retention" *American Journal of Nursing, Vol.102* No.6, June 2002, p. 26-34

[8]   Rosenstein, A.; Lauve, R., Russell. H. "Disruptive Physician Behavior Contributes to Nursing Shortage" The Physician Executive, November-December 2002, p. 8-11

[9]   Rosenstein, A., O'Daniel, M. "Disruptive Behavior and Clinical Outcomes: Perceptions of Nurses and Physicians" *American Journal of Nursing Publication Vol. 105* No.1 January 2005 p.54-64

[10] Rosenstein, A., O'Daniel, M. "Impact and Implications of Disruptive Behavior in the Peri-Operative Arena" *Journal of American College of Surgery Vol.203* No.1 p.96-105 July 2006

[11] Needleman, J., Buerhaus, P, Stewart, M., Zelevinsky, K. and Mattke, S. "Nurse Staffing In Hospitals: Is There A Business Case For Quality?" *Health Affairs, Vol.25* No.1 p. 204-211

[12] Baggs, J., Schmitt, M., Mushlin, A., Eldredge, D. et. al. "Association Between Nurse-Physician Collaboration and Patient Outcomes in Three Intensive Care Units" *Critical Care Medicine Vol.27* No.9 September 1999 p.1991-1997

[13] Knaus, W., Draper, E., Wagner, D., Zimmerman, J. "An Evaluation of Outcomes from Intensive Care in Major Medical Centers" *Annals of Internal Medicine Vol104* No.3 March 1986 p.410-418

[14] Boyle, d., Kochinda, C. Enhancing Collaborative Communication of Nurse and Physician Leadership in Two Intensive Care Units: *JONA Vol.34* No. 2 p.60-70 Feb. 2004.

[15] Reason, J. "Human Error: Models and Management" *British Medical Journal Vol.320* March 18, 2000

[16] Allesandra, T., O'Connor, M. *The Platinum Rule: Discover the Four Basic Business Personalities and How They Can Lead You to Succe*ss. Warner Books New York 1996

[17] Gray, J. *Men and Venus in the Workplace.* Harper Collins Publishers New York 2004

[18] Zelek, B., Phillips, S "Gender and Power: Nurses and Doctors in Canada International *Journal for Equity in Health Vol.2* No.1 February 11, 2003 p.1

[19] Lana caster, L., Stillman, D. *When Generations Collide.* Harper Collins Publishers New York 2002

[20] Peterson, Brooks. *Cultural Intelligence: A Guide to Working With People from Other Cultures.* Boston: Intercultural Press, 2004.

[21] Taylor SL, Lurie N. The Role of Culturally Competent Communication in Reducing Ethnic and Racial Healthcare Disparities. *American Journal of Managed Care.* 2004 Sep; 10 Spec No:SP1-4

[22] Early, P. Christopher and Ang, Soon. *Cultural Intelligence: Individual Interactions Across Cultures.* Stanford University Press, 2003

[23] Kohls, L. Robert and Knight, John M. A *Cross-Cultural training Handbook.* 2nd Edition. Boston Intercultural Press, 1994

[24] Webster's Ninth New Collegiate Dictionary Merrian- Webster Inc. Springfield, Massachusetts 19889

[25] Personal communication The Quint Studer Group Gulf Breeze, FL

[26] Leonard, M., Graham, S., Bonacum, D. "The Human Factor: The Critical Importance of Effective Teamwork and Communication in Providing Safe Care" *Qual Saf Health Care Vol.13* Suppl.1 2004 p.85-90

[27] Sutcliffe, K., Lewton, E., Rosenthal, M. "Communication Failures: An Insidious Contributor to Medical Mishaps" *Academic Medicine Vol.79* No.2 p.186-194 February 2004

[28] Grogan, E., Stiles, R., France, D., Speroff, T. et. Al. "The Impact of Aviation- Based Teamwork Training on the Attitudes of Health- Care Professionals" *The American College of Surgeons Vol.199* No.6 December 2004 p.843-848

[29] Leming-Lee, S., France, D., Feistritzer, N., Kuntz, A. et. al., "Crew Resource Management in Perioperative Services: Navigating the Implementation Road Map" *JCOM Vol.12* No.7 July 2005 p.353-358

[30] Sexton JB, Thomas EJ, Helmreich RL. "Error, Stress, and Teamwork in Medicine and Aviation: Cross Sectional Surveys. *BMJ Vol.320* March 2000 p.745–9.

[31] Naik, G. "A Hospital Races to Learn Methods of Ferrari Pit Stop" *WSJ* November 14, 2006 p.D1-D2.

[32] Personal communication Peachy Hains RN, Christopher Ng MD, Cedars-Sinai Medical Center Los Angeles, California

[33] "Silence Kills" American Association of Critical Care Nurses *www.silencekills.com* VitalSmarts Provo, UT 2005

[34] Patterson, K., Grenny, J., McMillan, R., Switzler, A. *Crucial Conversations: Tools for Talking When Stakes are High.* McGraw – Hill New York 2002

[35] "Building the Nurse- Physician Partnership: Restoring Mutual Trust, Establishing Clinical Collaboration" The Health Care Advisory Board Washington, D.C. 2005

In: Trends in Nursing Research   ISBN 978-1-60456-642-0
Editors: Adam J. Ryan and Jack Doyle   © 2009 Nova Science Publishers, Inc.

Chapter 10

A Preliminary Survey of Health Related Dietary Habits in Nursing Students, Registered Nurses and Older Persons In Hong Kong

***Mimi M.Y. Tse**[*]*
School of Nursing, The Hong Kong Polytechnic University, Kowloon, Hong Kong,
Iris F.F. Benzie
Department of Health Technology & Informatics, The Hong Kong Polytechnic
University, Kowloon, Hong Kong

Abstract

Diets rich in fresh fruits and vegetables protect against chronic, degenerative disease. This is suggested to be related to their high antioxidant content. Up to 40% of all cancers may be preventable by diet, and risk of other age-related diseases, such as heart disease, dementia, diabetes, has a strong dietary link also. Incidence of age-related disease is increasing, for most there is no cure, and treatment is difficult, expensive and often ineffective. Therefore disease prevention is a global issue of increasing importance.

Today's student nurses are tomorrow's primary healthcare professionals and role models for health promotion and good dietary habits. However, in a cross-sectional non-experimental dietary study of 274 nursing students (228 females, 46 males), results showed low daily intake of fluid, dairy products and fruits and vegetables (<2 portions) in the majority, and 40% never took breakfast. Interestingly, study of dietary habits of registered nurses yielded similar findings. Of 251 nurses (208 female, 43 male), >50% reported dining out and eating fast food regularly. Skipping meals, fewer family meals, and high intake of fast foods are habits that are likely to result in lower intake of 'healthy' food including fruits, vegetables and dairy products. Sixty-five percent of nurses studied ate <2 portions of fruits and vegetables per day, a worryingly low intake when the recommended intake for optimal health is 5 or more/day,

---

[*] Tel: 852 2766 6541; Fax: 852 2364 9663; email: hsmtse@inet.polyu.edu.hk

and 63% took no milk or other dairy products. Dairy products are a major source of dietary calcium, and low consumption of calcium is associated with higher risk of osteoporosis and bone fracture in later life. Interestingly, the self-perceived nutritional status was deemed satisfactory by most nursing students and nurses, even though study findings indicate dietary practices are far from optimal.

Thirty-six older persons in the local Chinese community were surveyed on dietary-related behaviour and lifestyle. Results showed that 40% lived alone and ate alone on a regular basis. They took few fruits and vegetable per day, no dairy or bean curd products, and inadequate fluid. Half were overweight or obese.

Results indicate low intake of antioxidant-rich food among nursing students, nurses and older persons in Hong Kong. Nurses must be trained to be knowledgeable about the relationship between diet and health and be ready and willing to lead by example, and therefore diet and health inter-relationships should be made explicit components of the nursing curriculum. Also, it is important to communicate to members of the public the importance of diet in prevention of age-related disease and promotion of healthy ageing.

Introduction

Diet and Health

One of the basic human needs is nutrition. Nutrition is the science that examines food and how food nourishes our bodies and affects our health (Thompson & Manore, 2005). Nutrition is a relatively new scientific discipline. It is noted that early research in nutrition mainly focused on making the connection between nutrient deficiencies and illness. Examples included the discovery of the lack of vitamin C in causing scurvy in mid-1700s. The discovery was confined to some ingredient found in citrus fruits that could prevent scurvy; yet, vitamin C had not been identified at that time. It was only in the twentieth century that the exact nutrient responsible for the deficiency symptoms was discovered (Thompson & Manore, 2005). Indeed, the majority of discoveries in the field of nutrition are relatively new, with more yet to be learned. These lessons are important because of the changing mortality patterns across the world.

In the twentieth century, the leading causes of death were infectious diseases, largely now preventable by vaccination or treatable by medication such as antibiotics. Currently, non-communicable, age-related diseases such as coronary heart diseases (CVD), cancer and stroke, are the leading causes of illness and death (Table 1). It is noted that health-compromising behaviors of the individual may contribute to the development of these non-infectious diseases. Health-compromising behaviors include high calorie and high cholesterol intake, sedentary lifestyle, cigarette smoking and excessive alcohol intake (Healthy People, 2004).

Incidence of chronic, age-related diseases including cancer, cerebrovascular disease (CVD; stroke), Type 2 diabetes mellitus and dementia is increasing. It is noted that there is no cure for most of these chronic-aged-related diseases, and that treatment is difficult, expensive and usually ineffective. Cancer and CVD are the leading causes of death world wide, Type 2 diabetes is reaching epidemic proportions and robs people of their health as well as bringing a high social cost in terms of treatment and working days lost, while osteoporosis badly affects the mobility and quality of life of many older persons (The International Council of Nurses, 2005; Anderson & Smith, 2003). These disorders are multifactorial in origin, but diet plays an important role in determining risk (Cox et al., 2000; Duthie et al., 2000). It is estimated that 30-40% of all cancers are diet related (World Cancer Research Fund & American Institute for Cancer, 1997; Tse & Benzie, 2005), and people who eat diets rich in fruits and vegetables have low risk of CVD (Pryor, 2000; Asplund, 2002). Beneficial effects of 'healthy' diets are suggested to be due, at least in part, to their antioxidant content (Benzie, 2003).

Table 1: Leading causes of death for all ages

1	Coronary heart disease
2	Cancer
3	Stroke
4	Chronic lower respiratory disease
5	Unintentional injuries
6	Diabetes
7	Influenza and pneumonia
8	Alzheimer's disease
9	Kidney disease

Source: National Center for Health Statistics, 2004

A healthy diet should be able to provide enough of all essential nutrients to avoid deficiencies. Yet, excessive calorie intake and obesity increases risk of chronic disease including heart disease, stroke and cancer (Dudek, 2006). It is clear that 'Healthy' diets comprise antioxidant-rich fruits and vegetables, wholegrain cereals and omega-3 fatty acids, and are low in saturated fat, in salt and in refined sugar. The World Cancer Research Fund International recommends taking 5 or more portions of fresh fruits and vegetables per day for health (World Cancer Research Fund, 1997). This level of intake provides a high antioxidant intake, especially when taken in conjunction with other plant based dietary agents including teas, herbs and red wine (Benzie & Strain, 2005).

Nurse: Health Promoter and Role Model for Healthy Diets

Nutrition is a basic human need throughout the life cycle, and a vital component of nursing care. Knowledge of nutrition principles and the ability to apply that knowledge are important for nurses working in home health, community wellness, outpatient settings, acute or long-term care facilities (Dudek, 2006). Nurses are ideally placed to play an important role in dissemination of health information to patients and the general public in relation to the role of diet in health enhancement. Because of their front line position across various healthcare settings, nurses have the opportunity to provide nutritional counseling, education and advice across the lifespan (St Leger, 1997; Williams & Lewis, 2002; Fowles, 2004; Rasanen et al., 2004; Pedersen, 2005). Seizing this opportunity can make a difference. For example, a positive correlation between maternal nutrition and birth outcome was demonstrated when pregnant women were closely monitored by nurses in regard to dietary habits and provided with nutrition education during their pregnancy (Fowles, 2004). In addition, nurses and dieticians together guided the supply of healthier food, with adequate and cheap fresh fruit being supplied, and limited or no access to high-sugar, low-fibre processed foods for children and adolescent at school (St Leger, 1997). Likewise, nurses provide various nutritional counseling and nutrient education programmes to children and their parents as well as young adults, with positive outcomes reported (Williams & Lewis, 2002; Rasanen et al., 2004). Older persons also need to be aware of the significant role of diet in health promotion. As such, nursing care based on active involvement of patients in their nutritional care was found to be an effective method to improve dietary habits and nutritional status among older persons (Pedersen, 2005).

Nurses should and can act as key players in health promotion, both as role models through healthy lifestyle practice and as informed advisors on dietary habits for health enhancement. This requires that nurses themselves increase their awareness, knowledge and understanding of interdisciplinary research findings relevant to health promotion. Nurses must be educated in what constitutes good dietary practice and a healthy lifestyle, otherwise, the opportunity to advise on and improve the diet of their clients and families will be lost.

Diet and Health Among Older Persons

There have been marked gains in life expectancy in the past 100 years. The number of people aged 65 and older has increased 11-fold since 1990 (Federal Interagency Forum on Aging Related Statistics, 2005), with a modern day average life expectancy of 79 years for men and 72 years for women (United Nations, 2001). The life expectancy in Hong Kong ranks second in the world (Hong Kong Policy Research Institute Ltd, 2006), at 78 for men and 84 for women. Therefore, one of the most important issues that Hong Kong is facing is the growing burden of disability and disease associated with its ageing population. In 2005, there were 836,400 elderly people in Hong Kong who were aged 65 years or over, representing 12.1% of the total population (Census and Statistics Department, 2006). By the year 2031, the proportion of the elderly in the population will grow to 24.3%, i.e. one in four people in Hong Kong will be aged 65 or over (Hong Kong Policy Research Institute Ltd, 2006).

The growth of the population age 65 and over will challenge policymakers, families and health care professions to meet the needs of ageing individuals. With increasing life expectancy, incidence of chronic diseases and illness that limits the self-caring ability of the older persons also increases (LEGCO Panel on Welfare Services, 2005). Aging brings various physiological changes including the loss of muscle mass and lean tissue, increased body fat, decreased bone density, a decline in immune function and impaired ability to absorb and metabolize various nutrients (Thompson & Manore, 2005). In light of the physiological changes associated with aging, older persons are more susceptible to disease of various kinds (Rosenthal & Kavic, 2004). Health care expenditure for the care of the elderly is expected to increase in this regard (Hong Kong Policy Research Institute Ltd, 2006). Likewise, quality of life for older persons is likely to be compromised because of existing chronic illnesses that may hinder self-caring ability and mobility (Koopman, 2001).

Therefore, it is important to educate the general public on the importance of primary care – development and maintenance of health promoting habits among community dwelling older persons in particular (Takahashi et al., 2004). It is noted that people with good health habits live longer and healthier, and reducing the chances of having to rely on the medical system during their old age (Hong Kong Policy Research Institute Ltd, 2006).

In short, most age-related diseases are largely preventable by dietary and lifestyle modification. Diet has a strong influence on the risk and progression of the most common chronic, age-related diseases including cardiovascular disease, dementia, diabetes and cancer (World Cancer Research Fund and American Cancer Institute, 1997; Hogstel, 2001; Yen, 2003; Benzie, 2005). Good dietary habits are important for health enhancement, while inadequate nutrition may increase susceptibility to and delay recovery from illness. Nutrition is a relatively new scientific discipline, and many older persons were not given formal nutrition education in their formative years (Hogstel, 2001). Therefore, older adults often lack adequate information on the importance of diet and dietary intervention in disease prevention. It is important to gain more information on diet and nutritional status of the elderly in the community in order for nurses to be able to direct appropriate nutritional advice and education to this group. Furthermore, it is important to ensure that nurses are adequately knowledgeable themselves, so that they can do this effectively. To this end, we need to explore the diet, lifestyle and self perceived health and nutritional status of nurses and community-dwelling older persons in Hong Kong. In this article we summarise data from three studies involving nursing students, practicing nurses and older people in the community.

Studies on Health and Dietary Behaviours of a Group of Nursing Students and Registered Nurses

Knowledge of nutrition principles and the ability to apply that knowledge in various clinical settings are important for nurses. It is a vital and integral component of nursing care. Nevertheless, education in relation to diet and health is not a usual competent of the nursing curriculum. In order for nurses to be able to seize the opportunity to provide nutritional advice and to act as role models for health promotion, it was of interest to explore the health related and dietary behaviours in a group of first year nursing students and a group of registered nurses working in the hospital in Hong Kong and to assess their self-perceived nutritional status in order to identify gaps in their knowledge base.

For the nursing students, a cross-sectional non-experimental study was performed. A convenience sample of 290 first year full-time university nursing students was approached and invited to complete a simple diet and lifestyle-related questionnaire. The questionnaire was based on the Nutrition Risk Assessment form (White et al., 1991). Questions focused on the number of portions of fruits and vegetables eaten daily, on intake of calcium-rich dairy foods, fluid intake and whether or not breakfast was taken daily. Study participants were also asked to describe their self-perceived nutritional status as one of the following: 'don't know'; 'poorer than others'; 'satisfactory'.

Table 2: Reported Dietary-related Behaviours and Self-Perceived Nutritional Status of a Sample of Nursing Students in Hong Kong (n=274)

	Number of participants	% of participants
Eating breakfast daily		
Never	110	40
Occasionally	54	20
Daily	110	40
Daily fluid intake (water, tea, juice. Soft drink)		
≥ 5	137	50
< 5 cups	137	50
Taking dairy products (milk, cheese, yoghurt) daily		
Never	163	60
Occasionally	82	30
Daily	28	10
Fruit & vegetable consumption per day		
≥ 5 portions	28	10
≥ 2 - 5 portions	71	26
< 2 portions	175	64
Self-perceived nutritional status		
Satisfactory	164	60
Poorer than others	41	15
Don't know	69	25

The purpose and procedure of the study were explained to all students, and then, informed consent was obtained from them. The questionnaire was distributed by hand along with verbal instructions and clarification as to the terms used in the questionnaire. For example, one portion of fruit was equivalent to one whole item of fruit (one apple, one banana), one portion of vegetable was equivalent to one rice bowl full. Fluid intake included juice, tea and water and soft drinks. Participants were asked to complete and return the questionnaire within 2 days.

A total of 274 nursing students (228 females, 46 males, aged 19-24 years) returned completed questionnaires, giving a response rate of 94.4%. Dietary related behaviours and self-perceived nutritional status among the participants is summarized in Table 2. Results showed low intake of fluid, dairy products and fruits and vegetable among the majority of the participants. Also, 40% of respondents reported never taking breakfast. The reported self-perceived nutritional status was deemed satisfactory by the majority of participants. However, 25% of the nursing students reported that they did not know whether their nutritional status was satisfactory or not.

For the study of practicing nurses, a stratified random sampling method of 25% (327 of the total of 1,306) of the registered nurses working in a large public hospital were invited to complete a diet and lifestyle-related questionnaire. These registered nurses worked in various fields including medical, surgical, geriatric, orthopedic, neurosurgical, pediatric, and gynecology services, surgical suite (operating theater), and accident and emergency room, represents a wide cross-section of work settings. The questionnaire was modified from a previous survey 'the Hong Kong Adult Dietary Survey 1995' (Leung et al., 1997). There were 34 questions in the questionnaire, measuring the demographic data, dietary habits, and self-perceived nutritional status and health status. To address the content validity among nurses, five experts including a medical officer, a dietitian, two advanced practice nurses and a nurse specialist reviewed the questionnaire. The content validity was 0.95. The content validity index (CVI) of more than 0.75 was considered to be satisfactory (Polit, Beck & Hungler, 2001), thus, the CVI was satisfactorily established in this questionnaire. Also, the test-retest reliability was established (r=0.88) by repeat testing among 10 registered nurses in Hong Kong. A value of over 0.8 was interpreted as excellent agreement (Polit et al., 2001), thus, the reliability tests showed the stability of this questionnaire.

Table 3: Demographic data of the registered nurses

Clinical experiences	% of respondents
Years	
0-5	38.65
6-10	30.28
11-15	17.53
16 or above	13.55
Qualification	
Certificate in Nursing	13.15
Diploma in Nursing	17.53
Degree in Nursing	62.95
Master in Nursing	6.37
Present Position	
Enrolled Nurse	6
Registered Nurse	89.2
Advanced Practice Nurse	0.4
Nursing Officer	4.4

A total of 251 nurses (43 male and 208 female) completed and returned the questionnaire. Of these, 89% were registered nurses, 5% were nursing officers and 6% were enrolled nurses. The median age was 26 to 30 years old. More demographic data is presented in table 3.

Result showed that 8.4% of the respondents were overweight, with the body mass index (BMI) greater than or equal to 23 according to the Asian threshold (World Health Organization, 2002) and 10.8% were obese. The BMI data are shown in table 4.

Regarding the amount of fruits intake, table 5 showed around 28% did not take any fruit on a regular daily basis, while 66% consumed 1 to 2 servings per day, 3.6% consumed 3 to 4 servings daily, only 2.4% (6 of the 251 nurses studies) consumed 5 or more servings per day. In terms of vegetable intake, 4.4% of subjects did not take any vegetables on a regular daily basis, while 78.5% reported taking 1 to 2 servings per day, 15.5% took 3 to 4 servings per day and only 1.6% (4 of the 251 nurses studied) reported taking 5 or more servings per day.

The antioxidant intake of this group of practicing nurses, therefore, was low. Interestingly, 50% reported having a 'good' nutritional status, even though the overall findings of the survey indicated dietary practices that were far from optimal.

Table 4: Body mass index data among the registered nurses

	Body Mass Index (for Asian) Kg/m2	% of participants fall within this group
Underweight	< 18.5	18.33%
Normal	18.5 - 22.9	62.55%
Overweight	≥23	8.37%
Obese	25 -30	9.96%
Obese	> 30	0.80%

Reference: World Health Organization (2002). WHO reassessed appropriate body-mass index for Asian populations. Lancet, 360 (9328), 235

Studies on Dietary-Related Profile of Older Persons in the Chinese Community

To gain more information on diet and nutrition status of the elderly in the community in order for nurses to be able to direct appropriate nutritional advice and education to this group, 36 older persons (25 female and 11 male; aged 58 to 93 years, with mean±SD age of 75±7.8 years) were recruited from a community centre in Hong Kong. A diet and lifestyle questionnaire was developed based on the Nutrition Risk Assessment form (White et al., 1991) and the Physical Activity Questionnaire (Hayslip et al., 1996). Information included household income, health and medical status, medications use, exercise pattern identifying the type, frequency, and duration of activities during the previous week, dietary habits and dietary-related behaviours were collected. Self-perceived nutritional status was assessed using a 4-point scale (4='good', 'satisfactory', 'poor', 'not sure'=1), and a self-perceived health status in comparison with other people of similar age was assessed using a 4-point scale (4='better than others', 'as good as others', 'not as good as others', 'not sure'=1) with reference from Guigoz et al., (1994). The body weight and height were measured and body mass index (BMI) was calculated. The test-retest reliability of the questionnaire was established (r = 0.85) by repeat testing among 5 elderly persons over a period of 2 weeks. Descriptive analysis of the demographic information and household income, health and medical status, medications used; exercise pattern, dietary habits, dietary-related behaviours was performed, and inter-relationships between the self-perceived nutritional status and self-perceived health status were explored using Spearman's *rho*.

Results showed that 62% (22 of the 36 subjects) lived with their spouse, 36% (n=13) lived alone, and one person (2%) lived with other family members. In terms of education lever, 50% had not received any formal education but were able to read, write and understand Chinese. The majority of them (75%) reported known medical problems and needed regular medication and follow up. Health problems of these older persons include hypertension (in 36%), cataract (in 29%), Type 2 diabetes mellitus (in 22%), and gout (in 18%). Monthly income was less than HK$1,999 (US$250) in 31% of the participants. The major sources of income were family members and a government elderly subsidy scheme.

Dietary habits and dietary-related profile are shown in Table 6. Almost one third of the participants reported financial constraints in obtaining food, and 30-40% reported having problems with dentition and eating alone most of the time. In terms of body weight (Table 7), over 50% were found to be either overweight or obese. All subjects took breakfast regularly, and only a few drank alcohol. For intake of dairy products, dairy or bean curd products were eaten daily by only half them, the reason stated being that these products are too expensive. Very few (n=3) of the subjects took the recommended 5 or more portions of fruits and vegetables per day. In regard to fluid intake, in around half the subjects fluid intake was quite low. Interestingly one third of participants reported never drinking tea of any type. In terms of physical activity (Table 8 & Figure 1) the majority reported participating in some type of regular physical activity, with 56% reporting physical activity on a daily basis.

Sixty-one percent of the participants perceived their current nutritional status to be satisfactory, while 44% considered their health status to be as good as others of their age. A positive correlation was found between perceived nutritional status and perceived health status (r = 0.749, p< 0.0001).

Table 5: Dietary habits of registered nurses

	% of respondents
Amount of fruits consumed (per day)	
None	27.89
1-2 serving(s)	66.14
3-4 servings	3.59
5 or more servings	2.39
Amount of vegetables consumed (per day)	
None	4.38
1-2 serving(s)	78.49
3-4 servings	15.54
5 or more servings	1.59
Times of dining out (per week)	
0	2.39
1	3.59
2	7.17
3	19.92
4	13.55
5	17.93
6	7.17
7	3.19
> 7	25.1
Self-perceived nutritional status	
Very good	3.19
Good	75.7
Fair	19.12
Poor	1.00

Table 6: Dietary intake and dietary-related profile of the older persons (n=36)

	% of participants	Number of participants
Financial constraints in buying food		
Yes	28	10
Eating alone most of the time		
Yes	40	14
Having tooth or dentures problem		
Yes	30	11
Number of prescription drugs taken per day		
0	25	9
1	17	6
2	56	20
When necessary	2	1
Servings of fruit & vegetables taken per day		
1 serving	17	6
2 serving	31	12
3 serving	39	13
4 serving	5	2
5 serving	8	3
Dairy or bean curd products (milk/cheese/yohurt/tofu/soya milk) taken per day		
0	50	18
1	50	18
Servings of meat/poultry taken per day		
0	11	4
1 serving	83	30
2 serving	6	2
Drinking alcohol		
Daily	3	1
Occasionally	6	2
Never	91	33
Amount of fluid (water, juice, coffee, tea, milk, soup) taken per day		
< 3 cups	14	5
3 - 5 cups	44.5	16
6 - 8 cups	41.5	15

Table 7: Body mass index among the older persons

	Body Mass Index (for Asian) Kg/m2	% of participants fall within this group
Underweight	< 18.5	6
Normal	18.5 - 22.9	45.5
Overweight	≥23	15.1
Obese	25 -30	30
Obese	> 30	3.4

Discussion

Much of the knowledge about the relationship between diet and health has been gained over the last century. There is now a wealth of knowledge in the area of nutrition, and, while much is still to be clarified, an important task is to transmit current knowledge to healthcare providers and the general public in regard to how to lower risk of chronic-and life-threatening diseases by changing dietary habits. With the movement of health care towards wellness and primary prevention, the importance of nutrition in maintaining health deserves to highlight. Nutrition is a basic human need, and good nutrition impacts all along the wellness-illness continuum (Dudek, 2006). In this regard, knowledge of the principles of good nutrition and the ability to apply these are required for general public and patients and their families in home healthcare, community wellness, outpatient settings, and acute or long-term care facilities.

Nurses are involved in all aspects of care, and are well placed to promote good nutritional habits. Nurses should advise patients on how to follow a healthy diet, and also should practice what they preach. Generally, it is the nurse who raises concerns in regard to nutritional problems in patients, and who interacts with the patient to reinforce dietary counseling and achieve dietary change. In acute care settings when the patient is recovering from illness or surgery, the requirements for calories, protein, and other nutrients are increased, and if these are not met prolonged recovery, lower response to medical treatment and drug therapy, and poorer outcome may result.

Table 8: Physical activity profile of the older persons

	% of Participants
Physical activity engaged in the previous week	
Yes	78
No	22
Frequency of Physical Activity	
Daily	56
1 or 2 days/week	24
3 or more days/week	20
Duration of Physical Activity	
15 - 30 minutes	38
31 - 60 minutes	41
>= 61 minutes	21

While good nutrition underpins recovery from illness, optimal nutrition is associated with disease prevention. It is important to ensure that dietary requirements are met, but for some dietary components, such as sodium, simple sugars, saturated fat, cholesterol, intake should be restricted. If the consequences of excess intake are known, such as high salt intake and increased risk of stroke, high caloric intake and risk of Type 2 diabetes, then better dietary behaviours are more likely to be adopted and maintained. This message of health promotion through good nutrition has to be reinforced by nurses and health care professions. Therefore, nurses must be both knowledgeable about the relationship between diet and health and be ready and willing to lead by example. It is worrying, therefore, the present studies have demonstrated that nursing students appear to show little knowledge or awareness of good dietary practice. Also, the health and dietary behaviours of registered nurses were found to be inadequate.

Type of Physical Activity among older persons

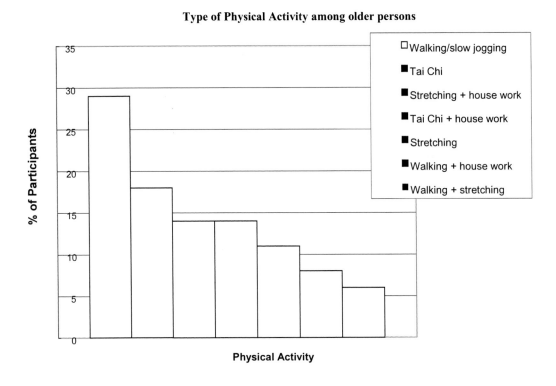

Figure 1: Types of physical activities engaged by older persons

Healthy eating has low priority among young adults (Neumark-Sztainer, et al., 1999). It is noted that consumption of total fat intake is increasing among adolescent and young adults, whereas intake of fruit, vegetables and milk is decreasing (Cavadini et al., 2000), and the prevalence of obesity is increasing (National Center for Health Statistics 1999-2002). The findings of present study are consistent with the literature suggesting an unhealthy eating pattern among young persons, even though the group studied was comprised of nursing students, who might be expected to be more health conscious and actively concerned about their nutrition.

Having breakfast is regarded as an important dietary habit for health; however, most of the nursing students in the present study omitted breakfast. This is in line with the skipping breakfast behaviour reported among young persons (Siega-Riz, et al., 1998; Neumark - Sztainer et al., 1999; Dwyer et al., 2001). Skipping meals, fewer family meals, and high intake of fast foods among adolescents is likely to lead to poor nutrition and increased risk of chronic disease, especially as the increased intake of 'restricted' items such as sodium and cholesterol, is likely to joined to decreased intake of 'healthy' food groups including antioxidant-rich fruits, vegetables and less dairy products (Neumark-Sztainer et al., 1997; Siega-Riz et al., 1998; Gillman et al., 2000; Videon & Manning, 2003).

In the present study, most participants took fewer than 2 portions of fruits and vegetables per day. The recommended daily intake for optimal health is five or more daily portions. Inadequate intake of fruits and vegetables places individuals at higher risk of various chronic diseases (World Cancer Research Fund, 1997; Khaw et al., 2001; American Heart Association, 2005). Another potentially worrying finding of this study was that 60% of the nursing students studied did not take dairy products of any kind. Dairy products are a major source of dietary calcium, and low consumption of calcium is associated with higher risk of osteoporosis and bone fracture in later life (Whitney & Rolfes, 2002).

Nutritional status was not objectively assessed in this study, but 40% of the students surveyed self-reported a poor or unknown nutritional status. This is not to say that these students were malnourished, but rather this result is a likely indicator of their lack of knowledge of nutrition. Perhaps more worryingly, 60% reported having a 'good' nutritional status, even though the overall findings of the survey indicated dietary practices that were far from optimal.

At the time of the study, the 274 first year students who participated in this study had received no formal theoretical input on nutrition as part of their undergraduate nursing programme. Findings of this study indicate that the pre-existing knowledge of nutrition in student nurses is poor, and without formal or structured theoretical input as part of their curriculum it is likely that the knowledge base and dietary behaviours of these students as they enter the workforce will remain so. However, nurses need to act effectively as both advisors and role models for health promotion, as well as for their personal wellbeing. Therefore, structured education on nutrition and the role of diet in health promotion is needed as a explicit and important part of nursing curricula. A holistic nursing educational curriculum that includes information on diet and health, nutritional supplements, the dangers of obesity and the benefits of certain dietary habits would be useful in health promotion at the individual level, and would also support the move toward nurses as promoters of health, and not simply carers of the sick. Such information would equip nurses to be both knowledgeable about the relationship between diet and health and be ready and willing to lead by example. Therefore, it is worrying that dietary habits and behaviours among registered nurses studied was less than satisfactory.

Among the registered nurse in the present study, almost 20% were considered as overweight or obese, and many reported dining out often instead of preparing their own meals, consuming fast food regularly, eating few fruits and vegetables, and low levels of physical exercise. It is noted that unhealthy diet habits, together with physical inactivity and the overweight situation among these group of nurses may contribute to the development of long-term health problems in later life. Apart from this, the credibility of the overweight or obese healthcare provider to provide dietary advice is low. Therefore, education needs on diet and health are not limited to the trainees only, and the finding presented here reinforce the view that health education and health promotion strategies in relation to lifestyle and dietary influences on disease risk should be incorporated in in-service training programmes for practising health care professionals.

In this study, the dietary habits and the physical activity profile of older, community living adults were examined also. Almost one third lacked a sense of food security, and had limited resources to buy nutritious food. It is noted that financial constraints may be exacerbated by the higher cost of food in shops accessible to the older persons, and because it is often impractical for an older person living alone to purchase and transport food in bulk, making catering for one person relatively more expensive (Blaylock et al, 1991). As a result, fresh nutritious food may be put at the bottom of the list, and such food as is eaten may be filling, such as bread or rice, but may not contain the protein, antioxidants and other micronutrients required for promotion of health.

In light of the very strong link between nutrition and health, the various dietary-related problems experienced by older persons is likely to make them more susceptible to a range of diseases, including cancer, coronary heart disease, osteoporosis, diabetes and dementia. In particular, the low consumption of fruits, vegetables, tea and calcium-rich dairy and bean curd products in the subjects studied gives cause for concern.

It was found that 36% of the older adults lived alone and they were likely to eat alone frequently. It would be undesirable for older persons to eat alone and on a regular basis. Lack of social support and eating alone often leads to poor diet quality and fewer scheduled meals, the use of more convenience foods and lower amounts and varieties of foods taken (Toner & Morris, 1992; McClelland et al, 2002). Indeed, older persons living alone were found to have a poorer nutritional status when compared to the counterparts who were living with family members (Huang et al., 2002). Social interaction encourages more healthful food patterns and improves food variety, and companionship during mealtimes enhances food consumption (Hodgson et al., 1994). To ensure the intake of a variety of food for nutrition and for health and to reduce costs, community-based services that facilitated bulk buying of fruits, vegetables, meat and dairy products would be helpful for older adults. Also, older adults could be encouraged to take a meal together with a companion as much as possible.

In addition to socioeconomic issues, other nutrition-related issues reported in this study include dental problems; inadequate fluid intake and polypharmacy. These contribute to inadequate nutrition in older persons, even when there are no financial constraints. Dental problems have been identified as an important factor affecting the nutritional status of older adults (Geissler & Bates, 1984).

Obesity is a serious problem in Hong Kong, as elsewhere in the developed world, as this markedly increases risk of Type 2 diabetes mellitus, cardiovascular disease and cancer. As noted above, almost 20% of nurses studied were overweight or obese, and almost 50% of the older person studied were in this category. In this regard, a well-balanced diet with more antioxidant rich foods, such as fruits and vegetables, along with increased physical activity could have a significant impact on public health in Hong Kong.

The question is how to get the message of 'eat well, feel well, stay well' across to all persons, to health care professions and to elders in an effective way. Education and increased awareness of the risks and benefits associated with certain dietary habits and factors can help improve food choices and nutritional status, even when income is low. It is important to disseminate the message on the importance of diet and dietary-related factors in the prevention of cancer, hypertension, cardiovascular disease, diabetes and osteoporosis, and in maintaining the immune system. Antioxidant rich foods are reported to lower risk of all these diseases. The World Health Organization recommendation for healthy eating is to enrich the diet with 5 or more servings of fruits and vegetables per day. Intake of other plant based agents such as teas, herbs, red wine is also beneficial to health, and calcium is needed to maintain bone health (Hogstel, 2001). Older persons are willing to make changes to maintain health and independence (US Department of Health & Human Services, 1990; Department of Health, 2004). As such, motivation to make such changes will be enhanced if the benefits are made clear. Motivation for behavioural change among older persons is greater still once they are aware they are at a great risk (McClelland et al., 2002). This further reinforces the need for vigorous nutritional education to all persons, nurses, patients, and community dwellers alike, for health maintenance and disease prevention.

References

[1]   American Heart Association. *Diet and Nutrition.* Available from *http://www.americanheart.org/presenter.jhtml?identifier*=1200010 Accessed Mar 31, 2005.

[2]   Asplund K. (2002) Antioxidant vitamins in the prevention of cardiovascular disease: a systematic review. Journal *of Internal Medicine* 251: 372-392.

[3]   Benzie IFF. (2003) Evolution of dietary antioxidants. *Journal of Comparative Biochemistry and Physiology* 136A:113-126.

[4]   Benzie IFF. (2005). Antioxidants: Observational Studies. *In The Encyclopedia of Human Nutrition, 2nd edition*. B Caballero, L Allen, A Prentice (eds) Academic Press London. pp 117-130.

[5]   Benzie IFF, Strain JJ. (2005). Diet and Antioxidant Defence. *In The Encyclopedia of Human Nutrition, 2nd edition*. B Caballero, L Allen, A Prentice (eds) Academic Press London. pp 131-137.

[6]   Blaylock, J., Smallwood, D. & Blisard, N. 1991. Per capita food spending. *Food Review*, July-September, 28-32.

[7]   Cavadini, C., Siega-Riz, A., & Popkin, B. (2000). U.S. adolescent food intake trends from 1965 to 1996. *Achieve Disorder Child* 83, 18-24.

[8]   *Census and Statistics Department.* (2006) "Population and vital events" (online). Available on line *http://www.censtatd.gov.hk/hong_kong_statistics /statistics_by_ subject/index.jsp* Accessed May 2, 2006.

[9]   Cox BD, Whichelow MJ, Prevost AT (2000) Seasonal consumption of salad vegetables and fresh fruit in relation to the development of cardiovascular disease and cancer. *Public Health Nutrition* 3, 19-29.

[10]   Department of Health 2004. Government of the Hong Kong Special Administrative Region Topical Health Report No. 3. Elderly Health. *Disease Prevention and Control Division and Elderly Health Services.* Available at: *http://www.info.gov.hk/dh/ diseases/acrobat/ehc_eng.pdf.* Cited 2-7-2004.

[11]   Dudek, S.G. (2006). *Nutrition Essentials for Nursing Practice. (5th ed.).* Philadelphia: Lippincott. (page 178)

[12]   Duthie GG, Duthie SJ, Kyle JAM (2000) Plant polyphenols in cancer and heart disease: implications as nutritional antioxidants. *Nutrition Research Reviews* 13, 79-106.

[13]   Dwyer, J. Evans, M., Stone, E.J. et al (2001). Adolescents' eating patterns influence their nutrient intakes. Journal of American Diet Association 101, 798-801.

[14] *Federal Interagency Forum on Aging related statistics.* Available on line. http://www.agingstats.gov/chartbook2004/population.html Accessed on 11 April 2005.

[15] Fowles, E.R. (2004). Prenatal Nutrition and Birth Outcomes. *Journal of Obstetric, Gynecologic & Neonatal Nursing* 33 (6), 809-822.

[16] Geissler, C.A.,& Bates, J.F. 1984. The nutritional effects of tooth loss. *American J. of Clinical Nutrition.* 39, 478-489.

[17] Gillman, M., Rifas-Shiman, S., Frazier, A. et al (2000). Family dinner and diet quality among older children and adolescents. *Achieve Family Medicine* 9, 235-240.

[18] Hayslip, B., Weigand, D., Weinberg, R., Richardson, P., & Jackson, A. 1996. The Development of New Scales for Assessing Health Belief Model Constructs in Adulthood. *Journal of Aging and Physical Activity.* 4, 307-323.

[19] Healthy People 2010: Progress Review. Nutrition and Overweight. U.S. Department of Health & Human Services. *Public Health Services* (2004) Available from URL: *http://www.cdc.gov/nchs/about/otheract/hpdata2010/focusareas/fa19-nutrition.htm* accessed on 12-9-2005.

[20] Hodgson, J.M., Hsu-Hage, B.H., & Wahlqvist, M.L. 1994. Food variety as a quantitative intake descriptor of food intake. *Ecology of Food and Nutrition,* 32, 137-148.

[21] Hogstel, M.O. 2001. Gerontology. *Nursing care of the older adult.* Australia: Thomson Learning.

[22] Hong Kong Policy Research Institute Ltd (2006). *Health Care for an ageing population – the challenge ahead for Hong Kong.* (on line) Available: http://www.hkpri.org.hk/ Accessed on 2 May 2006.

[23] Huang, L.H., Chen, S.W., Yu, Y.P., Chen, P.R., Lin, Y.C. 2002. The effectiveness of health promotion education programs for community elderly. *J of Nursing Research.* 10(4), 261-269.

[24] Khaw KT, Bingham S, Welch A, Luben R, Wareham N, Oakes S, Day N. (2001) Relation between plasma ascorbic acid and mortality in men and women in EPIC-Norfolk prospective study: a prospective population study. *Lancet* 357:657-663.

[25] Koopman WJ. (2001). *Arthritis and allied conditions.* Philadelphia: Lippincott Williams & Wilkins.

[26] LEGCO PANEL ON WELFARE SERVICES. *Implications of 2001 Population Census on the Provision of Social Welfare Services.* 11 March 2002. (online). Available at *www.hwfb.gov.hk/hw/english/archive/legco/W_11_3b/Cen-Eng.htm* Accessed January 6, 2005.

[27] Leung, S.F., Ho, S., Woo.J., Lam, T.H., & Janus, E.D. (1997). *Hong Kong adult dietary survey* 1995. Hong Kong: Chinese University of Hong Kong.

[28] McClelland, J.W., Bearon, L.B., Velzaquez, S., Fraser, A.M., Reid, H.M., & Mustian, R.D. 2002. Profiling rural Southern congregate nutrition site participants: implications for designing effective nutrition education programs. *Journal of Nutrition for the Elderly.* 22(2), 57-70. `

[29] National Center for Health Statistics (1999-2002). *Prevalence of Overweight Among Children and Adolescents: United States, http://www.cdc.gov/nchs/products/pubs /pubd/hestats/overwght99.htm#Table%201.* Accessed Mar 31, 2005.

[30] Neumark-Sztainer, D., Story, M., Dixon, L. et al (1997). Correlates of inadequate consumption of dairy products among adolescents. *Journal of Nutrition Education* 29, 12-20.

[31] Neumark-Sztainer, D., Story, M., Perry, C. et al. (1999). Factors influencing food choices of adolescents: Findings from focus-group discussions with adolescents. *Journal of American Diet Association* 99, 929-34, 937.

[32] Pedersen, P.U. (2005). Nutritional care: the effectiveness of actively involving older patients. *Journal of Clinical Nursing 14* (2), 247-255.

[33] Polit, D.F., Beck, C.T., & Hungler, B.P. (2001). *Essentials of nursing research: Methods, appraisal, and utilization (5th ed.).* Philadelphia: Lippincott.

[34] Pryor WA. (2000) Vitamin E and heart disease: basic science to clinical intervention trials. *Free Radical Biology & Medicine* 28,141-164.

[35] Rasanen, M., Keskinen, S., Niinikoski, H., Heino, T., Simell, O., Ronnemaa, T., Helenius, H., & Viikari, J. (2004). Impact of nutrition counseling on nutrition knowledge and nutrient intake of 7-to 9-y-old children in an atherosclerosis prevention project. *European Journal of Clinical Nutrition 58* (1), 162-172.

[36] Siega-Riz, A., Carson, T., & Popkin, B. (1998). Three squares or mostly snacks – What do teens really eat? *Journal of Adolescent Health* 22, 29-36.

[37] St Leger, L. (1997). Health promoting settings: from Ottawa to Jakarta. *Health Promotion International 12* (2), 99-101.

[38] Takahashi, P., Okhravi, H.R., Lim, L.S. (2004). Preventive health care in the elderly population: a guide for practicing physicians. *Mayo Clinic Proceedings* 79(3), 416-427.

[39] The International Council of Nurses. *ICN on Healthy Aging.* Available on line: *http://www.icn.ch/matters_aging.htm.* Assessed at 30-3-2005.

[40] Thompson, J., Manore, M. 2005. *Nutrition: An Applied Approach.* San Francisco: Pearson.

[41] Toner, H.M., & Morris, J.D. 1992. A social-psychological perspective of dietary quality in later adulthood. *Journal of Nutrition for the Elderly*, 11, 35-53.

[42] Tse, M.M.Y., & Benzie, I.F.F. (2004). Diet and health: Nursing perspective for the health of our aging population. *Nursing and Health Sciences* 6, 309-314.

[43] U.S. Department of Health & Human Services. 1990. Healthy People 2000: National health promotion and disease prevention objectives. *DHHS Publication No. (PHS)* 91-50212. Washington, D.C: U.S.Government Printing Office.

[44] United Nations, *2001 Report on the World Social Situation.* (on line) Available: *http://www.un.org/esa/socdev/rwss/overview.html* Accessed on 11 April 2005.

[45] Videon, T.M., & Manning, C.K. (2003). Influences on adolescent eating patterns: the importance of family meals. *Journal of Adolescent Health* 32, 365-373.

[46] White, J.V., Han, R.J., Lipschitz, D.A., Dwyer, J.T., & Wellman, N.S. 1991. Consensus of the Nutrition Screening Initiative: Risk factors and indicators of poor nutritional status in older Americans. *Journal of the American Dietetic Association*, 91, 783-787.

[47] Whitney, E., & Rolfes, S. (2002). Life cycle nutrition: infancy, childhood and adolescence. In *Understanding Nutrition* (9th ed.). Belmont, CA: Wadsworth/ Thompson Learing. P. 560-561

[48] Williams, D.R., & Lewis, N.M. (2002). Effectiveness of nutrition counselling in young adult males. *Nutrition Research* 22, 911-917.

[49] World Cancer Research Fund (WCRF) and American Institute for Cancer (AIC). (1997). *Food, Nutrition and the Prevention of Cancer: a Global Perspective.* London: WCRF/AIC.

[50] World Cancer Research Fund and American Cancer Institute Food, *Nutrition and the Prevention of Cancer: a Global Perspective* 1997. London:WCRF/AIC.

[51] World Health Organization (2002). WHO reassessed appropriate body-mass index for Asian populations. *Lancet*, 360 (9328), 235.

[52] Yen, P.K.Y. 2003. Vitamins and Disease Prevention. *Geriatric Nursing*, 23(5), 316-317.

Index

B

E

F

G

H

I

J

K

L

O

P

S

T

U